RXpert SERIES
Student's Companion

Pharmaceutical Analysis

Rxpert SERIES
Student's Companion

Pharmaceutical Analysis

C.N. Nalini,
M.Pharm., Ph.D,
Professor,
Head of the Department of Pharmaceutical Analysis
C.L. Baid Metha College of Pharmacy,
Chennai, Tamil Nadu.

Poorna Basuri
M.Pharm
Assistant Professor,
Department of Pharmaceutical Analysis
C.L.Baid Metha College of Pharmacy

Pharma Med PRESS
An Imprint of BSP Books Pvt. Ltd.

TM **PharmaMed Press**
An imprint of BSP Books Pvt. Ltd.
4-4-309/316, Giriraj Lane,
Sultan Bazar, Hyderabad - 500 095.

Pharmaceutical Analysis
***by* C.N. Nalini and Poorna Basuri**

Published by

PharmaMed Press ™
An imprint of BSP Books Pvt. Ltd.
4-4-309/316, Giriraj Lane, Sultan Bazar, Hyderabad - 500 095.
Phone: 040-23445688; Fax: 91+40-23445611
E-mail: info@pharmamedpress.net
www.bspbooks.net/www.pharmamedpress.net

ISBN: 978-93-49562-01-1 (Hardback)

eface

: science of pharmaceutical analysis is fundamental to ensuring the safety, efficacy, and lity of pharmaceuticals. In an industry where precision, accuracy, and reliability are -negotiable, the techniques and methodologies of pharmaceutical analysis serve as the kbone of quality control and drug development. This textbook is designed to provide an in-th, practical understanding of these essential analytical principles and techniques.

This book has been crafted to cater to students, educators, and professionals in the field of rmacy, and other related sciences. It encompasses the theoretical foundations as well as the ctical applications of analytical techniques used in pharmaceutical research, development, quality assurance. Each chapter has been carefully structured to introduce readers to specific hods and their application in analyzing drugs, formulations, and other pharmaceutical ducts.

The content is organized to facilitate a progressive understanding—from fundamental cepts to advanced techniques. We cover a wide array of topics including chromatographic niques, spectroscopy, electrical methods, and advanced instrumental methods. Additionally, emphasize regulatory standards and guidelines, aligning the analytical techniques discussed h the industry's compliance requirements, particularly with respect to Total Quality nagement (TQM), Good Laboratory Practice (GLP) and International Council for monisation (ICH) guidelines.

Our hope is that this textbook will not only serve as a valuable academic resource but also pire a deeper interest in pharmaceutical analysis. We recognize the essential role of analysis he advancement of pharmaceutical science, and we are committed to contributing to the cation and empowerment of the next generation of professionals in this critical field.

We extend our gratitude to the management of C.L. Baid Metha College of Pharmacy for r constant support. It is our sincere hope that this textbook meets the expectations of our lers and serves as a comprehensive guide in their journey through pharmaceutical analysis.

Suggestions and criticisms for the improvement of the book shall be highly appreciated.

-Authors

ntents

SECTION - I: QUALITY ASSURANCE

SECTION - II: CHROMATOGRAPHY

SECTION - III: ELECTROMETRIC METHODS

SECTION - IV: SPECTROSCOPY

ɔout the Authors

N. Nalini, is currently serving as Professor and Head of the Department of Pharmaceutical alysis in C.L.Baid Metha College of Pharmacy, Chennai, Tamil Nadu. She has a teaching ɔerience of 25 years along with two years of industrial experience as an analytical chemist. ɜ has also served as a Pharmacist in Christian Fellowship Hospital, Oddanchatram and as a ɪior Assistant Pharmacist for one year in Christian Medical College Hospital, Vellore.

She has completed her D.Pharm in 1985, B.Pharm in the year 1992, and M.Pharm in 1997. ɜ was awarded a Ph.D. by the Tamil Nadu Dr. M.G.R. Medical University in the year 2010. ɜ has been awarded the best teacher award from the Tamil Nadu Dr. M.G.R. Medical iversity in the year 2011.

She has held various positions like Member of Board of Studies, Research proposal eening committee, Screening committee for Research Grant, Inspection Committee, the ɔert Committee for Pharm D, B.Pharm and M.Pharm, Faculty at the TN Dr. M.G.R Medical iversity. She is also a member of the doctoral committee for research in various universities luding TNMGRMU. She is a guide and co-guide for many doctoral students. She has guided re than 50 postgraduate students and many undergraduate students. She is a Question paper ter, valuator, practical examiner, and UG/PG dissertation adjudicator in the TN Dr. M.G.R edical University and other universities including Anna University Chennai, Annamalai iversity, SRMCP, SRM, Mother Teresa, and Chettinad University.

She has more than 60 publications to her credit in peer-reviewed National and International rnals. Her areas of publication include Pharmaceutical Analysis and Pharmaceutical emistry.

s. Poorna Basuri is currently serving as an Assistant Professor in the Department of armaceutical Analysis at C.L. Baid Metha College of Pharmacy. She obtained her B.Pharm in 17 from Faculty of Pharmacy, Sri Ramachandra University, and her M.Pharm in 2019 from ..Baid Metha College of Pharmacy, affiliated to T.N.Dr.MGR Medical University. She has en teaching ever since. She has qualified GPAT in 2017. She is also a Certified Clinical search Personnel (CCRP). She is a recipient of the InSc Young Researcher Award 2022. She participated and presented in various conferences and seminars. She has also published ny articles to her credit. She also acts as a reviewer in various journals. She has also served Pharmacy Council of India as Technical Assistant.

SECTION – I: Quality Assurance

1. Introduction, Sources of Quality Variation, Control of Quality Variation
2. Concept of Statistical Quality Control
3. Validation Methods- Quality of Equipment, Validation of Equipment, and Validation of Analytical Instruments and Calibration
4. GLP, ISO 9000
5. Total Quality Management, Quality Review, and Documentation
6. ICH - International Conference on Harmonisation- Guidelines
7. Regulatory Control

CHAPTER 1

Introduction, Sources of Quality Variation, Control of Quality Variation

INTRODUCTION

Quality can be characterized in a variety of ways, such as "fitness for use" or "conformance to criteria". Quality assurance is a systematic procedure through which a product or service's compliance with predetermined specifications is determined. QA defines and upholds standards for developing or producing dependable products.

According to WHO, quality assurance in the pharmaceutical industry is a broad concept that encompasses all factors that either individually or collectively affect a product's quality. It is the totality of all the plans put in place to guarantee that pharmaceutical products are of the quality needed for their intended usage. GMP and other criteria like product design and development are thus included in quality assurance. Quality assurance, therefore, incorporates GMP and also other factors like product design and development.

Variation is the difference between the actual assessment of a product characteristic and the desired value. When the industry specifies the quality of a drug, any deviation from the norm is its fault. Any error made from the time the raw materials are received until the finished product is packaged can result in a quality variation. As the amount of material and the complexity of the process increase, the threat of error also rises.

TYPES OF ERRORS

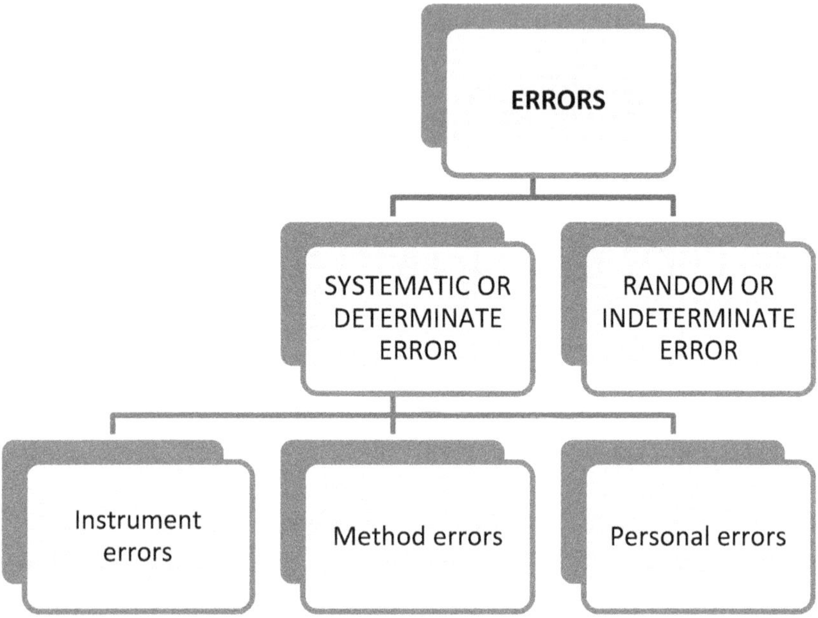

Systematic/Determinate Errors

The error is reproducible and can be discovered and corrected.

(a) Instrument errors

- ✓ Failure to calibrate, degradation of parts in the instrument, power fluctuations, variation in temperature, etc.,
- ✓ Can be corrected by calibration or proper instrumentation maintenance

(b) Method errors

- ✓ Errors due to no ideal physical or chemical behavior completeness and speed of reaction, interfering side reactions, sampling problems
- ✓ Can be corrected with proper method development

(c) Personal errors

- ✓ Occur where measurements require judgment, result from prejudice, color acuity problems

Random error/Indeterminate errors

Caused by uncontrollable variables, which cannot be defined/eliminated

1. Sources of Quality Variation

(i) Materials

(ii) Machines
(iii) Methods
(iv) Men
(v) Milieu (Environment or Premises)

(i) Materials

- Variations among suppliers of the same substances
- Variations among batches from the same suppliers
- Variations within a batch

(ii) Machines

- Variation of equipment of the same process
- Differences in adjustments of equipment
- Aging of machines and improper care

(iii) Methods

- Wrong procedure
- Inadequate procedure
- Negligence in the procedure by chance

(iv) Men

- Improper working conditions
- Inadequate training and understanding
- Lack of interest and emotional upheavals
- Dishonesty, fatigue, and carelessness

(v) Milieu (Environment or premises)

- The environment must be clean, dust-free, spacious, and properly designed to minimize the risk of errors and permit effective cleaning and maintenance to avoid cross-contamination.
- It must be suitable for the purpose for which it is used.

2. Control of Quality Variation

The variations in quality can be controlled by managing the mistakes and GMP variations. The mistakes can be minimized or eliminated by material control, and packaging control. GMP variations can be managed when Quality Control and Quality Assurance work side by side.

Control Procedure:

Controlling every step of the process can control variations. Control can be divided into:

(i) Material Control
(ii) Manufacturing practices control
(iii) Packing control
(iv) Distribution control

(i) Material Control

- It starts just after the reception of materials. Most of the materials that are: active substances, excipients, packaging, and printed materials are received by the industry from suppliers.
- Thus there should be an adequate established system for the receipt, testing, and storage of all these supplies. There should be a complete record of all the procedures and tests.
- In materials, the following things are included:
  - Drug substances.
  - Excipients.
  - Packaging and printed materials.
- After the reception of the material, it is kept in a definite area. Thus before laboratory testing, proper containers, labels, lot numbers, expiry dates, etc, all are checked.
- The material is stored properly, either they are arranged alphabetically or they are differentiated depending upon physical nature. Then samples are taken for laboratory testing and a label (Sampled) is fixed on the material.
- In the case of active constituents, percentage purity, adulteration, expiry date, lot number, exact packing, etc are checked.

(ii) Manufacturing Practices Control

Successful GMP is difficult to attain but to some extent, it can be modified and controlled. Specific procedures can be applied to attain the best quality. In the case of manufacturing, the following controls are important:

A. Personnel.

B. Equipment and building.

C. Control of record.

D. Production procedure control.

A. Personnel

Usually properly educated and well-trained persons should be in the industry.

(a) There should be proper selection and training in all departments i.e. production, packaging, labeling, etc.

(b) There should be general lectures for less educated persons who work in the labeling or packaging section in an understandable language.

(c) They should be made aware of the importance of life-saving.

(d) They should be warned about all the dangers of their mistakes and errors.

(e) There should be properly educated supervisors working above the workers.

(f) The supervisors should always be there so that in case of any trouble or question, they must be available.

B. Equipment and building

(a) The equipment and building used in storage, processing, checking, and packaging should be of a suitable design, size, construction, and location.

(b) In the case of equipment, these should be constructed in the proper size and proper way. The size should be such that the complete batch can be processed all at once.

(c) The surfaces of equipment should be non-reactive, non-absorptive, and non-additive.

C. Control of records

The records such as master formula records and batch production records must be maintained.

1. Master Formula Record:

(a) The master formula record must be prepared for each product.

(b) It must be signed by a competent and responsible person.

(c) The language must be simple and easy to understand so that it may not be misinterpreted.

(d) It should be checked by another competent person and must be countersigned.

(e) Master formula record includes the following information:

- ✓ Name of the product, dosage form, and strength.
- ✓ Complete list of ingredients including excipients.
- ✓ Quality by weight or volume of every ingredient.
- ✓ Standards or specifications of each ingredient.
- ✓ Any calculated excess of an ingredient.
- ✓ Theoretical yield and termination of the process.
- ✓ Manufacturing and control instructions, specifications, and precautions.
- ✓ Complete description of closures, containers, labeling, packaging, and other finishing material.

2. Batch Production Record:

(a) Batch production record must be prepared, maintained, and controlled for each batch of a product.

(b) It must be retained for about 5 years after product distribution.

(c) Batch production record should have the following information in addition to the master formula record:

- ✓ Batch number.
- ✓ Code number.
- ✓ Manufacturing date.
- ✓ Expiry date.

D. Production procedure control

The processes of manufacturing are operated according to the established rules from the reception of material up to the delivery of the final product.

(a) In the production procedure control, some tests are done during the process, which is called "In Process Quality Control (IPQC)"

(b) The IPQC is under Quality Control Department.

(c) Both the Quality Control and Production Departments are responsible for the production procedure control.

IPQC Tests for Different Dosage Forms are as Under:

1. ***IPQC tests for tablets:***

   (a) Drug contents determination.

   (b) Moisture, contents of granules.

   (c) Assay of active ingredients.

   (d) Weight variation of uncoated tablets.

   (e) Hardness test.

   (f) Disintegration test

2. ***IPQC tests for syrups and suspensions:***

   (a) Drug contents determination.

   (b) Assay of active ingredients.

   (c) pH.

   (d) Weight per ml.

   (e) Particle size

3. ***IPQC tests for semi-solids:***

   (a) Drug contents determination.

   (b) Assay of active ingredients.

   (c) Uniformity and homogeneity test.

(d) Viscosity and specific gravity test
(e) Filling test.
(f) Leakage test

4. ***IPQC tests for injectables:***
   (a) Drug contents determination.
   (b) Assay of active ingredients.
   (c) pH
   (d) Pyrogen test.
   (e) Stability test.
   (f) Leakage test.
   (g) Check up of particulate matters.

(iii) Packing Control

The packaging control is usually completed before manufacturing the product.

(a) When the product comes in the packaging section, it should be packed in recommended containers and there should not be any mistakes in the case of labelling and writing of batch number, etc.

(b) The packaging material is used according to the nature and distribution of the product.

(iv) Distribution Control

The responsibilities of the Quality Control Department are not finished even after the distribution of finished dosage forms in the market.

(a) The samples of each batch are kept in record and these samples are selected during packaging and are in the same packs as they are marketed.

These are kept for years to examine or test the material for any purpose or necessary demand.

CHAPTER 2

Concept of Statistical Quality Control

DEFINITION

Statistics means a good amount of data to obtain reliable results. The Science of statistics handles this data in order to draw certain conclusions. Its techniques find extensive applications in quality control, production planning and control, business charts, linear programming, etc.

Quality is a relative term and is generally explained with reference to the end use of the product. Quality is thus defined as fitness for purpose.

Control is a system for measuring and checking or inspecting a phenomenon. It suggests when to inspect, how often to inspect, and how much to inspect. Control as certains the quality characteristics of an item, compares the same with prescribed quality characteristics of an item, compares the same with prescribed quality standards, and separates defective items from non-defective ones.

Statistical Quality Control (SQC) is the term used to describe the set of statistical tools used by quality professionals. SQC is used to analyze quality problems and solve them. Statistical quality control refers to the use of statistical methods in monitoring and maintaining the quality of products and services. All the tools of SQC are helpful in evaluating the quality of services. SQC uses different tools to analyze the quality problem.

CHARACTERISTICS OF S.Q.C

- Designed to control the quality standard of goods produced for marketing.
- Exercise by the producers during production to assess the quality of goods.
- Carried out with the help of certain statistical tools like Mean Chart, Range Chart, P-Chart, C-Chart, etc.
- Designed to determine the variations in the quality of the goods & limits of tolerance.

CAUSES OF VARIATIONS IN QUALITY

Assignable causes: It refers to those changes in the quality of the products which can be assigned or attributed to any particular causes like defective materials, defective labor, etc.

Chance causes: These causes emerge by chance or randomly as a result of the compounding effects of numerous small, unrelated causes that are difficult to pin down. Every form of production has these causes by nature.

Elements of SQC: Statistical quality control can be divided into the following three broad categories.

- Descriptive statistics
- Statistical process control (SPC)
- Acceptance sampling

Descriptive statistics

These are the statistics used to describe certain quality characteristics such as the central tendency and variability of the observed data. It also describes the relationship. Descriptive statistics include statistics such as the mean, standard deviation, range, and a measure of the distribution of data.

1. **Mean**

   It is an important statistical tool that measures the central tendency of a set of data. The mean is computed by simply summing up all the observations and dividing by the total number of observations.

2. **Range and standard deviation**

   This information provides the variability of the data. It tells how the data is spread out around the mean. The range is the difference between the largest and the smallest observations in a set of data while standard deviation is a statistic that measures the amount of data dispersion around the mean. Small values of the range and standard deviation mean that the observations are closely clustered around the mean while large values of the range and standard deviation mean that the observations are spread around the mean.

3. **Distribution of data**

   It is a measure to determine the quality characteristics. When the distribution of data is symmetric then there are the same numbers of observations below and above the mean. This is what is commonly found when only normal variation is present in the data. When a disproportionate number of observations are either above or below the mean, then the data has a skewed distribution.

Statistical process control (SPC)

It consists of statistical tools that involve inspecting a random sample of the output from a process and deciding whether the process is producing products with characteristics that fall within a predetermined range. SPC answers the question of whether the process is functioning properly or not. These tools are very important for a process since they help in identifying and catching a quality problem during the production process. This is the most critical criteria compared to others.

TOOLS IN STATISTICAL PROCESS CONTROL

The seven major tools used for Statistical Process Control are,

1. Control charts
2. Checksheets
3. Pareto chart
4. Stratification
5. Cause and Effect diagram
6. Histogram
7. Scatter diagram

1. Control Charts

- ➢ A control chart is a time plot of a statistic, such as a sample mean, range, standard deviation, or proportion, with a center line and upper and lower control limits.
- ➢ The limits give the desired range of values for the statistic. When the statistic is outside the bounds, or when its time plot reveals certain patterns, the process may be out of control.
- ➢ A process is considered in statistical control if it has no assignable causes, only natural variation.

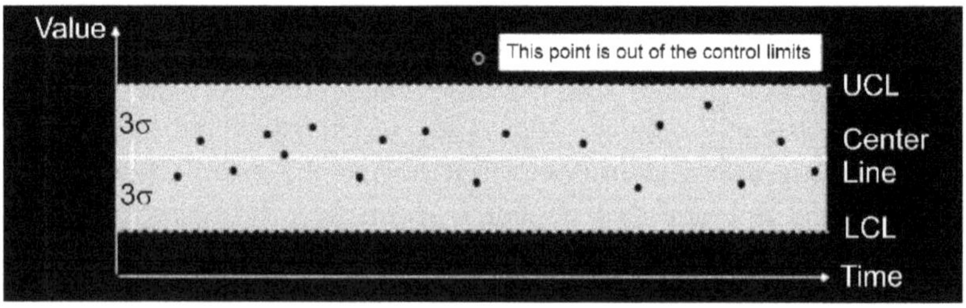

Purpose & uses of control charts:

1. Helps in determining the quality standard of the products.
2. Helps in detecting the chance & assignable variations in the quality standards by setting two control limits.
3. Reveals variations in the quality standards of the products from the desired level.
4. Indicates whether the production process is in control or not.
5. Ensures less inspection cost & time in the process control.

Types of Control Charts:

- **Variable**
  A product characteristic that can be measured and has continuum of values
- **Attribute**
  A product characteristic that has a discrete value and can be counted.

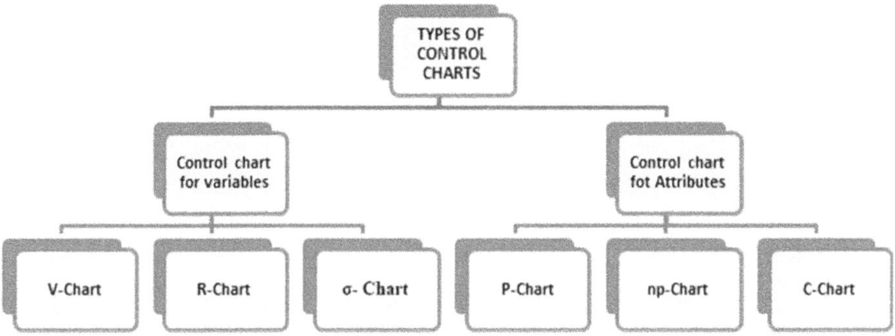

CONTROL CHARTS FOR VARIABLES

1. **V - Chart/ Mean chart**: This chart is constructed for controlling the variations in the average quality standard of the products in a production process.

$$\text{Mean} = \frac{x_1 + x_2 + x_3 + x_4 + \ldots.. + x_n}{n}$$

2. **R - Chart:** This chart is constructed for controlling the variations in the dispersion or variability of the quality standards of the products in a production process.
3. **σ- Chart:** This chart is constructed to get a better picture of the variations in the quality standard in a process than that is obtained from the range chart provided the standard deviation(σ) of the various samples are readily available.

CONTROL CHARTS FOR ATTRIBUTES

1. **P-chart:** This chart is constructed for controlling the quality standard in the average fraction defective of products in a process when the observed sample items are classified into defectives & non-defectives.
2. **np-chart:** This chart is constructed for controlling the quality standard of attributes in a process where the sample size is equal & it is required to plot the no. of defectives (np) in samples instead of fraction defectives (p).
3. **C-Chart:** This chart is used for the control of no. of defects per unit say a piece of cloth/glass/paper/bottle which may contain more than one defect. This inspection unit in this chart will be a single unit of product. The probability of occurrence of each defect tends to remain very small.

Uses:

The following are the field of application of C-Chart:

- Number of defects of all kinds of aircraft final assembly.
- Number of defects counted in a roll of coated paper, sheet of photographic film, bale of cloth etc.

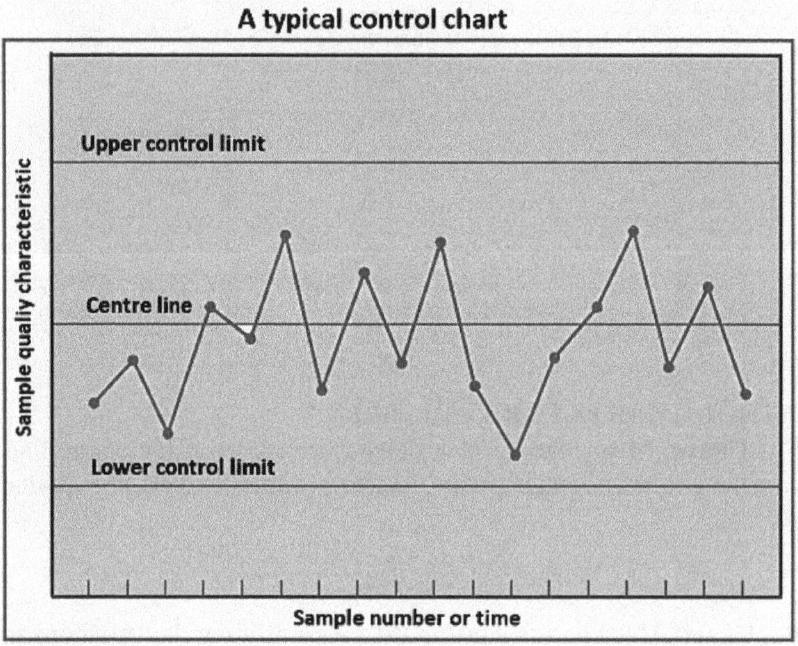

2. Checksheets

Check sheets are simple data gathering devices. They are used to collect data effectively and efficiently. They prepare data for further analysis. A check sheet is in the form of a designed format used to collect data in a systematic manner and in real time at the location where the data is generated. The data it captures can be either quantitative or qualitative. When the information is quantitative, the check sheet is sometimes called a tally sheet. The defining characteristic of a check sheet is that data are recorded by making marks (checks) on it. A typical check sheet is divided into regions, and marks made in different regions have different significance. Data are read by observing the location and number of marks on the sheet. Various types of check sheets are (i) process distribution check sheet, (ii) defect cause check sheet, (iii) defect location check sheet, and (iv) defect cause-wise check sheet.

3. Pareto chart

A Pareto chart, named after Vilfredo Pareto, is a type of chart that contains both bars and a line graph, where individual values are represented in descending order by bars, and the cumulative total is represented by a line.

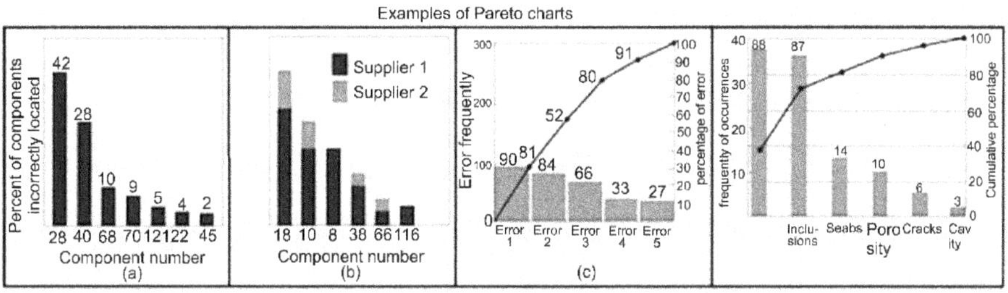

4. Stratification

Stratification is a technique used in combination with other data analysis techniques. When data from a variety of sources or categories have been lumped together, the meaning of the data can be impossible to see. The technique separates the data so that the pattern can be seen. Stratification can be used in cases (i) before collecting the data (ii) when data come from several sources or conditions such as shifts, days of the week, suppliers, materials, products, departments, equipment, or population groups, and (iii) when data analysis can need separating different sources or conditions. The stratification procedure consists of the following three steps.

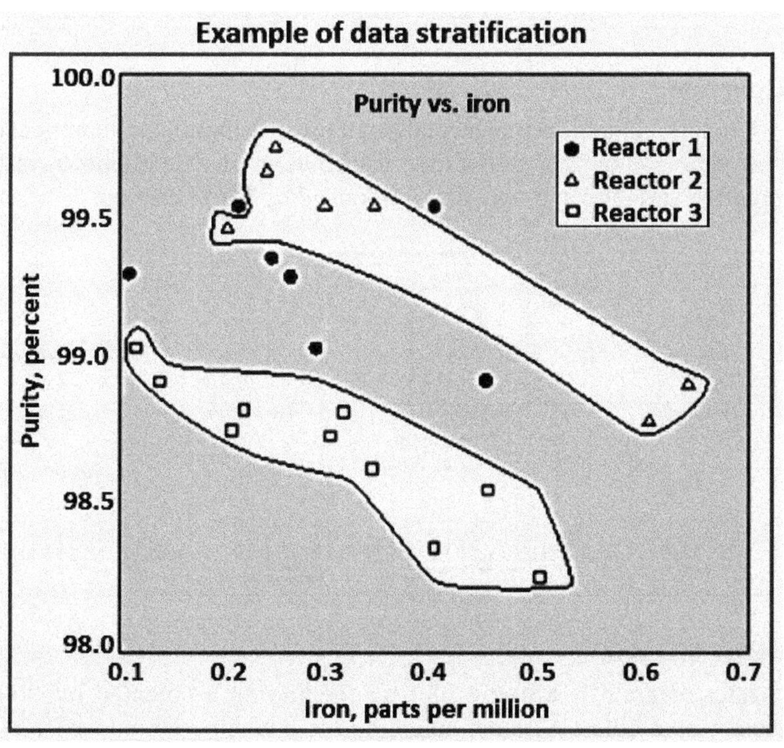

5. Cause and Effect diagram

A graphic tool that helps identify, sort, and display possible causes of a problem or quality characteristic.

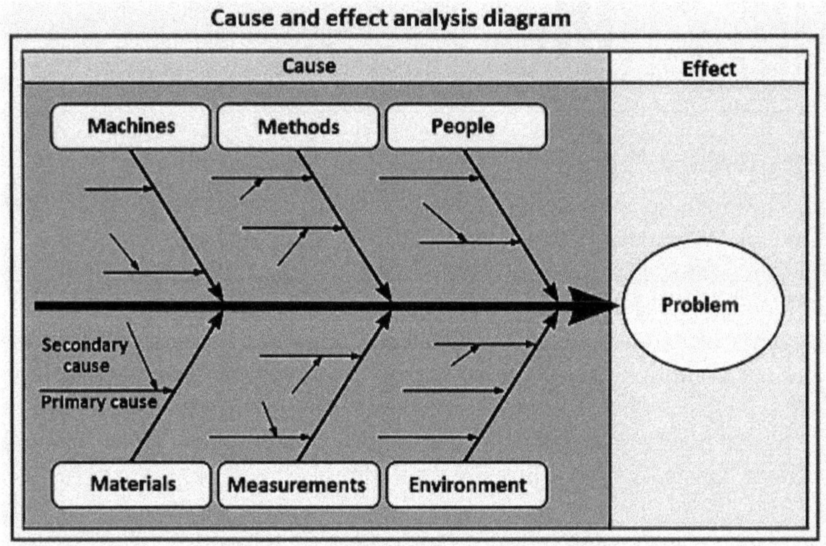

6. Histogram

A histogram is a graphical representation of the distribution of numerical data. It is an estimate of the probability distribution of a continuous variable (quantitative variable) and was first introduced by Karl Pearson.

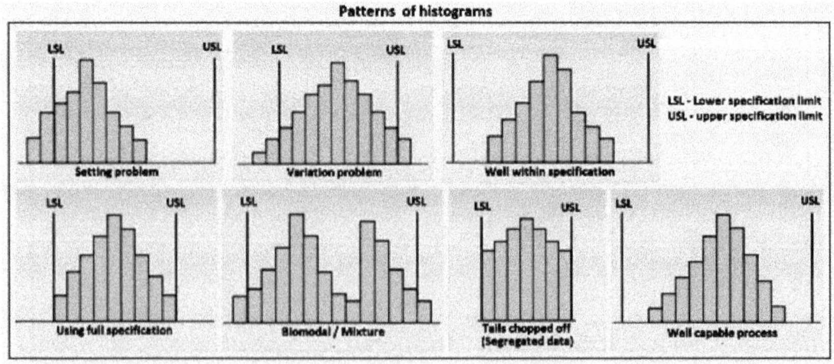

7. Scatter diagram

The scatter diagram is a useful plot for identifying a potential relationship between two variables. A scatter diagram is used when a variable exists which is below the control of the operator. If a parameter exists which is systematically incremented and / or decremented by the other, it is called the control parameter or independent variable and is customarily plotted along the x axis. The measured or dependent variable is customarily plotted along the y axis. If no dependent variable exists, either type of variable can be plotted on either axis or a scatter diagram illustrates only the degree of correlation (not causation) between two variables.

Typical scatter diagrams

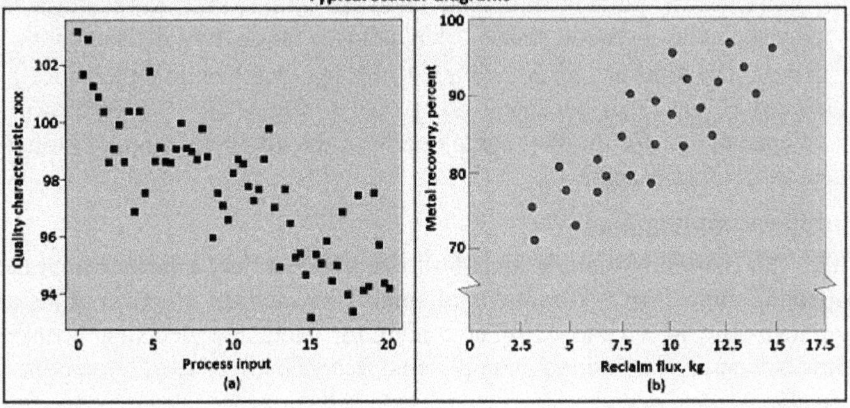

Acceptance sampling

It helps in evaluating whether there is a problem with quality and whether the desirable quality is being achieved for a batch of products. Accepting sampling consists of the process of randomly inspecting a sample of goods and deciding whether to accept the entire lot based on the results. This sampling decides whether a batch of goods is to be accepted or rejected.

Acceptance Sampling is concerned with the decision to accept a mass of manufactured items as conforming to standards of quality or to reject the mass as non-conforming to quality. decision is reached through sampling.

Single sampling plan:

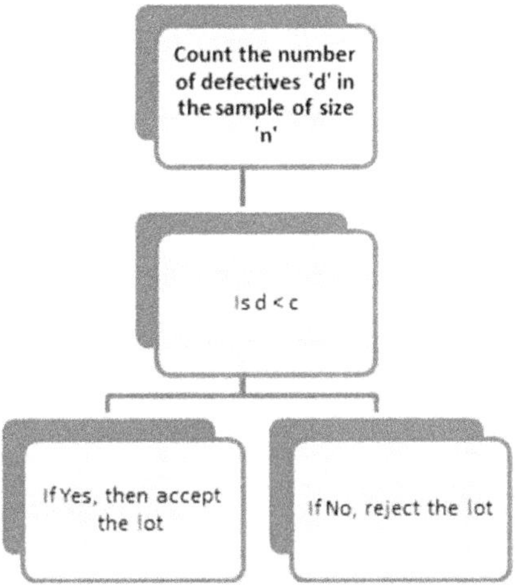

Double sampling plan:

- Under this sampling plan, a sample of 'n' items is first chosen at random from the lot of sizes 'N'
- If the sample contains, say, 'c' or few defectives, the lot is accepted.
- If it contains more than 'c' defectives, the lot is rejected.
- If however, the number of defectives in the sample exceeds 'c', but is not more than C2', a second sample of 'n' items is taken from the same lot.
- If now, the total no. of defectives in the two samples together does not exceed c', the lot is accepted; otherwise it is rejected. (*c,' is known as acceptance no. for the first sample & 'c' is the acceptance no. of both the samples taken together).

Multiple sampling plan:

Under this sampling plan, a decision to accept or reject a lot is taken after inspecting more than two samples of small size each. In this plan, units are examined one at a time & after examining each unit decision is taken. "However, such plan are very complicated & hence rarely used in practice."

Advantages of S.Q.C:

- ✓ Helpful in controlling quality of a product.
- ✓ Eliminate Assignable causes of variation.
- ✓ Better quality at lower inspection cost.
- ✓ Useful to both consumers & producers.
- ✓ It makes workers quality conscious.
- ✓ Helps in earn goodwill.

Limitations:

- ❖ Does not serve as a 'PANACEA' for all quality evils.
- ❖ It cannot be used to all production process.
- ❖ It involves mathematical & statistical problems in the process of analysis & interpretation of variations in quality.

Provides only an information services.

CHAPTER 3

Validation Methods- Quality of Equipment, Validation of Equipment, and Validation of Analytical Instruments and Calibration

DEFINITIONS

VALIDATION

Validation is the confirmation by examination and the provision of objective evidence that the particular requirements for a specific intended use are fulfilled. The validation of a test method is the process by which the relevance and reliability of the method are assessed for a particular purpose. It is an essential stage in the evolution of the method from its development to its acceptance and application for regulatory purposes.

According to USFDA, the goal of validation is to establish documented evidence that provides a high degree of assurance that a specific process will consistently produce a product meeting its predetermined specifications and quality attributes.

CALIBRATION

Calibration is the activity of checking, by comparison with a standard, the accuracy of a measuring instrument of any type. It may also include adjustment of the instrument to bring it into alignment with the standard.

Calibration achieves two main objectives -

(a) It checks the accuracy of an instrument

(b) It determines the traceability of the measurement

QUALIFICATION

"It is the action of proving and documenting that equipment or ancillary systems are properly installed, work correctly, and actually lead to the expected results."

Qualification is part of validation, but the individual qualification steps alone do not constitute process validation. Qualification of analytical instrumentation is essential for accurate and precise measurement of analytical data. If the instrumentation is not qualified, ensuring that the results indicated are trustworthy, all other work based upon the use of that instrumentation is suspect.

CALIBRATION VS VALIDATION

CALIBRATION	VALIDATION
Calibration is a demonstration that, a particular instrument or device produces results within specified limits by comparisons with those produced by a reference or traceable standard over an appropriate range of measurements.	Validation is a documented program that provides a high degree of assurance that a specific process, equipment, method, or system consistently produces a result meeting pre-determined acceptance criteria.
In calibration, performance of an instrument or device is compared against a reference standard	No such reference standards are used in the validation program.
Calibration ensures that instruments or measuring devices produce accurate results.	Validation provides documented evidence that a process, equipment, method, or system produces consistent results (in other words, it ensures that uniform batches are produced).
Shall be performed periodically, to identify the 'drift' of the measuring device or equipment and make them accurate.	No such requirements. Shall be performed when changes or modifications happen to the existing system or once the revalidation period is reached.
Shall be performed as per calibration SOP	Shall be performed as per validation protocol

Difference between Validation vs. Qualification	
Validation	**Qualification**
Validation is the documented act of demonstrating that a procedure, process, and activity will consistently produce results meeting predetermined acceptance criteria.	**Qualification** is the act of proving that the specific equipment or system and its ancillary components are correctly installed, work as expected and fit for intended use.
Validation shall be carried out to ensure the process can produce consistent results within the approved specifications.	**Qualification** shall be performed for all new/existing equipment, facility, system, and instruments
Validation incorporates the concept of qualification	**Qualification** is part of validation, but the individual qualification steps alone do not constitute validation
Validation is achieved	**Qualification** is a test or challenge that is performed
Validation is directly related to the process	**Qualification** is directly related to equipment, instruments, systems, or software
Methods/Process/Procedures (the way we use things) are validated	Things are qualified: equipment, instruments, software.

Validation examples
• Equipment validation
• Cleaning Validation
• Process Validation
   ○ Process Design
   ○ Process Qualification
   ○ Continued Process Verification
• Analytical method validation
• Computer system validation
	Qualification includes the following steps:
	• URS
	• DQ
	• FAT/SAT
	• IQ
	• OQ
	• PQ

All **validation** and **qualification** studies should be planned and take the life cycle of facilities, equipment, utilities, process, and product into consideration.	

VALIDATION

Validation is a documented evidence that provides a high degree of assurance to a desired result with the predetermined compliance. This term comes from the word “valid or validity” which means “legally defined”. The concept of validation was first proposed by the Food and Drug Administration (FDA) in 1970s to improve the quality of pharmaceutical products.

Adequate validation is beneficial to the manufacturer in many ways:

(i) It deepens the understanding of processes; decreases the risk of preventing problems and thus assures the smooth running of the process.

(ii) It decreases the risk of defect costs.

(iii) It decreases the risk of regulatory noncompliance.

(iv) A fully validated process may require fewer in-process controls and end-product testing.

Validation should thus be considered in the following situations:

(i) Totally new process;
(ii) New equipment;
(iii) Process and equipment which have been altered to suit changing priorities; and
(iv) Process where the end-product test is poor and an unreliable indicator of product quality.

Scope of validation

(a) Validation requires an appropriate and sufficient infrastructure including: organization, documentation, personnel, and finances
(b) Involvement of management and quality assurance personnel
(c) Personnel with appropriate qualifications and experience
(d) Extensive preparation and planning before validation is performed
(e) Validation should be performed:
    (i) for new premises, equipment, utilities and systems, and processes and procedures;
    (ii) at periodic intervals; and
    (iii) when major changes have been made.
(f) Validation in accordance with written protocols.
(g) Validation over a period of time, e.g. at least three consecutive batches (full production scale) to demonstrate consistency. (Worst case situations should be considered.)
(h) Significant changes (facilities, equipment, processes) - should be validated
(i) Risk assessment approach used to determine the scope and extent of validation needed

Importance of validation

1. Assurance of quality
2. Time-bound
3. Process optimization
4. Reduction of quality cost.
5. Minimal batch failures, improved efficiency, and productivity.
6. Reduction in rejections.
7. Increased output.
8. Fewer complaints about process-related failures.
9. Reduced testing in process and in finished goods.
10. More rapid and reliable start-up of new equipment
11. Easier maintenance of equipment.
12. Improved employee awareness of processes.
13. More rapid automation,
14. Government regulation (Compliance with validation requirements is necessary for obtaining approval to manufacture and introduce new products)

METHODS OF VALIDATION

The major methods of Validation:

1. Process validation.
2. Cleaning validation.
3. Equipment validation.
4. Analytical method validation.

1. Process validation:

As per FDA, "The collection of data from the process design stage throughout production, which establishes scientific evidence that a process is capable of consistently delivering quality products"

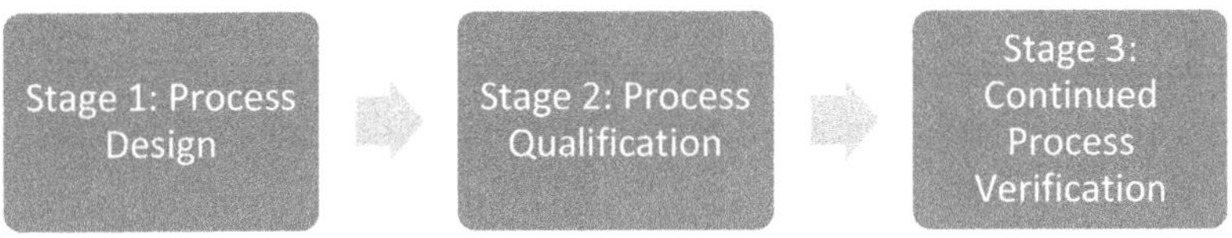

Types of Process Validation:

(i) Prospective Validation.
(ii) Retrospective Validation.
(iii) Concurrent Validation.
(iv) Revalidation.

(i) Prospective Validation:

Validation conducted prior to the distribution of either a new product or a product made under a revised manufacturing process is called prospective validation. It is evident that the system does what it purports to do based on the plan. (e.g process validation plan of first three commercial batches).

The objective of the prospective validation is to prove or demonstrate that the process will work in accordance with the validation protocol prepared for the pilot production trials. Prospective validation should normally be completed prior to the distribution and sale of the medicinal product. In Prospective Validation, the validation protocol is executed before the process is put into commercial use.

(ii) Retrospective Validation:

Validation of a process for a product already in distribution based upon accumulated production, testing, and control data or evidence that the system does what it purports to do based upon review and analysis of existing information is called retrospective validation. (e.g stability studies)

Retrospective validation is only acceptable for well-established processes and will be inappropriate where there have been recent changes in the composition of the product, operating procedures, or equipment. Validation of such processes should be based on historical data. For retrospective validation, generally, data from ten to thirty consecutive batches should be examined to access process consistency, but fewer batches may be examined if justified.

(iii) Concurrent Validation:

In-process monitoring of critical processing steps and end-product testing of current production is involved in concurrent validation or evidence that the system does what it purports to do based upon information generated during the implementation of the system is called Concurrent Validation. (e.g equipment validation)

It is a process where current production batches are used to monitor processing parameters. Concurrent Validation means establishing documented evidence a process does what it is supposed to be based on data generated during the actual implementation of the process.

(iv) Revalidation:

Revalidation should be performed to ensure that the analytical method maintains its characteristics. The degree of revalidation depends on the nature of the change i.e. a new dosage strength in a product may require validation of the method in terms of recovery and linearity at the new dosage strength; a new formulation would require revalidation in terms of selectivity, recovery, etc.

Re-validation becomes necessary in certain situations. Some of the changes that require validation are as follows:

(i) Changes in raw materials (physical properties such as density, viscosity, particle size distribution, etc., that may affect the process or product).

(ii) Changes in the source of active raw material manufacturers.

(iii) Changes in packaging material (primary container/closure system)

(iv) Changes in the process (e.g., mixing time, drying temperatures, and batch size)

(v) Changes in the equipment (e.g., addition of automatic detection system).

(vi) Changes in the plant/facility.

2. Cleaning validation:

Cleaning validation ensures that there is no cross-contamination in a multiproduct manufacturing plant and also prevents microbial contamination. Once a product is manufactured, the equipment is cleaned using appropriate established cleaning SOP's established during the IQ of the equipment.

Types of contamination to be considered in cleaning validation:

(i) Cross-contamination.

(ii) Microbial contamination.
(iii) Contamination by cleaning or sanitizing agent.
(iv) Contamination by other agents.

3. Equipment validation:

As per FDA,

- The action of proving that any equipment works correctly and leads to the expected result is equipment qualification.
- It is not a single-step activity but instead results from many discrete activities.

STEPS INVOLVED

1. Design qualification (DQ)
2. Installation qualification (IQ)
3. Operational qualification (OQ)
4. Performance qualification (PQ)

DESIGN QUALIFICATION	INSTALLATION QUALIFICATION	OPERATIONAL QUALIFICATION	PERFORMANCE QUALIFCATION
• Before purchasing a new instrument	• At documented installation of new or existing instruments	• After installation • After major changes **e.g.** repair, updates • At regular intervals (risk based)	• Whenever the instrument is used **e.g.** daily

1. *Design Qualification (DQ)*

It is the documented verification that the proposed design of the facilities, systems and equipment is suitable for the intended purpose. DQ should be performed when new equipment is being purchased, or when existing equipment is being used for a new application. DQ serves as the precursor to defining the equipment Installation Qualification (IQ) and OQ protocols.

The purpose is to ensure that all the requirements for the final systems have been clearly defined at the start. In other words,

"Has it been designed and selected correctly?"

DQ check items:

(i) GMPs and regulatory requirements
(ii) Performance criteria
(iii) Reliability and efficiency
(iv) Commissioning requirements
(v) Construct ability and installation of equipment
(vi) Safety and environmental impact
(vii) Description of the intended use of the equipment

(viii) Preliminary selection of the supplier
(ix) Final selection of the equipment

2. *Installation Qualification (IQ)*

It is documented evidence that the premises, supporting utilities, the equipment have been built and installed in compliance with design specifications. It verifies that the equipment has been installed in accordance with manufacturers recommendation in a proper manner and placed in an environment suitable for its intended purpose.

It involves the co-ordinate efforts of the vendor, the operating department, and the project team. The purpose of IQ is to check the installation site environment, confirms equipment specifications, and verify the condition of installed equipment; and also to ensure that all aspects (static attributes) of the facility or equipment are installed correctly and comply with the original design.

In other words,

"Has it been built or installed correctly?"

In IQ, connect each unit (Electrical system, Flow line system) and confirm that the connections are correct.

IQ check items:

(i) Equipment design features (i.e. material of construction cleanability, etc.)
(ii) Installation conditions (wiring, utility, functionality, etc.)
(iii) Calibration, preventative maintenance, cleaning schedules.
(iv) Safety features.
(v) Supplier documentation, prints, drawings and manuals.
(vi) Software documented.
(vii) Spare parts list.
(viii) Environmental conditions (such as clean room requirements, temperature, and humidity.

Any problems identified in IQ must be investigated and appropriate actions must be taken. All such actions must be documented and approved by a higher authority.

3. *Operational Qualification (OQ)*

It is defined as refers to "establishing by objective evidence within process control limits and action levels which result in a product that meets all predetermined requirements". OQ is the process of demonstrating that an instrument will function according to its operational specification in the selected environment. The purpose is to ensure that all the dynamic attributes comply with the original design. In other words,

"Does it work correctly?"

Prior to implementing OQ, check the system configuration, determine the items to be evaluated and record them in OQ record and have them approved.

OQ check items:

(i) Process control limits (time, temperature, pressure, line speed, setup conditions, etc.)

(ii) Software parameters.

(iii) Raw material specifications

(iv) Process operating procedures.

(v) Material handling requirements.

(vi) Process change control.

(vii) Training.

(viii) Potential failure modes, action levels and worst-case conditions.

(ix) The use of statistically valid techniques such as screening experiments to optimize the process can be used during this phase.

Any problems identified in OQ must be investigated and appropriate actions must be taken. All such actions must be documented and approved by higher authority.

4. *Performance Qualification (PQ)*

After the IQ and OQ have been performed, the instrument's continued suitability for its intended use is proved through performance qualification. It refers to establishing by objective evidence that the process, under anticipated conditions, consistently produces a product that meets all predetermined requirements.

PQ should always be performed under conditions that are similar to routine sample analysis. PQ should be performed on a daily basis or whenever the equipment is being used.

PQ considerations include:

(i) Actual product and process parameters and procedures established in OQ.

(ii) Acceptability of the product.

(iii) Assurance of process capability as established in OQ.

(iv) Process repeatability, long-term process stability.

The objective is to ensure that the instrument is performing within specified limits. The PQ represents the final qualification of equipment or system.

It is used to establish and or confirm;

1. Definition of performance criteria and test procedures.
2. Selection of critical parameters, with predefined specifications.
3. Determination of the test intervals, e.g.,

   (a) - Everyday.

   (b) - Every time the system is used.

   (c) - Before, between and after a series of runs.

4. Define corrective actions on what to do if the system does not meet the established criteria.

Re- Qualification:

Modification to, or relocation of equipment should follow satisfactory review and authorization of the documented change proposal through the change control procedure. This formal review should include consideration of re-qualification of the equipment.

Minor changes or changes having no direct impact on final or in-process product quality should be handled through the documentation system of the preventive maintenance program.

4. Analytical method validation:

Validation of an analytical procedure is the process by which it is established, by laboratory studies, that the performance characteristics of the procedure meet the requirements for the intended analytical applications. Method validation provides an assurance of reliability during normal use, and is sometimes referred to as "the process for providing documented evidence that the method does what it is intended to do." The main objective of the validation is to demonstrate that the analytical method is suitable for its intended purpose, and is accurate, specific, and precise over the specified range that an analyte will be analyzed.

Why to validate?

- ➢ Method validation provides a high level of assurance that such a method should consistently yield results that are accurate, reproducible, and they are within previously established specifications.
- ➢ Mandatory requirements for product registration and approval for marketing by the drug regulatory authorities of various countries.
- ➢ To minimize product quality complaints and product recall and quick release of the product batch.
- ➢ Validation provides a high degree of confidence that same level of quality is built into each unit of finished product from batch to batch.

When to validate?

- ➢ New method development.
- ➢ Established method revised to incorporate improvements.
- ➢ Established method used in a different laboratory, analysis or instrumentation.
- ➢ To demonstrate the equivalence between new and established method.

Validation parameters

(i) Accuracy

(ii) Precision

  (a) Repeatability

  (b) Intermediate Precision

  (c) Reproducibility

(iii) LOD (Limit of Detection)
(iv) LOQ (Limit of Quantification)
(v) Linearity
(vi) Range
(vii) Robustness
(viii) Specificity
(ix) SST (System Suitability Test)
(x) Ruggedness
(xi) Transferability
(xii) Sensitivity

PARAMETERS	DESCRIPTIONS
Accuracy **Known as "Trueness"**	➢ **"The closeness of agreement between real value and measured value"** ➢ Accuracy should be checked across the range of spiking 5 different concentration of the active ingredient in placebo (dummy medication) preparation. ➢ Drug recovery should be calculated. ➢ %RSD value should not bc more than 2.0 % and % recovery of the individual should be between 98-102 % for the active drug.
Precision **Known as "Degree of Scatter"** **Or** **"series of measurement"**	➢ **"the closeness of agreement between a series of measurements."** ➢ Means measurement of reproducibility of whole analytical method. ➢ System precision will be checked by 6 replicate injections of the same test concentration. ➢ Method precision will be checked by preparing 5 assay samples separately from the homogeneous sample % RSD should not be more than 2.0 %
Precision repeatability Known as Intra-assay precision	*Method:* 9 determinations covering the specified range or 6 determinations at 100 % of the test concentration.
Intermediate precision	➢ **"express within laboratory variation"** *Method:* ➢ Depends on circumstances of usage of the methods. ➢ Should include variations in days, analyst, columns.
Reproducibility	➢ **"precision between laboratories."** *Method:* ➢ Dependent on usage of method ➢ Should include inter laboratory study.

Contd...

PARAMETERS	DESCRIPTIONS
LOD (Limit Of Detection)	➢ "lowest amount of analyte that can be detected ". **Determination of LODs (limits of detection)** LOD's may also be calculated based on the standard deviation of the response (SD) and the slope of the calibration curve (S) at levels approximating the LOD according to the formula: LOD = 3.3(SD/S). The standard deviation of the response can be determined based on the standard deviation of y-intercepts of regression lines.
LOQ (Limit Of Quantification)	➢ **"lowest amount of analyte that can be detected and quantified"** ➢ The value derived shall be validated by injecting same concentration of solution and determining the signal to noise (S/N) ration & that should not be less than 3 in case of LOD, but in case of LOQ S/N ratio should not be less than 10. ➢ The calculation method is again based on the standard deviation of the response (SD) and the slope of the calibration curve (S) according to the formula: ➢ **LOQ = 10(SD/S).**
Linearity	➢ **"proportionality of measured value of concentration."** ➢ A linear relationship should be established by dilution of the stock solution. ➢ A minimum of 5 concentrations should be tested & correlation coefficient should be checked &which should not be less than 0.99
Range	➢ **"Concentration interval where method is precise, accurate and linear"** ➢ Interval between the upper and lower conc. Of analyte in the sample.
Robustness	➢ **"reproducibility under normal but variable laboratory conditions"** ➢ % RSD of assay results by small but deliberate variations should not be more than 2.0 %
Specificity	➢ **"Ability to measure the desired analyte in a complex mixture."** ➢ "it is the ability to assess unequivocally the analyte in the presence of components which may be expected to be present. typically, these might include impurities, degradants, matrix etc." ➢ Placebo interference will be checked by injection of assay preparation of placebo, [means dummy medications, No active ingredient but therapeutic effect,].

Contd...

PARAMETERS	DESCRIPTIONS
Ruggedness	➢ **"ruggedness should be established by 2 different system, columns and analyst.** ➢ Repeatability will be checked by minimum of 5 different concentration prepared separately from homogenous sample. ➢ % RSD of assay results of analyst-1 and analyst -2 should not be more than 2%
SST Known as System Suitability Test (SST).	➢ Check the theoretical plates, tailing factor, resolution and % RSD etc... ➢ This result should be within specification limits.
Transferability	➢ It is the ability of the method to be used correctly by others without seeking additional information
Sensitivity	➢ **"smallest quantity that can be detected-accurately measured"**

VALIDATION MASTER PLAN (VMP)

The VMP serves as the validation roadmap, setting the course, justifying the strategy, outlining the preliminary test and acceptance criteria, and documenting the necessary programs that ensure a continuing state of validation.

- The validation master plan should provide an overview of the entire validation operation, its organizational structure, its content, and its planning.
- It is a key document in GMP
- The main elements of it are the list/inventory of the items to be validated and the planning schedule.
- All validation activities relating to critical technical operations, relevant to the product and process controls within a firm should be included in the validation master plan.
- It should comprise all prospective, concurrent, and retrospective validations as well as revalidations.
- The Validation Master Plan should be a summary document and should therefore be brief, concise, and clear.
- It should not repeat information documented elsewhere but should refer to existing documents such as policy documents, SOP's and validation protocols and reports.
- The format and content should include:
    - ✓ *Introduction:* validation policy, scope, location and schedule.
    - ✓ *Organizational structure:* personnel responsibilities.

- ✓ *Plant/process/product description:* rational for inclusions or exclusions and extent of validation.
- ✓ Specific process considerations that are critical and those requiring extra attention.
- ✓ Key acceptance criteria.
- ✓ Documentation format.
- ✓ Reference to the required SOPs.
- ✓ Time plans of each validation project and sub-project.
- ✓ List of products/ processes/ systems to be validated, summarized in a matrix format, validation approach.
- ✓ Re-validation activities, actual status and future planning

CALIBRATION

Calibration of an instrument is the process of determining its accuracy. The process involves obtaining a reading from the instrument and measuring its variation from the reading obtained from a standard instrument. Calibration of an instrument also involves adjusting its precision and accuracy so that its readings come in accordance with the established standard.

Why calibration?

Calibration brings out the nature and magnitude of an error (if any) of testing measuring instruments. This error is the deviation from the reference standard and it is the hidden deficiency of the quality measuring system of an organization.

Advantages of calibration:

The knowledge of the nature and extent of errors of testing and measuring the instruments employed in the quality measuring system will help an organization in the following ways:

- ✓ One can take the error of an instrument into account while using it and hence correct measurements are recorded and reported. This will help an organization to set its process and quality control system correctly.
- ✓ Wherever possible, one can adjust or repair the instrument to minimize the error to the best extent.
- ✓ Any dispute arising with a customer due to instrument error can be resolved.

Scope/Purpose of Calibration:

Calibration is primarily done to achieve 5 main purposes which are:

- ➢ To make sure that the readings of equipment or instruments are consistent with other measurements and display the correct readings every single time.

- To determine the accuracy, precision, reliability and deviation of the measurements produced by all the instruments
- To establish the reliability of the instrument being used and whether it can be trusted to deliver repeatable results each time
- To map the 'drift' as documented. Instruments have a tendency to produce inaccurate measurements over a period of time, following repeated use.
- Ensuring that the industry standards, quality assurance benchmarks such as current good manufacturing practice (cGMP) and government regulations are adhered to.

Instrument calibration:

Instrument calibration can be defined as the process of comparing the measurements made by the instrument to be calibrated against a known measurement of either standards or an instrument known to be making measurements that exceed the acceptable limits of accuracy and precision.

Usually, calibration labs prefer a standard with 10 times the accuracy; however, most regulating organizations and authorities also accept a 3: 1 accuracy ratio.

Frequency of Instrument Calibration:

How often you conduct instrument calibration mainly depends upon its tendency to drift from the true measurement and how it impacts the quality of the end product. Examine each instrument being used and study its behaviour. Based on this information, you can design a calibration schedule for each instrument. The interval between calibrations can vary as.

- Weekly
- Monthly or bi-monthly
- Quarterly, semi-annually or annually
- After every heavy usage of the instrument

Commonly Used Calibration Methods and Procedures:

There are different ways that are used to calibrate an instrument. These methods are chosen based on the desired results of the calibration and regulatory authorities' requirements, like FDA guidelines. Let us look at three such procedures:

Standard Calibration: This method is mostly preferred for calibrating instruments that are non-critical to quality or are not required for accreditation and license purposes. Use traceable standards and document its performance.

Calibration with Data: Procedures for calibrations with data are similar to that of accredited calibration. The only exception is that these procedures are not accredited to the ISO standard. Moreover, they are not accompanied by data on measurement uncertainties.

ISO 17025 Accredited Calibration: This has to be the strictest method of calibration. Generally, it requires a measurement report which has the details of the measurements that are made against a standard of 'as found' (before calibration is started) and 'as left' (once the calibration is completed). If the calibration is done by a calibration service provider, they must issue a certificate of the same.

Importance of Regular Calibration:

- Calibration is responsible for defining the accuracy of any measurement and its quality that is recorded by any instrument.
- When you start working with any instrument, it must be calibrated well, thus assuring you of accurate results. However, over a period of time you will start observing a drift. Calibration minimizes such uncertainties by assuring the accuracy of the test equipment.
- When you regularly calibrate your equipment, you can eliminate the drift at its budding stage instead of allowing it to grow till it affects the measurements in significant ways.
- Calibration helps in quantifying and controlling errors and uncertainties within various measurement processes to an acceptable level.
- Further, it helps in improving the accuracy of the measuring device, which in turn improves the quality of the end product.
- In short, regular calibration allows pharmaceutical companies to have confidence in their results which they can record, monitor and control.

CHAPTER 4

GLP, ISO 9000

GOOD LABORATORY PRACTICE (GLP)

GLP is a formal regulation created by USFDA as these regulations were proposed on November 19,1976 and designated as a new part of Chapter 21 of the Code of Federal Regulations (CFR) as 21 CFR Part 58 in 1979. In 1981 an organization named OECD (Organization for Economic Cooperation and Development) produced GLP principles that are international standards.

GLP in OECD principles is defined as *"a quality system concerned with the organizational process and the conditions under which non-clinical health and environmental safety studies are planned, performed, monitored, recorded, archived and reported"*.

When & Why was GLP Created?

GLP was first introduced in New Zealand and Denmark in 1972, and later in the US in 1978 in response to the Industrial Bio Test Labs scandal. In the early 70's FDA became aware of cases of poor laboratory practice all over the United States. They discovered a lot of fraudulent activities and a lot of poor lab practices. Examples of some of these poor lab practices found were:

1. Equipment has not been calibrated to standard form, therefore giving wrong measurements.
2. Incorrect/inaccurate accounts of the actual lab study.
3. Inadequate test systems.

Why GLP was created?

GLPs were initially invoked in reaction to malpractices in the laboratories conducting safety experiments of medicine. In the early 1970s, research laboratories in the USA were found doing work in unethical ways like

- data generation without conduct of the study
- falsification of the laboratory work
- replacement of dead animals and fabrication of test results, etc.

Advantages of GLP

- Assures that the data are a true reflection of results obtained from studies.
- Preclinical safety and residue safety.

- Generate high-quality and reliable test data.
- Mutual acceptance of data ~ Increases public confidence.
- Shortens the time to market for new products.

Disadvantages of GLP

- More manpower is required.
- Expensive process.
- Time-consuming process.

Objectives of GLP

- GLP makes sure that the data submitted or a true reflection of the results obtained from the study.
- GLP makes sure that the data is traceable
- Promote international acceptance of tests

Principles of GLP

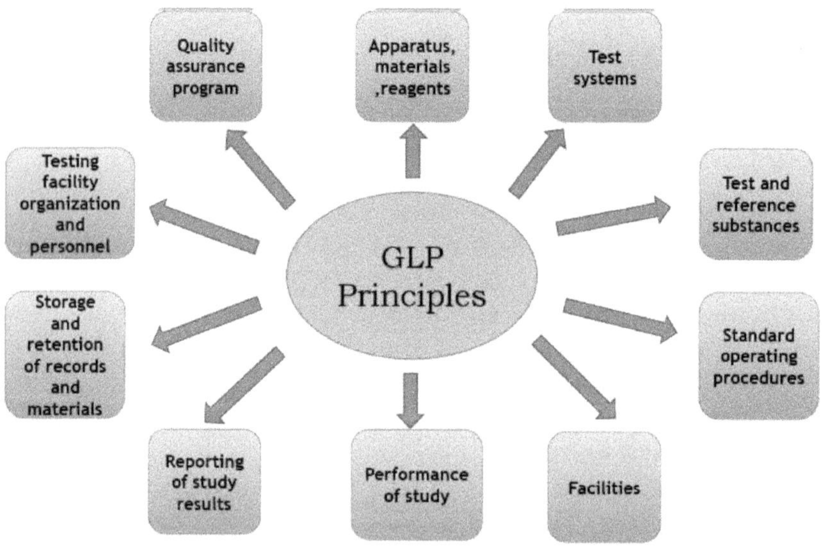

How to practice GLP?

A. General provisions
B. Organization and Personnel
C. Facilities
D. Equipment
E. Testing facilities operation
F. Test and control articles
G. Protocol for and the conduct of the nonclinical laboratory study
H. Records and Reports

A. General provisions

- ✓ It prescribes GLP for conducting non-clinical laboratory studies that support research and marketing permits of products regulated by the FDA
- ✓ Applicability to studies performed under grants and contracts
- ✓ Inspection of the testing facility
- ✓ Statements of compliance or non-compliance
- ✓ Effects of non-compliance

B. Organization and Personnel

- ➢ Personnel
- ➢ Testing facility management
- ➢ Study director
- ➢ Quality assurance unit

Organization- Functions:

1. Identification of quality activities.
2. Dividing the jobs among the personnel.
3. Define the authority and responsibility of each job and the relationship of each job with other jobs
4. Coordinate the work of internal departments and outside agencies

Personnel

Each individual engaged in the conduct or supervision of non-clinical laboratory study shall have:

1. Education
2. Training
   - General training
   - Specific training
3. Experience or combination
4. Personal sanitation and health precautions

Testing facility management

1. A sufficient number of qualified personnel, appropriate facilities, equipment, and materials available for conducting of the study
2. Maintenance of records of qualifications, training, and experience of personnel and their job description
3. New appointment of study, Director
4. Quality assurance program with designated personnel

Study Director

A scientist or other professional with appropriate education, training, and experience.

The responsibilities of the study director are:

1. Approval of protocol and study plans including amendments.
2. Technical conduct of the study.

3. Ensure that the QA personnel and study personnel are updated with the study plan and SOPs.
4. Interpretation, analysis, documentation, and reporting of the results.
5. Also checks that experimental data is accurately recorded and verified.
6. Sign and date the final report for acceptance of data.

Quality Assurance Unit

1. An individual or a group designated by management to assure that the studies are in compliance with GLP principles.
2. Monitors the study to assure management that the facilities, equipment, personnel, methods, practices, records, and controls are in conformance with the regulations.
3. Maintain the copies of master schedule sheet, protocols, and SOPs
4. Access to updated study plans and SOPs
5. Document, and verification of compliance of the study with GLP principles
6. Inspections to determine the compliance of the study with GLP principles and three types of inspections are:
   (a) Study-based inspections
   (b) Process-based inspections
   (c) Facility-based inspections
7. Determines any deviation from the approved protocol and reports to SD (Study Director), PI (Principal Investigator), and management.
8. Prepare statements to be included in the final report containing dates and types of inspection.

C. Facilities

1. General facilities:
   - Testing system facilities
   - Archive facilities
   - Waste disposal
2. Animal care facilities

General facilities

(a) Testing system facilities

- Suitable size, construction, and location.
- An adequate degree of separation of different activities.
- Laboratories should be well-ventilated, and free of dust, drafts, and extreme temperatures.
- A minimum of 150sq.feet of floor space and a minimum of 6 linear feet of usable bench space should be provided for each analyst.

(b) Archive facilities

Secure storage and retrieval of study plans, raw data, final reports, and specimens to prevent untimely deterioration.

(c) Waste disposal

Appropriate collection, storage, and disposal facilities and decontamination procedures.

Animal care facilities

1. Located away from testing laboratories preferably in a separate building.
2. Contamination risk is reduced by a "barrier" system as well as by providing "clean" and "dirty" corridors
3. Separate areas for animals of different species and studies.
4. Separate areas for diagnosis, treatment, and control of laboratory animal diseases.
5. Lighting should be proper as light intensity and noise level is sufficient
6. Maintain room temperature, humidity, and air changes in animal quarters.

D. Equipment

1. Appropriate design and adequate capacity.
2. Equipment shall be adequately inspected, cleaned, and maintained.
3. Equipment used for the generation, measurement, or assessment of data shall be adequately tested, calibrated, and standardized.
4. Log books for each equipment should be there.

E. Testing Facilities Operation

1. Standard Operating Procedures (SOPs)
2. Reagents and solutions
3. Animal care

Standard Operating Procedures (SOPs)

1. Written documents specifying procedures for laboratory programs.
2. Testing facility should have a written SOP approved by management.
3. SOPs should be available wherever applicable e.g. test and reference items, apparatus, materials and reagents, record keeping, and reporting. storage and retrieval, test systems, and quality assurance procedures.
4. Any deviation from SOP should be authorized by SD and documented in the raw data.
5. Routine inspection, cleaning, maintenance, testing, and calibration.
6. Actions to be taken in response to routine failure.

Reagents and solutions

1. Reagents used in the operation should be specified in the SOPs.
2. Reagents and solutions should be labeled.
3. Deteriorated or outdated reagents and solutions should not be used.
4. Store under ambient temperature.

Animal care

1. SOPs - for housing, feeding, handling, and care of animals

2. Animals should be free of any disease and if during the course of study, animals contract a disease then the diseased animals shall be isolated
3. Diagnosis, authorization of treatment, description, and date of treatment shall be documented and retained,
4. Animals of different species shall be housed in separate rooms when necessary.
5. The animal cages, racks, and accessory equipment shall be cleaned and sanitized at appropriate intervals

F. Test and Control Articles

1. Test and control article characterization
2. Test and control article handling
3. The Mixture of articles with carriers

Test and control article characterization

1. The identity, strength, purity, and composition or other characteristics of the test and control article shall be determined and
2. Methods of synthesis, fabrication, or derivation shall be documented by the sponsor or the testing facility.
3. Stability of each test and control article is determined.
4. Storage conditions are maintained and each storage container shall be labeled by name, chemical abstract number, or batch number

Test and control article handling

Handling procedures of test and control articles ensures:

1. Proper storage.
2. Minimum risk of contamination and deterioration or damage.
3. Receipt and distribution of each batch are documented.
4. Documentation includes the date and quantity of each batch distributed or returned.

The mixture of articles with carriers

1. Appropriate analytical methods shall be conducted for determination of uniformity of mixture and concentration of test or control article in the mixture.
2. Stability of the mixture is determined.
3. Expiration date should be written on the container.

G. Protocol for and Conduct Study

1. Protocol
2. Conduct of a nonclinical laboratory study

Protocol

Contents of protocol

1. Identification
2. Title and statement of purpose
3. Identification of test (or control) items
4. Names and addresses of the sponsor, test facility, and test site

5. Name of the study director and other personnel
6. Proposed dates
7. Justification for selection of the test system
8. Description of the test system
9. Experimental design

Conduct a nonclinical laboratory study

1. Study shall be conducted in accordance with the protocol.
2. Information on the specimens should be present on the container to avoid errors in the recording and storage of data.
3. All the data generated shall be recorded directly, promptly, and legibly by ink.

H. Records and Reports

1. Reporting of non-clinical laboratory results
2. Storage, retrieval, and retention of records and data

Reporting of non-clinical laboratory study results

The final report shall contain:

1. Information on sponsor and test facility.
2. Experimental starting and completion dates
3. Objectives and procedures stated in the protocol (including the changes in the protocol).
4. Description of materials and test methods.
5. A Quality Assurance Program statement.
6. Storage (specimens, reference items, raw data, and final report).

Storage, retrieval, and retention of records and data

1. Archives should be there for orderly storage and expedient of all raw data, documentation, protocols, specimens, and final reports.
2. Index of materials retained.
3. Master schedule sheet, copies of protocols, and records of Quality Assurance inspections shall be maintained by QAU (Quality Assurance Unit).
4. Wet specimens and samples of test and control articles shall be retained until the quality of preparation affords evaluation.
5. If any study plan is disposed of before expiry the reason to be justified and documented.

ISO 9000

ISO (International Organization for Standardization) is the world's largest developer and publisher of International Standards. ISO is a network of the national standards institutes of 157 countries, one member per country, with a Central Secretariat in Geneva, Switzerland, that coordinates the system.

In 1946, delegates from **25 countries** met in **London** and decided to create a new international organization, of which the object would be "to facilitate the international coordination and unification of industrial standards". The new organization, ISO, officially began operations on **23 February 1947, in Geneva, Switzerland**.

ISO is a **non-governmental organization** that forms a bridge between the public and private sectors. On the one hand, many of its member institutes are part of the governmental structure of their countries or are mandated by their government. On the other hand, other members have their roots uniquely in the **private sector**, having been set up by national partnerships of industry associations.

ISO Standards are voluntary. As a non-governmental organization, ISO has **no legal authority** to enforce the implementation of its standards. ISO does not regulate or legislate. However, countries may decide to adopt ISO standards - mainly those concerned with health, safety or the environment - as regulations or refer to them in legislation, for which they provide the technical basis. In addition, although ISO standards are voluntary, they may become a **market requirement**, as has happened in the case of ISO 9001 quality management systems, or of dimensions of freight containers and bank cards.

MEMBERS

Three types of members are available.

- Member Body

  It is a national body. Only one body in each country is admitted. Gives financial support to ISO through fees. Has full rights on technical and policy committees.
- Subscriber Membership

  A country with a small economy. Pay small fees. Nevertheless, can be in contact with ISO.
- Correspondence member

  An organization in a country not fully developed for national standards activity. Receive required information only.

Principal Officers of ISO

Elected

President

Appointed

Vice-President (Policy)

Vice-President (Technical Management)

Treasurer

Acting Secretary General

Organization of ISO

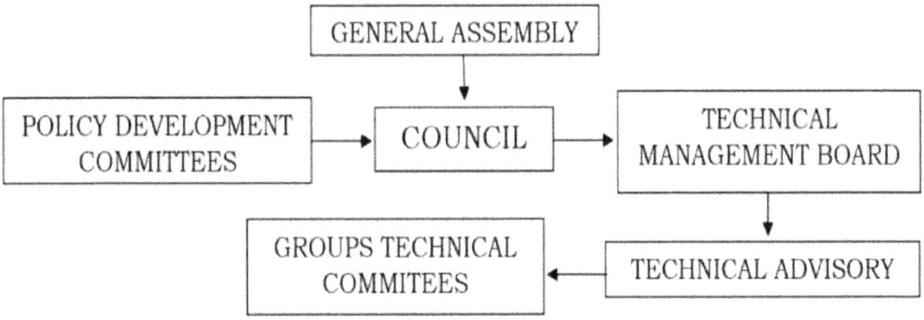

Importance of Standards

- Standards make an enormous and **positive contribution** to most aspects of our lives.
- Standards ensure desirable characteristics of products and services such as **quality, environmental friendliness, safety, reliability, efficiency, and interchangeability - and at an economical cost.**
- When products, systems, machinery, and devices work well and safely, it is often because they meet standards. And **the organization responsible** for many thousands of the standards which benefit the world is **ISO**.

ISO standards:

- make the development, manufacturing, and supply of products and services **more efficient, safer, and cleaner.**
- **facilitate trade** between countries and make it **fairer**.
- **share** technological advances and good management practices
- to disseminate **innovation**.
- **safeguard consumers**, and users in general, of products and services.
- make life simpler by providing **solutions** to common problems

Benefits of ISO Standards

ISO standards provide technological, economic, and societal benefits.

For **businesses**, the widespread adoption of International Standards means that **suppliers can develop and offer products and services meeting specifications** that have wide international acceptance in their sectors. Therefore, businesses using International Standards can compete in many more markets around the world.

For **innovators** of new technologies, International Standards on aspects like **terminology, compatibility, and safety** speed up the dissemination of innovations and their development into manufacturable and marketable products.

For **customers**, the worldwide compatibility of technology which is achieved when products and services are based on International Standards gives them a **broad choice** of offers. They also benefit from the **effects of competition** among suppliers.

For **trade officials**, International Standards create **"a level playing field"** for all competitors in those markets. The existence of divergent national or regional standards can create technical barriers to trade. International Standards are the technical means by which **political trade agreements can be put into practice.**

For **developing countries**, by defining the characteristics that products and services will be expected to meet on **export** markets, International Standards give developing countries a basis for making **the right decisions** when **investing** their scarce resources and thus avoid squandering them.

For **consumers**, conformity of products and services to International Standards provides **assurance about their quality, safety, and reliability.**

For **everyone**, International Standards contribute to the **quality of life** in general by ensuring that the transport, machinery, and tools we use are safe.

For **the planet** we inhabit, International Standards on air, water, and soil quality, on emissions of gases and radiation, and environmental aspects of products can contribute to **preserving the environment**.

STAGES OF THE DEVELOPMENT OF INTERNATIONAL STANDARDS

An International Standard is the result of an agreement between the member bodies of ISO. International Standards are developed by ISO technical committees (TC) and subcommittees (SC) through a six-step process:

Stage 1: Proposal stage

Stage 2: Preparatory stage

Stage 3: Committee stage

Stage 4: Enquiry stage

Stage 5: Approval stage

Stage 6: Publication stage

Stage 1: Proposal stage

The first step in the development of an International Standard is to confirm that a **particular International Standard is needed.** A new work item proposal (NP) is submitted for **vote** by the members of the relevant **TC or SC** to determine the inclusion of the work item in the program of work. The proposal is accepted if a **majority** of the members of the TC/SC votes in favour.

Stage 2: Preparatory stage

Usually, a working group of experts, the chairman (convener) of which is the project leader, is set up by the TC/SC for the preparation of a **working draft.** Successive working drafts may be considered until the working group is satisfied that it has developed the best **technical solution to the problem** being addressed. At this stage, the draft is forwarded to the working **group's parent committee** for the consensus -building phase.

Stage 3: Committee stage

As soon as a first committee draft is available, it is registered by the ISO Central Secretariat. It is **distributed for comment and, if required, voting**, by the members of the TC/SC. Successive committee drafts may be considered until a consensus is reached on the technical content. Once consensus has been attained, the text is finalized for submission as a **draft International Standard (DIS).**

Stage 4: Enquiry stage

The draft International Standard (DIS) is circulated to all ISO member bodies by the ISO Central Secretariat for voting and comment within a **period of five months.** It is approved for submission as a **Final Draft International Standard** (FDIS) if a two-thirds majority of the members of the TC/SC are in favor and not more than one-quarter of the total number of votes cast are negative. If the approval criteria are not met, the text is returned to the originating TC/SC for further study and a **revised document** will again be circulated for voting and comment as a **draft International Standard.**

Stage 5: Approval stage

The final draft International Standard (FDIS) is circulated to all ISO member bodies by the ISO Central Secretariat for a final Yes/No vote **within a period of two months.** If technical comments are received during this period, they are no longer considered at this stage but registered for consideration during a future revision of the International Standard. The text is approved as an International Standard if a two-thirds majority of the members of the TC/SC is in favor and not more than one-quarter of the total number of votes cast are negative.

Stage 6: Publication stage

Once a final draft International Standard has been approved, only minor editorial changes, if and where necessary, are introduced into the final text. The final text is sent to the ISO Central Secretariat which publishes the International Standard.

ISO 9000

The **ISO 9000** family addresses **"quality management"**. This means what the organization does to fulfill:

- the customer's quality requirements, and
- applicable regulatory requirements, while aiming to enhance customer satisfaction, and
- achieve continual improvement of its performance in pursuit of these objectives

Core Principles of ISO 9000

The seven quality management principles are:

QMP 1 – Customer focus

QMP 2 – Leadership QMP

QMP 3 – Engagement of people

QMP 4 – Process approach

QMP 5 – Improvement

QMP 6 – Evidence-based decision making

QMP 7 – Relationship management

1. ***Customer focus***

   The primary focus of quality management is to meet customer requirements and strive to exceed customer expectations. This principle includes,

   - ➢ To recognize the needs of existing and future customers
   - ➢ Aligning organizational objectives with customer needs and expectations
   - ➢ Meet customer requirements
   - ➢ Assess customer satisfaction
   - ➢ Handle customer relationships

2. ***Leadership QMP***

   Leaders at all levels establish unity of purpose and direction as well create conditions in which people are engaged in achieving the organization's quality objectives. This principle includes,

   - ➢ Establish a vision and direction for the organization
   - ➢ Set demanding goals
   - ➢ Model organizational values
   - ➢ Establish trust
   - ➢ Train and empower employees
   - ➢ Identify employee contributions

3. ***Engagement of people***

   Competent, empowered and engaged people at all levels throughout the organization are essential to enhance its capability to create and deliver value. This principle concentrates on,

- Ensure that people's skills are used and valued
- Make people responsible
- Enable participation in continual improvement
- Evaluate individual performance
- Facilitate learning and sharing of knowledge
- Enable open discussion of problems and constraints

4. ***Process approach***

   Consistent and predictable results are achieved more effectively and efficiently when activities are understood and managed as interrelated processes that function as a coherent system. This includes,

   - Supervise activities as processes
   - Assess the capability of activities
   - Identify linkages between activities
   - Prioritize improvement opportunities
   - Organize resources effectively

5. ***Improvement***

   Successful organizations have an ongoing focus on improvement. This includes,

   - Develop organizational performance and capabilities
   - Align advanced activities
   - Empower people to make improvements
   - Measure improvement consistently
   - Celebrate the improvements

6. ***Evidence-based decision making***

   Decisions based on the analysis and evaluation of data and information are more likely to produce desired results. This principle includes,

   - Guarantee the accessibility of accurate and consistent data
   - Use suitable methods to analyze data
   - Make decisions based on analysis
   - Balance data analysis with practical experience

7. ***Relationship management***

   For sustained success, an organization manages its relationships with interested parties, such as suppliers. This principle includes,

   - Identify and select suppliers to manage costs, optimize resources, and create value
   - Establish relationships considering both the short and long term
   - Share expertise, resources, information, and plans with partners
   - Collaborate on improvement and development activities
   - Recognize supplier successes.

CHAPTER 5

Total Quality Management, Quality Review, and Documentation

TOTAL QUALITY MANAGEMENT

TQM is a management system and philosophy that strives towards constant organizational improvement to achieve excellence and ensure customer satisfaction and loyalty. It is the continued process of detecting/reducing/eliminating errors in manufacturing, streamlining the process of supply chain management, improving customer experience, and ensuring employees are well-trained.

TQM is a structured approach to organizational management with a process focused on improving the quality of outputs of an organization, including services and goods, by the constant improvement of its internal practices. TQM is an organizational management philosophy seeking to continuously improve the quality of processes and products.

Using a set of management and quality tools, the TQM approach seeks to increase business even as it reduces loss due to improper practices. Being a highly adaptable concept, it has been widely applied in several industries in the production and service sectors.

MAJOR COMPONENTS OF THE TQM APPROACH

- ✓ Focus on consumer
- ✓ Analysis of the process
- ✓ Work in quality teams
- ✓ Systematic analysis of problems
- ✓ Implement planned changes and evaluate results
- ✓ Use data to identify problems and solutions
- ✓ Implement changes

TQM IMPLEMENTATION IN PHARMACEUTICALS

TQM can be difficult to accomplish and maintain whether an organization is endeavouring to retain its quality of products or be in line with regulations from the respective authorities. It can't be effectively accomplished without significant and relevant resources like funds and workforce.

TQM is a strategy through which managers, as well as employees, can be engaged in the constant process of quality improvement of products. It is a blend of value and managerial techniques focused on business expansion and the reduction of losses because of inefficient practices.

BENEFITS OF TOTAL QUALITY MANAGEMENT

TQM is the coordination of management efforts with the intention of improving quality at all levels within the organization. Thus, the TQM approach has various benefits. It comes with monetary benefits which incorporate lowered costs of production, increased investment and sales profits, and also the power to increase product prices to the quality involved.

Additional benefits may incorporate facilitated entry to worldwide markets, higher client maintenance levels, development of new innovations within a short period, and a good company reputation.

Just a few organizations implement the TQM approach on the grounds that a powerful program actualization is time-consuming and costly. In any case, organizations with the appropriate assets may gain the upper hand in their enterprises by actualizing the TQM.

CAUSE OF FAILURE IN TQM IMPLEMENTATION

TQM has yielded tremendous monetary benefits in various pharmaceutical manufacturers, while struggles for quality fizzled and yielded peripheral outcomes in some different manufacturers.

The following are reasons which can be behind a failed TQM implementation process:

- Concentrating solely on momentary financial-related outcomes while turning a blind eye to the improvement of systems (Improvement in quality calls for a change of thought in the management of the basic systems).
- Managers' interference in teamwork,
- Unclear strategies and procedures,
- Failure to understand the TQM approach, inadequate training as well as insufficient education resources

KEY ELEMENTS OF TQM

There are eight key elements on which an organization must focus to implement TQM with success:

1. Ethics
2. Integrity
3. Trust
4. Training
5. Teamwork
6. Leadership
7. Recognition
8. Communication

These eight elements are further clubbed into four groups as follows, based on their function:

(i) *Group I* – Foundation – Ethics, Integrity, and Trust
(ii) *Group II* – Building Bricks – Training, Teamwork, and Leadership
(iii) *Group III* – Binding Mortar – Communication
(iv) *Group IV* – Roof – Recognition

Foundation: A foundation of ethics, integrity, and trust helps to create an open and fair environment that fosters involvement by everyone in the organization. Ethics deals with what is good and bad in a given situation, both at the individual and the organizational levels. Integrity refers to the honesty with which one adheres to facts. When ethics are followed with integrity, it leads to the development of trust, the third element of the 'foundation', which creates an environment of cooperativeness.

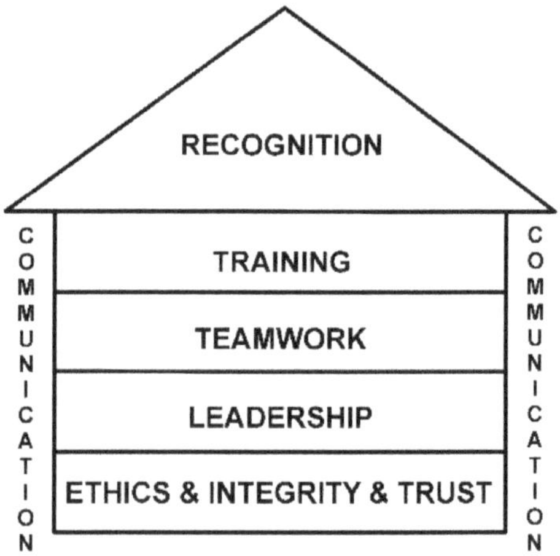

Building Bricks: Employees need to be trained in performing their duties right and in problem-solving. They must also be trained in interacting with others, to do their job better through teamwork. Any team is only as good as its leader, though, and so, there has to be inspirational leadership by someone who understands TQM and is committed to it in daily practice.

Binding Mortar: The link which binds all elements of TQM is communication which refers to a common understanding of the message by both the sender and receiver. Openness in communication between members of an organization, and with vendors, and customers is key to the success of TQM.

Roof: Recognizing the contributions of people in an organization, whether for teams or individuals, is the final element in TQM. When employees receive recognition, it brings about a leap in their self-esteem and such employees are more motivated which ultimately leads to better productivity and quality of work they do.

PHILOSOPHIES OF TQM

Several quality experts have given their viewpoints on how to achieve quality. Some of the most important concepts have been summed up in the table below:

Walter A. Shewhart	Understanding variability, the concept of statistical control charts
W. Edwards Deming	Management's responsibility for the quality, 14 points for quality improvement
Joseph M. Juran	Concept of quality cost, quality trilogy (quality planning, quality control, quality improvement)
Armand E. Feigenbaum	Total quality control
Philip B. Crosby	Concept of zero defects, do it right the first time
Kaoru Ishikawa	Concept of the internal customer, quality circles
Genichi Taguchi	Concept of product design quality, developed Taguchi loss function

TOOLS USED IN TQM

Tool	Purpose
Cause and effect diagram/Fishbone diagram	Identify and analyze causes of a problem
Checklists	Gathering of data
Flowcharts	Document detailed steps of a process
Scatter diagrams	Relation between two variables
Control charts	Identify variations in process
Histograms	Graphical display of frequency distribution of data
Pareto analysis	Degree of importance of each element

QUALITY REVIEW AND DOCUMENTATION

A Quality Review (QR) is a record of the performance against the Quality Goal at regular intervals. A Quality Review is an inspection with a specific structure, defined roles, and procedure designed to ensure a product's completeness and adherence to quality standards. The Quality Review is used to check if all Objectives of a Quality Goal have been achieved.

Quality review is planned and documented inspections of a review system. The review item may be a product, a group of related products, or a part of a product. The earlier an error is identified the less costly the implications and the penalty for failing to conduct adequate reviews. The US Food and Drug Administration proposed the requirement on 13 February 1976 rewriting of the GMPs. The purpose was to provide reliable procedures for a drug manufacturer to review the quality standard. Quality Review was published in September 1978. Final current GMP's (cGMP)regulation for drug products and became effective on 28 March 1979.

Objectives of Quality Review

1. Product Specification.
2. Identification of improvement.
3. Highlighting trends.
4. Appropriateness of starting material requirement specifications.

Principle

- ➢ QR studies indicate the product is within the specified limits.
- ➢ QR examines all documents to be sure there are no loose ends and also examine testing data to confirm that the product meets specifications.
- ➢ If there is a significant problem with the product, GMPs require the QC group to reject the product and investigate.

Phases in QR:

QR should be seen as a 3- Phase process

1. Phase – 1: Preparation
2. Phase – 2: Review meeting
3. Phase – 3: The Follow-up

Phase -1:

- ✓ It is the responsibility of the chairman and presenter to organize the Q.R. and notify all reviewers invited.
- ✓ Invitations and copies of the products being reviewed should be issued, allowing sufficient time for each reviewer to compile an error list.

Phase -2:

- ✓ Error lists and copies of annotated products should be brought to the meeting by each reviewer.
- ✓ During the review meeting the emphasis should be on error detection, in line with the criteria, and only limited discussion of corrective action should occur.
- ✓ It is important that 'personalities' and 'politics' are kept out of the review.
- ✓ For reviews that are 'complete' the action list tasks are allocated along with designated reviewers, to verify that the work is done.

- ✓ A project exception report should be raised for any errors detected in non-review items.

Phase 3:

- ✓ Follow-up period during which the errors identified at the review that was committed to the follow-up action list are rectified and signed off.
- ✓ At the end of the follow-up period which is typically restricted to one week, the follow up action list should be signed off by the chairman.

CHAPTER 6

ICH- International Conference on Harmonisation- Guidelines

ICH is the "International Council for Harmonization of Technical Requirements of Pharmaceuticals for Human Use". It is a joint initiative involving both regulators and research-based industry representatives of the EU, Japan and the US in scientific and technical discussions of the testing procedures required to assess and ensure the safety, quality, and efficacy of medicines. The ICH Secretariat is based in Geneva. The biennial meetings and conferences of the ICH Steering Committee rotate between the EU, Japan, and the USA.

OBJECTIVES OF ICH

- To increase international harmonization of technical requirements to ensure that safe, effective, and high-quality medicines are developed.
- To harmonize technical requirements for registration or marketing approval.
- To develop and register pharmaceuticals in the most efficient and cost-effective manner.
- To promote public health.
- To prevent unnecessary duplication of clinical trials on humans.
- To minimize the use of animal testing without compromising the safety and effectiveness of the drug.

GOALS OF ICH

- To promote international harmonization by bringing together representatives from the three ICH regions (EU, Japan, and USA)
- To discuss and establish common guidelines.
- To make information available on ICH, ICH activities, and ICH guidelines to any country or company that requests the information

- To promote a mutual understanding of regional initiatives in order to facilitate harmonization processes related to ICH guidelines regionally and globally
- To strengthen the capacity of drug regulatory authorities and industry to utilize them.

MEMBERS OF ICH

- ICH is comprised of representatives from **six parties** that represent the regulatory bodies and research-based industry in the European Union, Japan, and the USA.
- In Japan, the members are the **Ministry of Health, Labour and Welfare** (MHLW), and the **Japan Pharmaceutical Manufacturers Association** (JPMA).
- In Europe, the members are the **European Union** (EU), and the **European Federation of Pharmaceutical Industries and Associations** (EFPIA).
- In the USA, the members are the **Food and Drug Administration** (FDA), and the **Pharmaceutical Research and Manufacturers of America** (PhRMA).
- Additional members include **Observers** from the **World Health Organization** (WHO), **European Free Trade Association** (EFTA), and **Canada**. The Observers represent **non-ICH countries** and regions.

ICH STRUCTURE

The ICH structure consists of the ICH Steering Committee, ICH Coordinators, ICH Secretariat, and ICH Working Groups.

ICH Steering Committee

The Steering Committee is the body that governs the ICH, determines the policies and procedures for ICH, selects topics for harmonization, and monitors the progress of harmonization initiatives. Each of the six ICH parties has two seats on the ICH Steering Committee.

ICH Coordinators

The Coordinators are fundamental to the smooth running of the ICH and are nominated by each of the six parties. An ICH Coordinator acts as the main contact point with the ICH Secretariat.

ICH Secretariat

The Secretariat is primarily concerned with preparations for, and documentation of, meetings of the Steering Committee as well as coordination of preparations for Working Group and Discussion Group meetings.

Information on ICH Guidelines and the general ICH process can be obtained from the ICH Secretariat.

ICH Working Group

Depending on the type of harmonization activity needed, the Steering Committee will endorse the establishment of one of three types of working groups i.e., Expert Working Group (EWG), Implementation Working Group (IWG), or Informal Working Group.

ICH OPERATION

ICH operates through the ICH Steering Committee with administrative support from the ICH Secretariat and ICH Coordinators.

The Steering Committee meets at least twice a year. During these meetings, new topics will be considered for adoption, reports are received on the progress of existing topics, and maintenance and implementation of the guidelines are discussed.

The topics identified for harmonization by the Steering Committee are selected from Safety, Quality, Efficacy, and Multidisciplinary matters.

STEPS IN THE ICH PROCESS

Step 1: Drafts are prepared and circulated through many revisions until a "final harmonized draft" is completed

Step 2: This draft is signed by the EWG as the agreed-upon draft and forwarded to the Steering Committee for signing which signifies acceptance for consultation by each of the six co-sponsors

Step 3: The three regulatory sponsors initiate their normal consultation process to receive comments.

Step 4: This step is reached when the Steering Committee agrees that there is sufficient scientific consensus on the technical issues. This endorsement is based on the signatures from the three regulatory parties to ICH affirming that the Guideline is recommended for adoption by the regulatory bodies of the three regions.

Step 5: The process is complete when the guidelines are incorporated into national or regional internal procedures (implementation in the 3 ICH regions.)

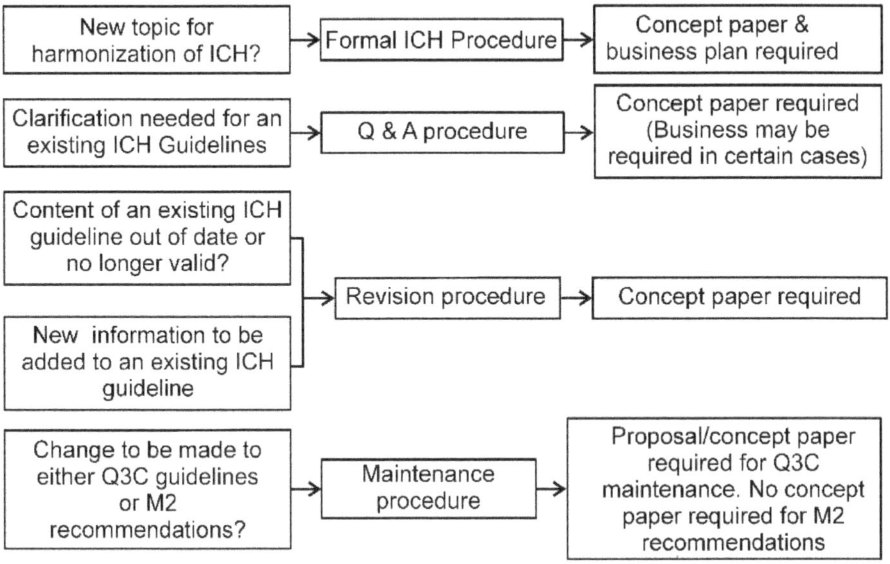

ICH GUIDELINES

- Quality guidelines – Q1 to Q14
- Safety guidelines – S1 to S12
- Efficacy guidelines – E1 to E21
- Multidisciplinary guidelines – M1 to M15

OVERVIEW OF QSEM

Q:"Quality" Topics, i.e., those relating to chemical and pharmaceutical Quality Assurance (Stability Testing, Impurity Testing, etc.)

S:"Safety" Topics, i.e., those relating to in vitro and in vivo pre-clinical studies (Carcinogenicity Testing, Genotoxicity Testing, etc.)

E:" Efficacy" Topics, i.e., those relating to clinical studies in the human subject (Dose-Response Studies, Good Clinical Practices, etc.)

M: "Multidisciplinary" Topics, i.e., cross-cutting topics which do not fit uniquely into one of the above categories.

QUALITY GUIDELINES

S. No.	Guidelines	Description
1	Q1A(R2)	Stability Testing of new drug substances and products (2nd revision)
2	Q1B	Stability Testing: Photostability Testing of New Drug Substances and Products
3	Q1C	Stability Testing for New Dosage Forms
4	Q1D	Bracketing and Matrixing Designs for Stability Testing of New Drugs
5	Q1E	Evaluation of Stability Data
6	Q2(R1)	Validation of Analytical Procedures: Text and Methodology (The Addendum dated November 1996 has been incorporated into the core guidelines in November 2005)
7	Q3A(R2)	Impurities in New Drug Substances
8	Q3B(R2)	Impurities in New Drug Products
9	Q3C(R9)	Impurities: Guidelines for Residual solvent
10	Q3D(R2)	Guidelines for Elemental Impurities
11	Q4B	Evaluation and Recommendation of Pharmacopoeial Texts for use in the ICH Regions
12	Q4B Annexe 4B (R1)	Microbiological Examination of Non-Sterile Products: Tests for specified Microorganisms General Chapter
13	Q4B Annexe 4C (R1)	Microbiological Examination of Non-Sterile Products: Acceptance Criteria for Pharmaceutical Preparations and Substances for Pharmaceutical use General Chapter
14	Q4B Annexe 5 (R1)	Disintegration Test General Chapter
15	Q4B Annexe 6	University of Dosage Units General Chapter
16	Q4B Annex 7 (R2)	Dissolution Test General Chapter
17	Q4B Annex 8 (R1)	Sterility General Chapter
18	Q4B Annex 9(R1)	Tablet Friability General Chapter
19	Q4B Annex 10 (R1)	PolyacrylamideGel Electrophoresis General Chapter

Contd...

S. No.	Guidelines	Description
20	Q4B Annex 11	Capillary Electrophoresis General Chapter
21	Q4B Annex 12	AnalyticalSieving General Chapter
22	Q4B Annex 13	Bulk Density and Tapped Density of Powder General Chapter
23	Q4B Annex 14	Bacterial Endotoxins Test General Chapter
24	Q5A (R2)	Vital Safety Evaluation of Biotechnology Products Derived from Cell Lines of Humans or Animal Origins
25	Q5B	Quality of Biotechnological Products: Analysis of the Expression Construct in cells Used for Production of r-DNA Derived Protein Products
26	Q5C	Quality of Biotechnological Products: Stability Testing of Biotechnological/Biological Products
27	Q5D	Derivation and characterization of cell substances used for production of Specification: Test Procedures and Acceptance criteria for Biotechnological/Biological Products
28	Q5E	Comparability of Biotechnological/Biological Products subject to changes in their manufacturing process
29	Q6A	Specification: Test Procedures and Acceptance criteria for New drug substances and New drug Products: chemical Substances
30	Q6B	Specification: Test Procedures and Acceptance criteria for Biotechnological / Biological Products
31	Q7	Good Manufacturing Practice Guide for Active Pharmaceutical Ingredients
32	Q8 (R1)	Pharmaceutical Development
33	Q9	Quality Risk Management
34	Q10	Pharmaceutical Quality System
35	Q11	Development and Manufacture of Drug Substances (Chemical Entities and Biotechnological/ Biological Entities)
36	Q12	Life Cycle Management
37	Q13	Continuous Manufacturing of Drug Substances and Drug Products
38	Q14	Analytical Procedure Development

SAFETY GUIDELINES

S. No.	Guidelines	Description
1	S1A	Guideline on the need for Carcinogenicity Studies of Pharmaceuticals
2	S1B	Testing of Carcinogenicity in pharmaceuticals
3	S1C (R2)	Dose selection for carcinogenicity studies of pharmaceuticals
4	S2(R1)	Guidance on Genotoxicity Testing and Data Interpretation for Pharmaceuticals Intended for Human Use
5	S2A	Guidance on Specific Aspects of Regulatory Genotoxicity Tests for Pharmaceuticals
6	S2B	A Standard Battery for Genotoxicity Testing for Pharmaceuticals
7	S3A	Note for Guidance on Toxicokinetic: The Assessment of Systemic Exposure in Toxicity Studies
8	S3B	Pharmacokinetics: Guidance for Repeated Dose Tissue Distribution Studies
9	S4	Duration of Chronic Toxicity Testing in Animals (Rodent and Non-Rodent Toxicity Testing)
10	S5	Detection of Toxicity to Reproduction for Medicinal Products & Toxicity to Male Fertility
11	S6	Preclinical Safety Evaluation of Biotechnology-Derived Pharmaceuticals
12	S7A	Safety Pharmacology Studies for Human Pharmaceuticals
13	S7B	The Nonclinical Evaluation of the Potential for Delayed Ventricular Repolarization (QT Interval Prolongation) By Human Pharmaceuticals
14	S8	Immunotoxicity Studies for Human Pharmaceuticals
15	S9	Nonclinical Evaluation for Anticancer Pharmaceuticals
16	S10	Photo-safety Evaluation
17	S11	Nonclinical Paediatric safety
18	S12	Nonclinical Biodistribution Considerations for gene therapy products

EFFICACY GUIDELINES

S. No.	Guidelines	Description
1	E1	Clinical Safety for Drugs used in Long-Term Treatment
2	E2A	Clinical Safety Data Management: Definitions and Standards for Expedited Reporting
3	E2B (R3)	Clinical Safety Data Management: Data Elements for Transmission of Individual Case Safety Reports (ICSRs)
4	E2B (R3) EWG/IWG	Electronic Transmission of Individual Case Safety Reports (ICSRs)
5	E2C (R2)	Periodic Benefit-Risk Evaluation Report

Contd...

S. No.	Guidelines	Description
6	E2D	Post-Approval Safety Data Management: Definitions and Standards for Expedited Reporting
7	E2E	Pharmacovigilance Planning
8	E2F	Development Safety Update Report
9	E3	Clinical Study Reports
10	E4	Dose-Response Studies
11	E5	Ethnic Factors
12	E6	Good Clinical Practice
13	E7	Clinical Trials in Geriatric Population
14	E8	General Considerations for Clinical Trials
15	E9	Statistical Principles for Clinical Trials
16	E10	Choice of Control Group in Clinical Trials
17	E11	Clinical Trials in Paediatric Population
18	E12	Clinical Evaluation by Therapeutic Category
19	E14	Clinical Evaluation of QT
20	E15	Definitions in Pharmacogenetics / Pharmacogenomics
21	E16	Qualification of Genomic Biomarkers
22	E17	Multi-Regional Clinical Trials
23	E18	Genomic Sampling
24	E19	Safety Data Collection
25	E20	Adaptive Clinical Trials
26	E21	Inclusion of Pregnant and Breastfeeding Individuals in Clinical

MULTIDISCIPLINARY GUIDELINES

S. No.	Guidelines	Description
1	M1	MedDRA Terminology
2	M2	Electronic Standards
3	M3	Nonclinical Safety Studies
4	M4	Common Technical Document
5	M5	Data Elements and Standards for Drug Dictionaries
6	M6	Gene Therapy
7	M7	Mutagenic impurities
8	M8	Electronic Common Technical Document (eCTD)
9	M9	Biopharmaceutics Classification System-based Biowaivers
10	M10	Bioanalytical Method Validation and Study Sample Analysis
11	M11	Clinical electronic Structured Harmonised Protocol (CeSHarP)
12	M12	Drug Interaction Studies
13	M13	Bioequivalence for Immediate-Release Solid Oral Dosage Forms
14	M14	Use of real-world data in pharmacoepidemiological studies
15	M15	General Principles for Model-Informed Drug Development

CHAPTER 7

Regulatory Control

Drugs play an important role in the health of both people and the economy of a country. Pharmaceutical drugs are available from a large number of sources. People and governments are willing to spend money on drugs for many reasons, they must be safe, effective and good quality, and used appropriately. This means, in turn, that the development, production, importation, exportation, and subsequent distribution of drugs must be regulated to ensure that they meet prescribed standards. Therefore, effective drug regulation is required to ensure the safety, efficacy, and quality of drugs as well as the accuracy and appropriateness of the drug information available to the public.

The drug regulatory authority (DRA) is the agency that develops and implements most of the legislation and regulations on pharmaceuticals. Its main task is to ensure the quality, safety, and efficacy of drugs, and the accuracy of product information. This is done by making certain rules that the manufacture, procurement, import, export, distribution, supply, and sale of drugs, product promotion, advertising, and clinical trials are carried out according to specified standards.

NEED FOR REGULATORY CONTROL

In an ideal world, the need for analysis should be driven by the desire to assure the quality of a drug product. However, in the real world, the need for pharmaceutical drug analysis is driven largely by regulatory requirements. A team consisting of R&D, QC, and QA unit members develop these quality and compliance systems. It should be one of the highest priorities of top management and QA units to develop and monitor these systems to comply with the cGMP and GLP expectations. Compliance documents are needed, in addition to the regulatory and research documents, to demonstrate the integrity of the data. Compliance documents refer to those reports required by GMP and/or utilized during the course of inspection by a health authority.

KEY FUNCTION OF REGULATORY AGENCIES

- Product registration (drug evaluation and authorization, and monitoring of drug efficacy and safety);
- Regulation of drug manufacturing, importation, and distribution;
- Regulation & Control of drug promotion and information.
- Adverse drug reaction (ADR) monitoring.
- Licensing of premises, persons, and practices.

The main goal of a regulatory agency is to guarantee the safety, efficacy, and quality of drugs available to the public.

DRUG REGULATION

The regulatory control is carried out by:

- Drug Laws
- Drug Regulatory Agencies
- Drug Regulatory Boards
- Quality Control
- Drug Information Centres etc.

DRUG REGULATORY SYSTEM IN INDIA

Drugs and Health are in the concurrent list of the Indian Constitution. It is governed by both Centre and State Governments under the Drugs & Cosmetics Act, of 1940.

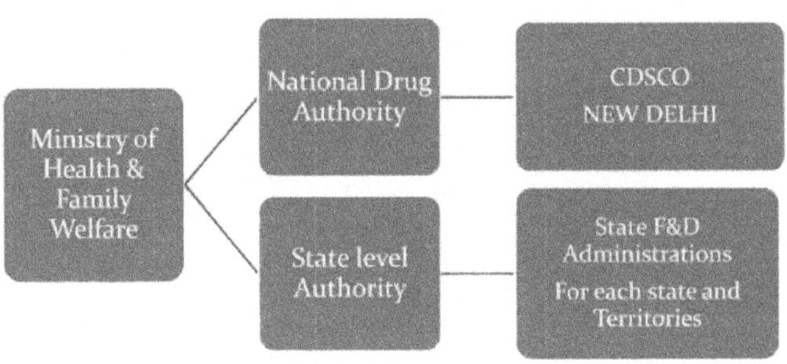

Distribution of powers Between State Government. & Central Government:

Regulatory control over the quality, safety, and efficacy of drugs in the country is exercised through central legislation called the Drugs and Cosmetics Act, of 1940 and the Rules made there under

- ✓ State Governments -Licensing of manufacturing and sales premises
- ✓ Central Government-Imports, permissions for marketing of New Drugs in the country, and for the conduct of Clinical Trials

APPROVAL OF INVESTIGATIONAL NEW DRUG

An investigational new drug is a substance that has been tested in the laboratory and is eligible for testing in people. The approval for testing is given by DCGI (Drug Controller General of India) after complete examination.

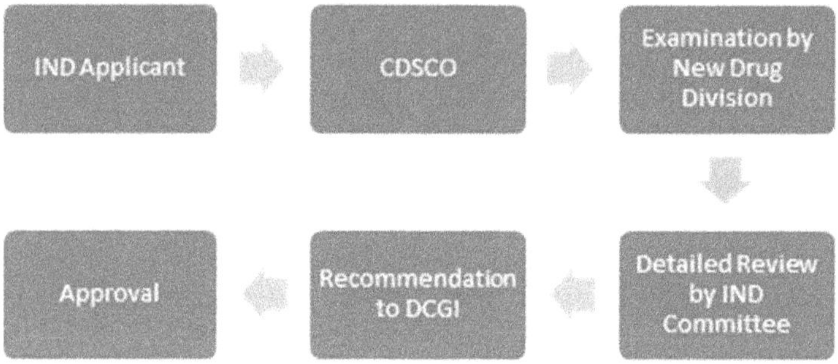

CENTRAL LICENSING

License for manufacturing has to be obtained from Central License Approving Authority (CLAA). CLAA issue license after complete examination.

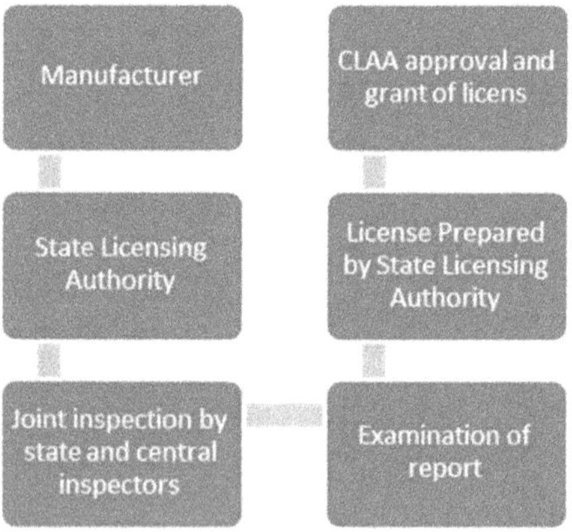

MAIN BODIES

- Central Drug Standard Control Organization (CDSCO)
- Ministry Of Health & Family Welfare (MHFW)
- Indian Council of Medical Research (ICMR)
- Indian Pharmaceutical Association (IPA)
- Drug Technical Advisory Board (DTAB)
- Central Drug Testing Laboratory (CDTL)
- Indian Pharmacopoeia Commission (IPC)
- National Pharmaceutical Pricing Authority (NPPA)

WELL-DEFINED DRUG REGULATORY SYSTEM (GOVT. OF INDIA)

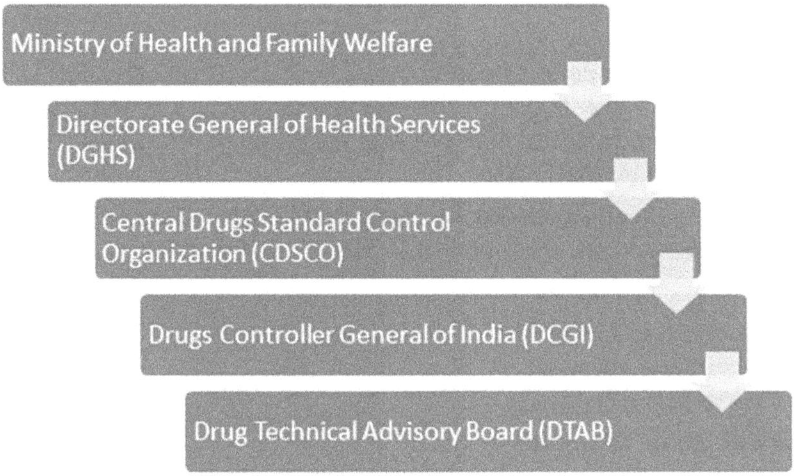

MINISTRY OF HEALTH AND FAMILY WELFARE

The Ministry of Health and Family Welfare (MHFW) is an Indian government ministry charged with health policy in India. It is also responsible for all government programs relating to family planning in India. The ministry is composed of two departments:

1. Departments of Health and Family Welfare.
2. Department of Health Research.

Department of Health-

It encompasses:

- ✓ 13 National Health Programmes
- ✓ Medical Council of India
- ✓ Food Safety and Standards Authority India (FSSAI)
- ✓ Central Drugs Standard Control Organisation (CDSCO)

Department of Welfare-

It includes:

- ✓ Central Drug Research Institute (CDRI) Lucknow
- ✓ Indian Council of Medical Research (ICMR) New Delhi

DEPARTMENT OF HEALTH RESEARCH-(DHR)

It has a scheme that provides advanced training in India and abroad to medical and health research personnel in cutting-edge research areas concerning medicine and health to create trained human resources for carrying out research activities.

CENTRAL DRUG STANDARD CONTROL ORGANIZATION (CDSCO)

It is a national regulatory body for Indian Pharmaceuticals and Medical Devices. Within CDSCO, DCGI (Drug Controller General of India) regulates pharmaceutical and medical devices under the gamut of the Ministry of Health and Family Welfare (MHFW).

CDSCO is **headquartered in New Delhi** and comprised of 6 Zonal offices, 2 sub zonal offices, 7 port offices, and 6 laboratories.

Zonal offices

- North Zone: Ghaziabad
- West Zone: Mumbai
- South Zone: Chennai
- East Zone: Kolkata
- Other zonal offices- Ahmedabad and Hyderabad.

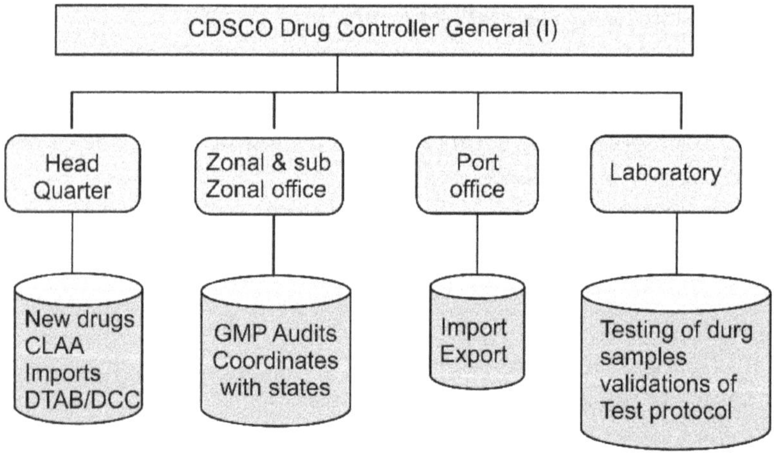

Functions of CDSCO

1. To protect and promote public health
2. Laying down standards of drugs, cosmetics, diagnostics, and devices.
3. Laying down regulatory measures, amendments to Acts, and rules.
4. To regulate market authorization of new drugs.
5. To regulate the manufacture, sale, and distribution of drugs
6. To regulate clinical research in India
7. To approve licenses to manufacture certain categories of drugs as
8. Central License Approving Authority (CLAA) i.e., for Blood Banks, Large Volume Parenteral, and Vaccines & Sera.
9. To regulate the standards of imported drugs.

10. Work relating to the Drugs Technical Advisory Board (DTAB) and Drugs Consultative Committee (DCC).
11. Testing of drugs by Central Drugs Labs.

NATIONAL INSTITUTE OF HEALTH AND FAMILY WELFARE (NIHFW)

NIHFW is an Apex Technical Institute, funded by the Ministry of Health and Family Welfare, for the promotion of health and family welfare programmers in the country through education, training, research, evaluation, consultancy, and specialized services. The NIHFW was established on March 9, 1977, by a merger of the National Institute of Health Administration and Education (NIHAE) with the National Institute of Family Planning (NIFP). There are 18 governing body members in NIHFW.

Activities and responsibilities

- Measuring the weight of children to assess their nutritional status.
- Assessment of diseases like level of anemia.
- Testing of food material like cooking salt for level iodine.
- To release funds on the advice of the Ministry.
- It is responsible for all government programs relating to family planning in India.

INDIAN COUNCIL OF MEDICAL RESEARCH (ICMR)

Structure and organization

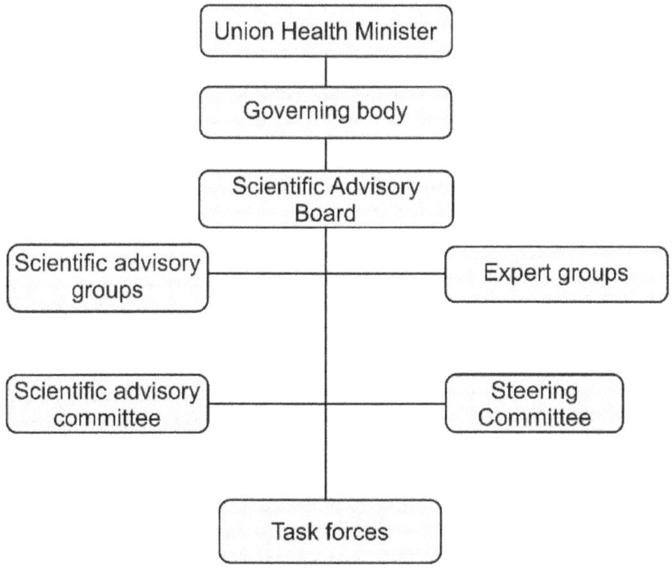
Union Health Minister
Governing body
Scientific Advisory Board
Scientific advisory groups
Expert groups
Scientific advisory committee
Steering Committee
Task forces

Activities and responsibilities

Extramural research is promoted by ICMR by establishing

- Centers for Advanced Research in different research areas.
- Open-ended research is conducted on the basis of applications for grants-in-aid received from scientists in non-ICMR Research Institutes, Medical colleges, and Universities located in different parts of the country.
- Balancing research efforts between different competing fields, especially when resources are severely limited, is a typical problem encountered in the management of medical research, particularly in developing countries

INDIAN PHARMACEUTICAL ASSOCIATION (IPA)

The Indian Pharmaceutical Association (IPA) has demanded to amend the Drugs &Cosmetics Act and Rules 1945 to make only pharmacy graduates eligible to become expert staff in the pharma manufacturing units. In the resolutions passed during the just concluded IPA Convention, the IPA also urged the government to expedite action to amend the Rules in such a way that all regulatory positions in the country must be an exclusive area for experienced and qualified pharmacists. Indian Pharmaceutical Association (IPA) is the premier professional association of pharmacists in India. The association has more than 10,000 members from various parts of the country and it operates in India through 17 state branches & more than 33 local branches. The association represents various facts of the pharmaceutical profession and in managing several academic programs.

DRUG TECHNICAL ADVISORY BOARD (DTAB)

- The Central Government constitutes a Board (to be called the Drugs Technical Advisory Board) to advise the Central Government and the State Governments on technical matters arising out of the administration of the D&C, Act 1940
- The Board shall consist of the following members, -20 members

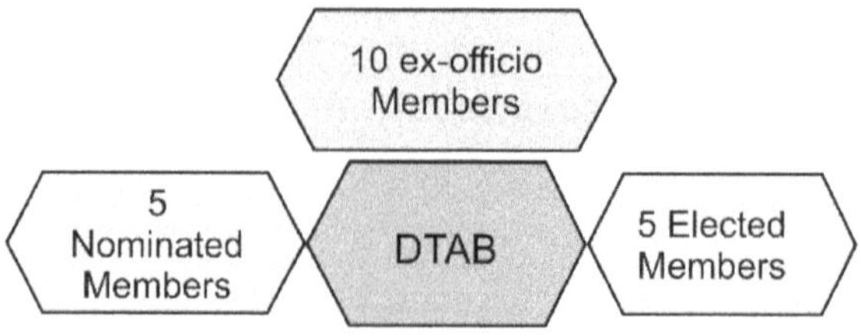

Members:

Ex-Officio:

(i) Director General of Health Services (Chairman)
(ii) Drugs Controller, India
(iii) Director of the Central Drugs Laboratory, Calcutta
(iv) Director of the Central Research Institute, Kasauli
(v) President of Medical Council of India
(vi) President of the Pharmacy Council of India
(vii) Director of Central Drug Research Institute, Lucknow

Nominated:

(i) Two persons by the Central Government.
(ii) One person by the Central Government from the pharmaceutical industry
(iii) Two persons holding the appointment of Government Analyst under this Act,

Elected:

(i) One person, to be elected by the Executive Committee of the Pharmacy Council of India,
(ii) One person, to be elected by the Executive Committee of the Medical Council of India,
(iii) One pharmacologist to be elected by the Governing Body of the Indian Council of Medical Research;
(iv) One person to be elected by the Central Council of the Indian Medical Association;
(v) One person to be elected by the Council of the Indian Pharmaceutical Association

Activities and responsibilities

- It advises on matters related to Drugs.
- The nominated and elected members of the Board shall hold office for three years, but shall be eligible for re-nomination and re-election.
- The Board may, subject to the previous approval of the Central Government, regulate its own procedure.

CENTRAL DRUG TESTING LABORATORY (CDTL)

The central drug laboratory, Kolkata is a national statutory laboratory of the government of India for quality control of drugs and cosmetics and was established under the D&C act, of 1940.Oldest quality control laboratory of the drug control authorities in India. Function under the director general of Health Services in the Ministry of Health and Family Welfare.

Statutory Function:

- To Act as an Appellate authority.
- To function as Government Analyst for such states who do not have their own testing facilities.
- Analytical quality control of the majority of imported drugs.
- Analytical quality control of drug formulations manufactured within the country on behalf of the Central & State Drug standard control organization

Other Functions:

- Procurement, establishment, maintenance, Storage, and distribution of I.P & International Reference standards.
- Preparation and standardization of I.P. reference standards against USP, BP primary standards.
- To undertake analytical research in standardization and methodology development of drugs.
- Training to drug analysts.
- Training to WHO fellows from abroad on modern methods of drug analysis.

Other laboratories:

- ✓ CDTL, Mumbai
- ✓ CDTL, Tamil Nadu
- ✓ CDTL, Hyderabad
- ✓ RDTL, Guhawati
- ✓ CDL, Kasauli
- ✓ RDTL, Chandigarh
- ✓ CDL, Kasauli

INDIAN PHARMACOPOEIA COMMISSION (IPC)

Activities and responsibilities

- Development of comprehensive monographs.
- Accord priority to monographs of drugs included in the national Essential Drug List and their dosage forms.
- Preparation of monograph for products that have normally been in the market for not less than 2 years.
- Collaborate with pharmacopeias like the BP, USP, JP and International Pharmacopoeia with a view to harmonizing with global standards.

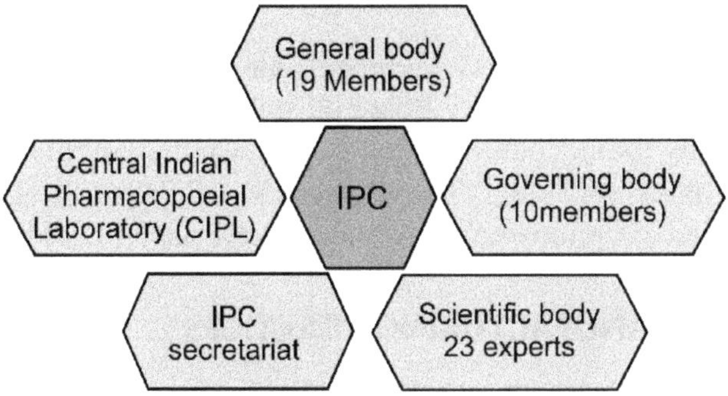

NATIONAL PHARMACEUTICAL PRICING AUTHORITY (NPPA)

NPPA was established, to fix/revise the prices of controlled bulk drugs and formulations and to enforce prices and availability of the medicines in the country, under the Drugs Prices Control Order (DPCO), 1995.Pricing policy and industry regulation constitute the key responsibility of the NPPA. Drugs with high sales and a market share of more than 50% are subjected to price regulation.

For the purpose of implementing provisions of DPCO, powers of the Government have been vested in the National Pharmaceutical Pricing Authority (NPPA). Drugs have been declared as essential and accordingly put under the Essential Commodities Act. Only 74 out of 500 commonly used bulk drugs are kept under statutory price control. However, the prices of other drugs can be regulated, if warranted in the public interest. The NPPA was established on 29th August 1997 as an independent body of experts following the Cabinet Committee's decision in September 1994 while reviewing the Drug Policy.

Features

- Ceiling and Non-Ceiling Prices of drugs and medicines in the controlled category regulated.
- Ceiling Price is the single maximum selling price fixed that is applicable throughout the country in the case of each bulk drug, which is under price control.
- Non-Ceiling Prices fixed by NPPA are specific to a particular pack size of scheduled formulation of a particular company

THE DRUGS CONSULTATIVE COMMITTEE (DCC)

It is also an advisory body constituted by central government.

Constitution:

- Two representatives of the Central Government
- One representative of each State Government

Functions:

- ✓ To advise the Central Government, the State Governments, and the Drugs Technical Advisory Board on any other matter tending to secure uniformity throughout India in the administration of this Act.
- ✓ There is a separate "The Ayurvedic, Siddha, & Unani Drugs Consultative Committee" constituted under sec 33 D of the Act.

GMP-GOOD MANUFACTURING PRACTICES

GMP guidelines are not prescriptive instructions on how to manufacture products. They are a series of general principles that must be observed during manufacturing. When a company is setting up its quality program and manufacturing process, there may be many ways it can fulfill GMP requirements. It is the company's responsibility to determine the most effective and efficient quality process.

Requirements

- ➢ To ensure that their products are safe, pure, and effective.
- ➢ To minimize or eliminate contamination, mix up and errors.
- ➢ Issues including record keeping, personnel qualifications, sanitation, cleanliness, equipment verification, process validation, and complaint Handling.
- ➢ GMP is also sometimes referred to as "cGMP".
- ➢ Failure of firms to comply with GMP regulations can result in very serious consequences including recall, fines, and even imprisonment.

WHO GUIDELINES (WORLD HEALTH ORGANIZATION):

- WHO is an agency of the United Nations. It is a specialized agency and its primary responsibility includes international health matters so that the goal, of health for all, can be achieved.
- The WHO GMP and the certification scheme were accepted by WHA (World Health Assembly) in resolution number WHA 28.65, as the revised version in 1975.
- With the appearance of ISO (International Organization for Standardization) the WHO GMP needed the next revision. The revised text contains 3 parts.

Part I: Outlines the general concepts of quality assurance and salient components of GMPs.

Part II: Outlines actions to be taken by production & quality control personnel separately for implementing general principles of quality assurance.

Part III: Supporting and supplementary guidelines.

The revised text of GMP appears as annex.

ANNEX I: Quality Management in the Drug Industry – Philosophy & Essential Elements

- Quality Assurance
- Good Manufacturing Practice
- Quality Control
- Sanitation & Hygiene
- Validation
- Complaints
- Product recalls
- Contract Production & Analysis
- Self inspection and quality audits
- Personnel
- Premises
- Material
- Documentation

ANNEX II:

- Good Practices – Production & Quality Control
- Good Practices in Production
- Good Practices in Quality Control

ANNEX III:

- Supporting and Supplementary Guidelines
- Sterile pharmaceutical Products
- Good Manufacturing Practice for Active
- Pharmaceutical Ingredients

WHO GMP Certification

Originally established in 1969 and revised in 1975.

Main objectives were:

- To inspect drug manufacturing facilities
- To assess compliance of GMP
- This would facilitate implementation of the scheme.

WHO GMP ensures the following:

- Avoidance of Cross- Contamination
- Prevention of Mix-ups
- Provide Traceability
- Accountability of actions
- Responsibility
- Product Performance Guarantee

IMMUNITIES IN DRUG CASES

1. **Officers**
   Officers acting in the discharge of their duties in good faith under the Act are immune from suits, prosecution, and other legal proceedings (Section 69).
2. **Addicts**
   Addicts charged with the consumption of drugs (section 27) or with offenses involving small quantities will be immune from prosecution if they volunteer for de-addiction. This immunity may be withdrawn if the addict does not undergo complete treatment (Section 64 A).
3. **Offenders**
   Central or state governments can tender immunity to an offender in order to obtain his evidence in the case. This immunity is granted by the government and not by the court (Section 64).
4. **Minors**
   All assess committed under any law by persons under the age of 18 will be covered by the Juvenile Persons (Care and Protection) Act. This Act seeks to reform such juveniles rather than punish them under the respective Acts. It prevails over any other Act in respect of persons below the age of 18.

DEFICIENCIES & LIMITATIONS OF THE DRUG REGULATORY SYSTEM

- The proliferation of spurious and sub-standard drugs in the Indian market.
- Lack of transparency in licensing procedures.
- Inadequate regulatory expertise and testing facilities to implement uniform standards.
- Need for greater coordination and transparency in functioning among different ministries concerned with drug regulation.

SECTION – II: Chromatography

CHAPTER 8

Introduction to Chromatography

INTRODUCTION

Chromatography is a separation technique used to separate a mixture of various components into individual components using equilibrated distribution between two phases (stationary phase and mobile phase). The basis of chromatography is the rate differences in the movement of the components of a mixture through the stationary phase (porous medium) against the mobile phase (solvent or gas).

The steps involved in chromatographic separation are

1. Adsorption or retention of the analyte components in the stationary phase.
2. Isolation of the adsorbed/retained components by the mobile phase.
3. Elution of the isolated substances by the flow of the mobile phase.
4. Qualitative and quantitative estimation of eluted substances.

HISTORY OF CHROMATOGRAPHY

Chromatography, which literally means "color writing" in Greek, is a versatile method for separating mixtures into their individual components. The history of chromatography dates back to the early 20th century, with significant contributions from various scientists. Here's a brief overview:

Mikhail Tsvet (1900s): A Russian-Italian botanist, Tsvet is often credited with the invention of chromatography. In 1906, he separated plant pigments using a glass column packed with calcium carbonate, marking the first instance of chromatography. He called this technique "chromatography" due to the colorful bands produced during separation.

Richard Kuhn (1930s): The German biochemist Richard Kuhn made significant advancements in chromatography, particularly in the separation of complex mixtures of organic compounds. He developed methods for separating amino acids and other organic compounds using paper chromatography.

Archer Martin and Richard Synge (1940s): British chemists Martin and Synge made groundbreaking developments in chromatography, for which they were awarded the Nobel Prize in Chemistry in 1952. They introduced the technique of partition chromatography, which used a liquid stationary phase supported on a solid matrix. This led to the development of gas chromatography and high-performance liquid chromatography (HPLC) in the future.

Gas Chromatography (GC) Development (1950s-1960s): The introduction of gas chromatography revolutionized analytical chemistry. It involves the separation of volatile compounds in the gas phase. Martin and Synge's work laid the foundation for this technique, which became widely used for analyzing organic compounds.

High-Performance Liquid Chromatography (HPLC) (1970s): HPLC emerged as a powerful analytical technique for separating and analyzing complex mixtures of compounds. It utilizes high-pressure pumps to move a liquid solvent containing the sample through a column packed with a stationary phase.

Advancements and Applications (1980s-present): Since the 1980s, chromatography techniques have continued to evolve with advancements in technology, instrumentation, and methodology. Various types of chromatography have been developed, including ion chromatography, affinity chromatography, and size-exclusion chromatography, each with specific applications in different fields such as pharmaceuticals, forensics, environmental analysis, and biochemistry.

Today, chromatography remains an indispensable tool in scientific research and various industries for qualitative and quantitative analysis, purification, and characterization of substances. Its versatility and wide range of applications continue to drive innovation in the field of analytical chemistry.

TYPES OF CHROMATOGRAPHY

Different methods of classification are available for chromatography. The classifications are

1. **Based on the nature of the stationary and mobile phase:** Depending on the type of the stationary and mobile phases used, the chromatographic methods can be classified as given below.

Table 8.1 Classification of chromatography based on stationary and mobile phase.

Mobile Phase	Stationary Phase	Name of the Technique
Gas	Solid	Gas Solid Chromatography (GSC)
Gas	Liquid	Gas Liquid Chromatography (GLC)
Liquid	Solid	Thin Layer Chromatography (TLC) Adsorption Column Chromatography High Performance Liquid Chromatography (HPLC)
Liquid	Solid matrix(Gel)	Gel Permeation Chromatography
Liquid	Liquid	Paper Partition Chromatography Column Partition Chromatography
Liquid	Solid-resin	Ion Exchange Chromatography

2. **Based on the principle of separation:** The principle of separation in chromatography can be adsorption or partition
   (i) Adsorption chromatography
   (ii) Partition chromatography
   (i) Adsorption chromatography: The separation of components in adsorption chromatography is based on the relative affinities of the components towards the stationary phase. The principle of separation is called adsorption, which is a surface phenomenon. The mixture (adsorbate), which is dissolved in the mobile phase, moves through the stationary phase (adsorbent) of the column. The component with more affinity for the stationary phase travels slower, and the component with more affinity for the mobile phase travels faster down the column. Thus the components are separated based on their affinity difference for the stationary phase. Under defined conditions, no two components will have the same affinity for the given set of the stationary, mobile phase.
   If the stationary phase is solid, then the principle of separation is adsorption
   E.g., GSC, TLC, column adsorption chromatography, HPLC
   (ii) Partition chromatography: In this mode of chromatography, the separation of components is based on the partition coefficients of the individual components. Partition coefficient (*P*) is the ratio of concentrations of a compound in a mixture of two immiscible solvents at equilibrium. The solute gets distributed between the two immiscible liquids based on its partition coefficient. The more soluble component in the stationary phase travels slower than the component that is soluble in the mobile phase. The components are

separated based on their differences in partition coefficient since no two components will have the same partition coefficient for the given set of conditions, including the stationary and mobile phases. The stationary phase is a liquid coated as a thin film over solid support.

If the stationary phase is a liquid, then the principle of separation is partition.

E.g., Gas-liquid chromatography, paper partition chromatography, column partition chromatography etc.

3. **Based on the modes of chromatography:** Modes of chromatography depend upon the polarities of the stationary and mobile phase. The interaction between solute, stationary and mobile phases are,
   (i) Polar-Polar interactions
   Polar solute dissolves in a polar solvent.
   (ii) Non –polar- Non-polar interactions
   Non-polar solute dissolves in Non-polar solvent
   These interactions are based on "like dissolves like"
   (iii) Polar – Non- Polar interactions are very weak.
   In this classification, two modes of separation are available.
   (a) Normal Phase chromatographic mode
   (b) Reverse phase chromatographic mode

   (a) Normal Phase Chromatography mode
   Stationary phase is polar (silica gel)
   Mobile phase is Non-polar
   Polar components interact more with the polar stationary phase and are retained in the column for a longer time. Non-polar components exhibit the least interaction with the stationary phase and are eluted fast. This mode is **not much** used in **pharmaceutical applications** because the nature of most **drug molecules are polar** and are **retained more**, making the elution time longer.

   (b) Reverse phase chromatography mode
   Stationary phase is Non -polar (ODS- C_{18} or C_8 etc.)
   Mobile phase is Polar
   In this mode, polar components are eluted faster, and the non-polar components are retained for a longer time in the stationary phase. This is the most **commonly used** technique in **pharmaceutical analysis**.
   The distinction between reverse phase and Normal phase mode is given in Table 8.2.

Table 8.2 Distinction between reverse phase and Normal phase mode.

Parameter	Normal Phase	Reverse Phase
Stationary phase	Polar	Non-polar
Mobile phase	Non-polar	Polar
Less retained (first eluted compound)	Non-polar	Polar
More retained (last eluted compound)	Polar	Non-polar
E.g. of stationary phase	Silica gel	ODS(C_{18}),C_8,C_4-bonded phases

4. **Other types of chromatographic techniques**
    1. **Ion exchange chromatography:** The principle involved is the reversible exchange of ions. The stationary phase used is an ion exchange resin. Anion exchange resin is used to separate anions, and cation exchange resin is used to separate cations. Acids, alkalis and buffers are used as mobile phase.
    2. **Ion–pair chromatography:** In this technique, ion-pairing agents like octane sulphonic acid, Tetraethyl ammonium hydroxide are used to convert a reversed-phase column into a temporary ion exchange column.
    3. **Size exclusion /gel permeation chromatography:** This technique is also called as Gel filtration or Gel permeation chromatography. The stationary phase is a porous matrix made up of porous materials like cross-linked polystyrene, cross-linked dextrans, polyacrylamide gels, agarose gels, etc. The separation is based on the analyte molecular sizes since the gel behaves like a molecular sieve. This technique is used to separate proteins, polysaccharides, enzymes, and synthetic polymers. The solvents used are aqueous buffers or organic solvents.
    4. **Chiral chromatography:** Chiral chromatography is used to separate enantiomers (dextro and levo form) using either chiral stationary or mobile phase.

Theories of chromatography

There are two theories of chromatography which deal with the rate of solute migration and peak development in the chromatogram.

(i) Plate theory

(ii) Rate theory

(i) Plate theory: This theory was developed by Martin and Synge in 1941. In plate theory, the column is divided into a number of adjacent imaginary segments called theoretical plates. In each theoretical plate, a complete equilibration of the solute occurs between the stationary and mobile phases.

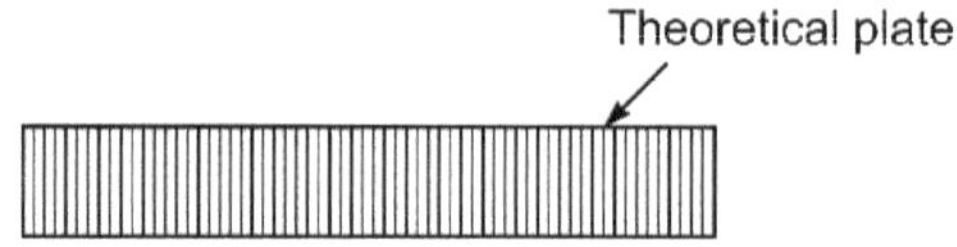

Fig. 8.1 Column showing imaginary theoretical plates.

The equal interaction of the solute components of the mixture with the mobile phase and stationary phase leads to the retention of the molecules (slow rate of movement).

Each solute molecule interacts with the mobile phase and stationary phase in a different manner and they will have different rates of migration leading to the separation of the components.

Significance of theoretical plates

Efficiency (good separation of the components) of the column increases with

1. Increase in the number of theoretical plates. (N)
2. Decrease in HETP (Height equivalent to theoretical plates)

   H = L/N where

   L - Length of the column

   N - Number of plates

   H - HETP or Height of the theoretical plates.

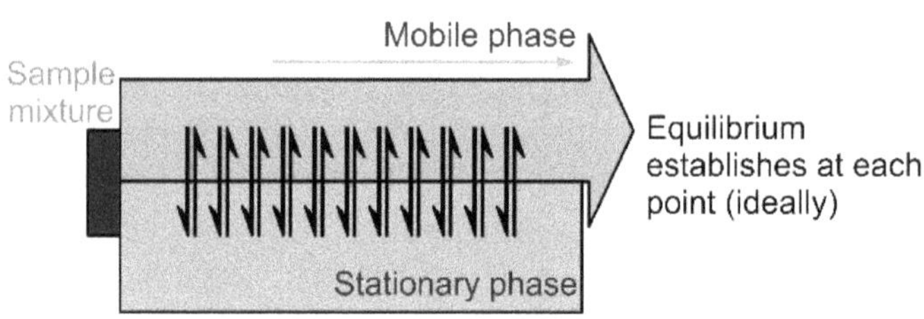

Fig. 8.2 Diagrammatic representation of Theoretical plates.

HETP is defined as the height of the theoretical plate in which a complete equilibration of the solute occurs between the stationary and mobile phase.

The molecules of the mixture interact with the molecules of the stationary and mobile phase leading to retardation of the molecular movement. Each molecule interacts differently with the mobile and stationary phase due to the **difference in their distribution coefficients and this causes net difference in rates of migration**

(ii) Rate theory: This theory was proposed by Van Deemter in the year 1956. This theory describes the processes that are working inside the column. The time taken for the equilibration of the solute between the stationary phase and the mobile phase is taken into account in this theory. The resulting band shape or chromatographic peak is affected by various factors that lead to band broadening.

Van Deemter equation explains the various factors leading to band broadening.

$$HETP = A + (B/u) + Cu$$

where A - Eddy diffusion
B - Longitudinal diffusion
C - Mass transfer
u - Average mobile phase velocity

Eddy diffusion – (A term) – is caused by turbulence in the solute flow path and is unaffected by flow rate (velocity of mobile phase).

Longitudinal diffusion – (B term) – is the movement of the analyte molecules outwards from the centre to the edges of its band.

Increased flow rate can control B term, and peak broadening can be avoided.

Mass transfer – (C term) – is the movement of the analyte or mass transfer between mobile and stationary phases.

Increased flow rate increases the resistance to mass transfer leading to band broadening.

A consensus has to be arrived between these three terms to get the optimum flow rate with minimum HETP so that the efficiency of the column can be increased with good resolution of the peaks.

The van Deemter plot below indicates the desired plate height (H or HETP) and flow rate as optimum efficiency and flow rate, respectively.

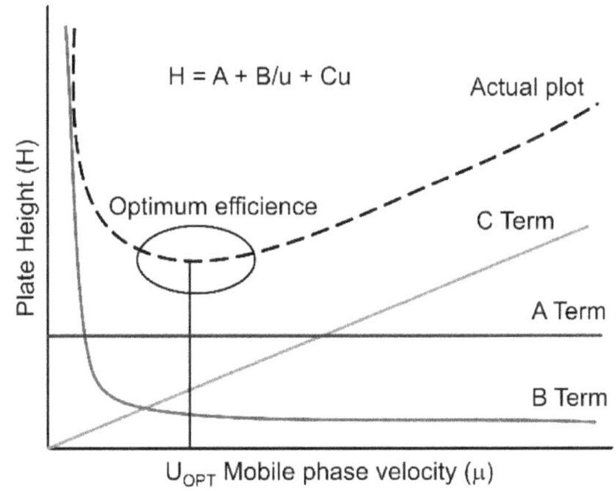

Fig. 8.3 Van Deemter plot.

Another equation given by the rate theory is $\mathbf{H = \sigma^2/L}$ where

σ - Standard deviation of band

H - HETP and is equal to H/dp,

Where dp is the particle size

H = (σ^2/L) × dp

This equation gives the relationship between stationary phase particle size and efficiency of the column (HETP)

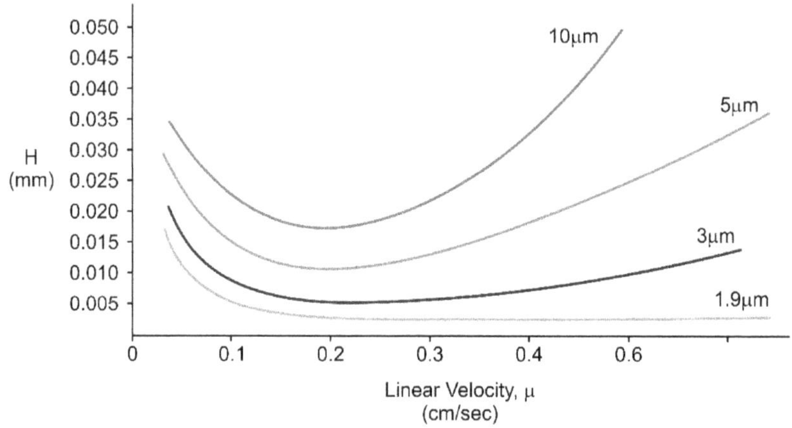

Fig. 8.4 Effect of particle size on Plate Height.

From the figure, it can be understood that **decreasing the particle size of the stationary phase yield better overall efficiency across a wide range of flow rates.**

We will discuss about different chromatographic techniques in detail in the forthcoming chapters.

CHAPTER 9

Adsorption Column Chromatography

The process of separation of a mixture into individual components is called chromatography. Column chromatography was developed by American chemist D.T Day in 1900, and M.S.Tsweet, a Polish botanist in 1906, used it for the separation of plant pigments. It is the most useful and common method for separating solids and liquids. In adsorption column chromatography, the stationary phase is solid, and the mobile phase is a liquid.

PRINCIPLE

Adsorption is the principle behind adsorption column chromatography. Adsorption is a surface phenomenon where a solute adheres to the surface of another material, forming a thin layer. This layer is often only one molecule thick. The solute molecule that gets adsorbed on the surface is known as adsorbate, and the surface on which adsorption occurs is known as adsorbent. The separation of the compounds depends on the interaction between adsorbents and adsorbates. The stationary phase is the adsorbent and the sample to be separated is the adsorbate.

The stationary phase used is packed in a column, and hence the name column chromatography. The principle behind column chromatography is **adsorption**, and the components are separated based on **differential adsorption**. The mixture of samples to be separated is dissolved in the mobile phase and introduced into the column. The rate at which the components move along the column depends on their relative affinities for the stationary or mobile phases. More affinity for the stationary phase makes the components to move slow, and the components with more affinity for the mobile phase move fast and gets eluted rapidly. Because of this difference in the affinities, the components are separated. This kind of adsorption interaction between the stationary phase and the solute is reversible in nature.

COMPONENTS OF COLUMN CHROMATOGRAPHY

1. Stationary phase
2. Mobile phase
3. Column

1. **Stationary phase:** The adsorbent is used as a stationary phase. The requirements of the adsorbent are
   1. The particle should have a uniform particle size. 60-200μ
   2. The particle should be spherical in shape.
   3. It should not be soluble in the solvent and mobile phases used.
   4. It should be colourless.
   5. It should be able to separate a wide variety of compounds.
   6. It should be inexpensive and readily available.

   Selection of stationary phase

   The proper stationary phase is selected based on the factors like

   (i) Nature of the compounds to be separated.

   E.g., the polar components can be separated on silica, and non-polar compounds are separated using alumina.

   (ii) Length of the column: For shorter columns, a strong adsorbent is used. For longer columns, a weak adsorbent is used.

   (iii) Difference in affinities between components: For components with similar affinities, a stronger adsorbent is used.

   The weaker adsorbent is used when there is a large difference in affinities of components.

   (iv) Adsorbent quantity: Adsorbate: adsorbent ratio - 1:20 or 1:30

   Types of adsorbents: The important adsorbents used in column chromatography are silica, alumina, calcium carbonate, calcium phosphate, magnesia and starch, etc

   Polar compounds are separated using silica, and alumina is used for non-polar compounds. The adsorbents can be classified as given in Table 9.1.

Table 9.1 Classification of adsorbents.

Weak	Medium	Strong
Sucrose	$CaCO_3$	Activated silica gel
Starch	Ca phosphate	Activated alumina
Inulin	Mg carbonate	Activated charcoal
Talc	Mg oxide	Activated magnesia
Sodium carbonate	Calcium hydroxide	Fuller's earth

2. **Mobile phase:** The mobile phase in the column is very important because it performs several functions. The functions of the mobile phase are:
   (i) as a solvent- introduces the sample into the column.
   (ii) as a developing agent- to develop the bands in the column
   (iii) as an elute – to elute the components from the column.

   Selection of mobile phase

   (i) The sample components must be soluble in the solvent system.
   (ii) The mobile phase should have a low boiling point so that the sample can be recovered.
   (iii) The solvent of appropriate polarity should be selected because the polarity of the solvents affects the relative rates of movement of the components.

   The mobile phase is chosen based on these properties.

   The common solvents used as mobile phases are given in the increasing order of polarity (elution strength): Petroleum ether, carbon tetrachloride, cyclohexane, Carbon disulphide, ether, acetone, benzene, toluene, ethyl acetate, chloroform, methanol, ethanol, water, pyridine, organic acids like acetic acid, etc.

   The mobile phase can be a single solvent or a mixture of solvents.

3. **Column:** The column is usually made up of neutral glass since it should not be affected by solvents. It is used as a support for the stationary phase. Column dimensions are Length: Diameter ratio- 10:1; 30:1 or 100:1

   The length of the column used depends on the following factors:

   1. The affinity of the solute (adsorbate) towards the adsorbent used.
   2. No. of components to be separated.
   3. Nature of the adsorbent.
   4. Sample quantity.

   Longer columns are used for better separation.

Methodology of column chromatography

The different steps involved in column chromatography are

I. Preparation of the column
II. Sample introduction
III. Elution (Development technique)
IV. Detection.

I. Preparation of column: Before packing into the column, the adsorbent is activated by heating to increase the adsorption capacity. Heating removes the adsorbed water from the adsorbent. Activation of adsorbent is done by heating silica gel to 110°C and alumina to 400°C for one hour. To start with the preparation, a glass wool/ cotton or asbestos pad is inserted at the bottom of the clean glass column. Then the column is packed with adsorbents to get a uniform packing. A paper disc is placed on top of the packing to avoid the disturbance of the packing during the introduction of the sample or mobile phase. Disturbance in the adsorbent packing causes irregular band separation.

The packing of the column is done by two methods

1. Dry packing
2. Wet packing

1. **Dry packing:** In this technique, the dry adsorbent is filled in the column by tapping, and the mobile phase is added till the equilibrium is reached in the column.

   Demerits:

   1. Air bubbles are trapped in the column, and the column is tapped to remove air bubbles.
   2. Cracks appear in the packed adsorbent.
   3. Clear band separation may not be obtained.

2. **Wet packing:** This is the most commonly used ideal technique. The adsorbent is made as a slurry by mixing with the solvent and pouring it into the column in portions. Slurry should be added carefully to avoid cracks and get a uniform adsorbent setting without the air bubbles. The solid adsorbent settles at the bottom, and the solvent covers the adsorbent layer on top.

   Advantages:

   1. The packing is uniform and suitable for separation.
   2. The resolution of the bands is good.

II. Sample introduction: The sample mixture is dissolved in a small volume of the mobile phase or suitable solvent. The entire sample is added at once into the column, and the sample gets adsorbed onto the top of the column to form a zone. The individual components are separated from this zone by elution.

III. Elution (Developmental technique): The recovery of the components is carried out by a process called elution. The development of the chromatograph zone of the separated components from the column is called elution. The solvent used is called eluent. The components are the eluates.

There are two elution techniques:

1. Isocratic elution
2. Gradient elution

1. **Isocratic Elution:** The same solvent or same solvent composition is used throughout the chromatographic separation.

E.g., chloroform throughout the separation, Pet ether: Benzene in the ratio 1:1 throughout separation

2. **Gradient elution:** In gradient elution, the composition of the eluting solvent can be varied gradually during the separation according to the nature of the components being separated. Solvents of increasing polarity/elution strength are used during the separation. A low polar solvent is used initially, and the polarity of the eluent is increased gradually by using more polar solvents.

   e.g., elution starting with benzene, chloroform, ethylacetate, and then changing to methanol.

   Developmental techniques other than elution are **frontal analysis** and **displacement analysis**.

   In frontal analysis, the original solution containing the sample is used for displacement. The sample is fed continuously into the chromatographic bed, and no additional mobile phase is used. The sample components displace each other in the order of least affinity for the chromatographic medium.

   In displacement analysis, another solvent that is more strongly adsorbed than the original solvent is used. It is a procedure in which the mobile phase contains a more strongly retained compound (the displacer) than the components of the sample. The sample is fed as a finite slug.

   Chromatograms are plots of the concentration of the components in the eluents against time.

IV. **Detection:** The coloured components can be observed visually, and they can be collected individually and detected. If the isolated components are colourless, anyone of the following detectors can detect the compounds. Sometimes developers like hydrogen sulphide and potassium ferrocyanide are used to visualize the separation as bands.

1. Optical detectors
   (a) UV- visible detector – If the sample absorbs UV/ visible light
   (b) Fluorescence detectors: For the samples which are emitting radiations.
2. Refraction index detector

   It detects the components based on the RI difference between the mobile phase with compound and without compounds.
3. Flame ionization detector/ argon detector
4. The other simple technique is collecting the fractions, evaporating the solvent and weighing the residue.
5. Conducting detectors used for ionized substances.
6. Thin-layer chromatography is used to monitor the fractions.

Factors affecting column chromatography

1. **Column dimensions:** Column efficiency can be improved by increasing the length: diameter ratio. E.g., 20:1 or 30:1 ratio can be increased to 100:1
2. **Adsorbent particle size:** Adsorbent activity depends on the surface area of adsorbent. Surface area increases with the decrease of particle size.

   Thus by decreasing particle size, adsorbent activity can be increased.
3. **Column temperature:** Elution speed increases with an increase in temperature, but the adsorbent activity decreases. Hence a compromise should be made between the elution and adsorbent activity. Room temperature is used for all samples.
4. **Column packing:** Uniform column packing leads to better separation of components.
5. **Solvent Nature:** More viscous solvents have less flow rate. Viscosity is inversely proportional to flow rate. Solvents of low viscosities give better separation.
6. **Pressure:** By increasing pressure above the column, the retention time of the analyte can be decreased.
7. **Adsorbent activity:** Adsorbent should be activated by heating to remove water.

Methodology of column chromatography

A tubular column similar to a burette is used. The column is packed with adsorbents like finely divided silica, alumina, charcoal, and calcium carbonate. The mixture to be separated is applied to the top of the column. Then the mobile phase is allowed to pass through the column under the influence of gravity. Equilibrium is established between the solute, adsorbent and the mobile phase. Different components have different interactions with the stationary and mobile phases. They move at different rates according to their affinity towards the stationary phase along the column, and separation is achieved. The least adsorbed component moves faster and gets eluted faster. Most adsorbed components move slower and get eluted later. The eluting solvent may be the same as the mobile phase or different from the mobile phase. The elution order of organic compounds with the increasing polarity of the solvent is given as

Alkanes < Alkenes < Ethers < halogenated hydrocarbons < Aromatic hydrocarbons < aldehydes and ketones < esters < alcohols < amines < carboxylic acids.

Normal phase chromatography (NP)

In the normal phase, the stationary phase is polar in nature, and the mobile phase is non-polar. Based on the 'like dissolves like' principle, the more polar component interacts more strongly with the stationary phase, moving slowly. The non-polar compound moves rapidly and gets eluted faster.

Reversed-phase column chromatography (RP)

In RP column chromatography, the stationary phase is non-polar, and the mobile phase is polar. Here, the non-polar compound moves slowly because of the increased interaction with the stationary phase. Polar compounds get eluted faster in the polar mobile phases (like dissolves like). Column chromatography mostly uses RP type of separation.

APPLICATIONS

(i) Column chromatography is used for the separation of
   1. Inorganic ions (cation and anions)
   2. Organic molecules (dyes, diastereoisomers)
   3. Tautomers
   4. Racemic mixtures
   5. Geometrical isomers
   6. Plant extracts
   7. Drugs
   8. Pharmaceuticals

(ii) Used in the purification process to remove impurities

(iii) Isolation of active constituents from plant extracts.

(iv) Estimation of drugs in formulations

CHAPTER 10

Thin Layer Chromatography

Thin layer chromatography (TLC) is a type of planar chromatography used for the separation and identification of organic compounds and also to test the purity of the compounds. The separation and identification of a mixture of components into individual components in TLC is carried out using finely divided adsorbent, solid/liquid spread over a glass plate and a liquid mobile phase. The history of Chromatography is described as given below.

Michael Tswett is credited as the father of liquid chromatography. Tswett developed his ideas in the early 1900s. In 1938 Izmailov & Shraiber described the basic principle and used it to separate plant extracts. Consden, Gorden & Martin started using filter papers to separate amino acids in 1944. In 1950 Kirchner used impregnated glass plate coated with alumina to identify terpenes. Ergon Stahl introduced standard equipment in 1958 for preparing TLC plates with uniform thin layers of known thickness.

PRINCIPLE

The principle of separation in TLC is **adsorption**. Adsorption is a surface phenomenon where a solute adheres to the surface of another material, forming a thin layer. This layer is often only one molecule thick. The solute molecule that gets adsorbed on the surface is known as adsorbate, and the surface on which adsorption occurs is known as adsorbent. The separation of the compounds depends on the interaction between adsorbents and adsorbates. The stationary phase is the adsorbent and the sample to be separated is the adsorbate.

A thin layer (0.25 mm) of adsorbent is coated onto solid support made of materials like glass, plastic and aluminium. The mixture of compounds to be separated is spotted on the adsorbent layer. **The mobile phase** solvent **rises** through the adsorbent (**against gravity**) by capillary action. The movement of the components is based on their affinities towards the adsorbent. **The**

component with more affinity for the stationary phase travels slowly and the component with lesser affinity moves faster, leading to the separation of components.

A binder like plaster of Paris is mixed with the adsorbent to facilitate the binding of the adsorbent with the support.

COMPONENTS AND METHODOLOGY OF TLC

1. **Stationary phase:** The selection of stationary phase in TLC depends on the nature of the components of the sample mixture. To obtain satisfactory separation efficiency, the factors to be considered are particle size, size distribution and morphology of the particles. The various adsorbents available are **Silica gel H** (without binder), **silica gel G** (silica gel+ calcium sulphate), **silica gel GF** (Silica gel +binder+ Fluorescent indicator), **Alumina**-without binder (Neutral, Basic, Acidic), **Alumina with the binder**, **Cellulose** with and without binder, Kieselguhr G, Diatomaceous earth+ binder and polyamide.
2. **Support for the adsorbent:** The support on which the adsorbent coated, is made up of **glass plates** of dimensions 20cm × 20cm, 20 × 10 cm or 20 × 5 cm. **Aluminium foil, plastic film or sheets** are also used as supporting plates for adsorbents like silica gel, alumina and cellulose. Ready to use TLC plates are available with adsorbent layer of varying thickness coated on aluminium foil. The thickness of these plates varies from 0.1 to 0.2mm. The glass TLC plates are prepared using a TLC spreader.
3. **Preparation and activation of TLC Plates:** The slurry of the adsorbent in water is made and using this slurry, the TLC plates are prepared. The different methods used for the preparation of TLC plates are
   (a) Pouring
   (b) Dipping
   (c) Spraying
   (d) Spreading

   (a) Pouring: The prepared slurry is poured onto the glass plate placed on a levelled surface. It is spread uniformly on the glass plate. The plates are allowed to be set, then dried in an oven.

   Disadvantage: Uniformity in thickness not obtained.

   (b) Dipping: This technique is used for small plates. Two plates are held back to back and dipped into the slurry of the adsorbent at the same time. The slurry is prepared in chloroform or in other volatile solvents. The plates are allowed to set, then dried

***Disadvantages*:**

1. The thickness of the adsorbent layer cannot be controlled.
2. Uniformity in thickness may not be there.
3. Large quantity of slurry is required even for the preparation of few plates

(c) **Spraying:** The slurry is diluted, and the suspension of the adsorbent(slurry) is sprayed over the glass plate using a sprayer.
Disadvantage: Difficult to get a uniform layer.

(d) **Spreading:** This is the most suitable technique to get a uniform thin layer of adsorbent on glass plates. The operation of the spreading technique with the spreader is shown below.
There are two types of spreaders.

(i) **Moving spreader type:** In this type, after pouring the slurry, the spreader is moved over the plates spreading the adsorbents.

(ii) **Moving plate type:** The plates are made to move under the adsorbent reservoir, so that they are coated with adsorbent.
In both methods, the plates are air-dried to avoid cracks developing on the surface of the adsorbent.

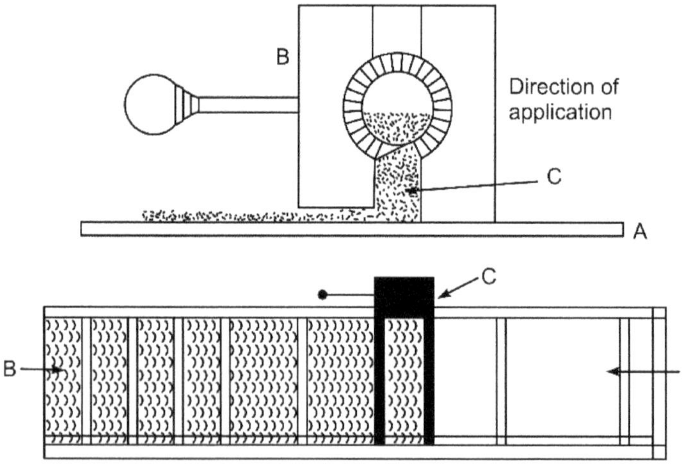

Fig. 10.1(a) Operation of thin layer spreader, **(b)** Tray alignment with partially coated plates A = Glass plate, B = Spreader, C = Slurry of the adsorbent.

Here, the slurry (C) is put in the spreader (B) and then moved along the direction of application onto the surface of the glass plate (A) to obtain a uniform layer.
In Fig (b), the slurry of the adsorbent is introduced into the aligning tray (C), which is then moved onto the glass plate (A) to obtain a uniform layer of adsorbent (B).

The glass plates are stacked on a base plate. The prepared slurry is poured into the reservoir of the TLC spreader. A knob is provided in the spreader to adjust the thickness of the adsorbent layer. The process is shown diagrammatically in Figures 10.1a and 10.1b.

For analytical purposes, 0.25mm thickness plate and 2mm thickness plate is used for preparative purposes.

After setting, the plates are activated by heating in an oven at 100°C to 120°C for one hour. Activation of the TLC plate is the removal of water/moisture from the surface of the adsorbent. This helps in retaining the adsorbent activity of the adsorbent.

4. **Mobile phase:** The choice of the mobile phase is dependent on
   (a) Nature of the component to be separated
   (b) Nature of the stationary phase
   (c) Chromatographic mode
   (d) Sample size

   Mobile phases used are either pure solvents or a mixture of solvents. Solvents of increasing polarity are used.

   An **elutropic series** ranks solvents by their relative abilities to displace solutes from a given adsorbent. The order of the elutropic series (increasing polarity) is given as

   Pet.ether<Carbon tetra chloride<cyclohexane< carbon disulfide<Ether<acetone<Benzene Toluene<Ethyl acetate<Chloroform<Alcohol<water<Pyridine<organic acids<acid mixtures with pyridine or alcohol.

   Usually the mobile phase composition is decided by trial and error method or sometimes from the literature.

5. **Sample application:** The sample solution should be of minimum concentration. Usually, 2-5µl of 1% solution of sample and standard are spotted on the plate using capillary for qualitative analysis and micropipette for quantitative analysis. Spots are placed 2cm above the base of the plate, and the spots should be as small as possible. When placing the plate inside the development chamber for elution, the spots should not be immersed in the mobile phase.

6. **Plate development:** For developing the plates, development chambers or glass beakers can be used. Nowadays, twin trough chambers are available, which are economical in using solvents (Fig 10.6). After pouring the mobile phase into the development tank, the tank is lined inside with a filter paper to saturate the atmosphere inside the tank with solvent vapours to avoid the **edge effect**. Reasons for the presaturation of the chamber is shown in fig 10.4a and figure 10.4b.

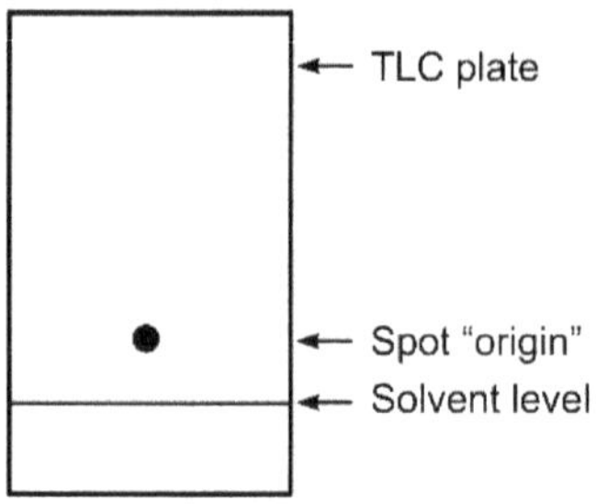

Fig. 10.2 Preparation & spotting of the TLC plate.

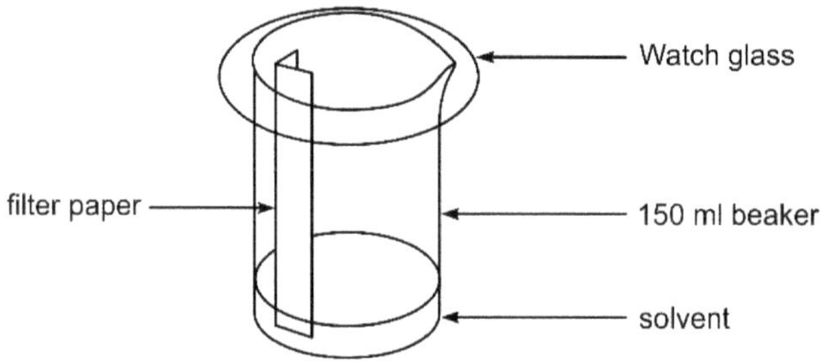

Fig. 10.3 Preparation of developing chamber.

The solvent front in the middle of the TLC plate moves faster than that of the solvent front in the edge as the mobile phase moves on the plate. This is called as **edge effect,** which makes the spots distorted. The Migration distance is more with the pre-saturated chamber than the non-saturated chamber. This is because, in a non-saturated chamber, the solvent migrating in the adsorbent layer vaporizes, leading to an edge effect. The edge effect is compared with normal TLC in figure 10.5.

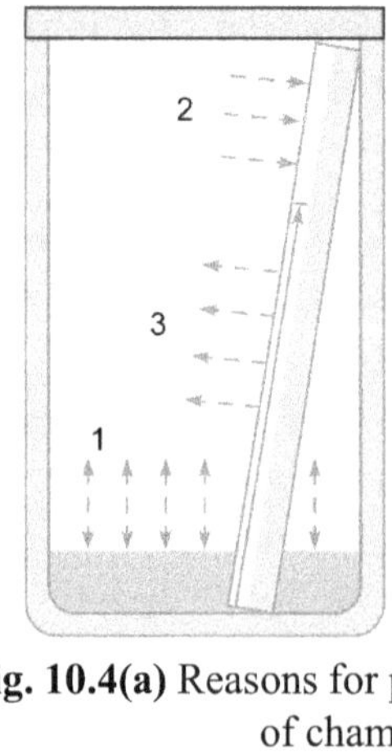

Fig. 10.4(a) Reasons for presaturation of chamber.

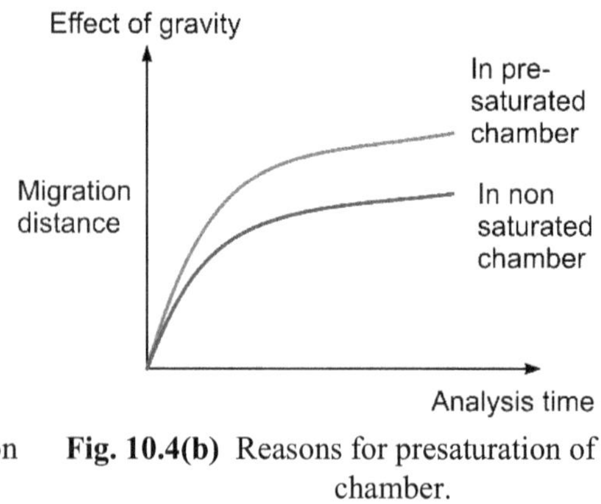

Fig. 10.4(b) Reasons for presaturation of chamber.

1. Solvent in Liquid-Vapour equilibrium
2. Solvent Vapour adsorbs on the layer
3. Solvent migrating from the layer vaporizes

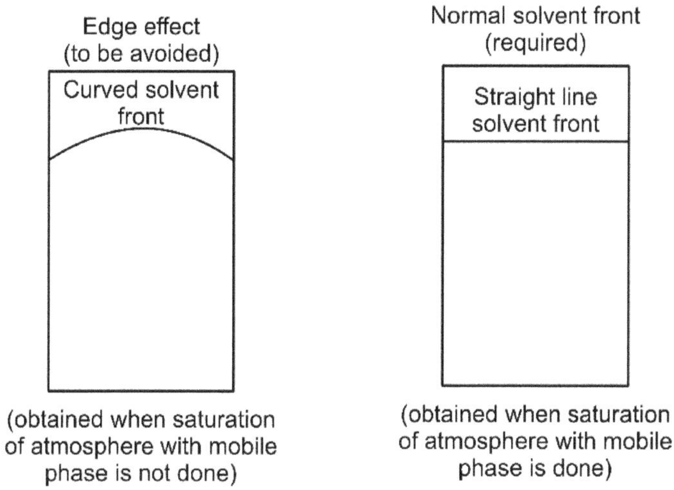

Fig. 10.5 Edge effect and normal TLC.

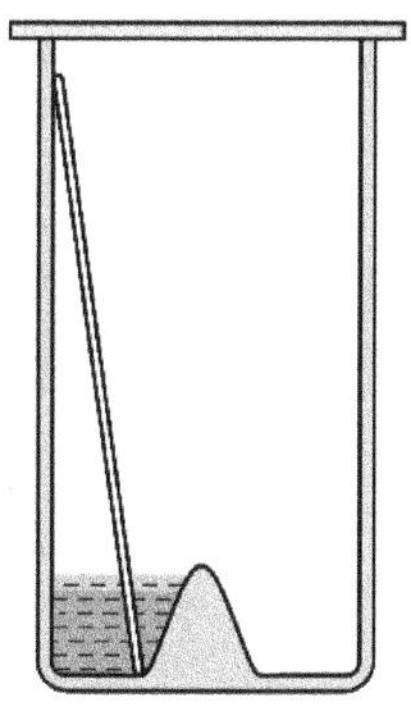

Fig. 10.6 Twin trough chamber.

After saturating the tank with solvent vapours, the prepared TLC Plate is placed in the development chamber and covered with a watch glass. The spots should be above the level of the mobile phase. It is kept aside undisturbed. The solvent rises up in the plate by capillary action. The solvent front is allowed to move up to ¾ th of the plate. The plate is removed from the tank, and the solvent front is marked with a pencil immediately.

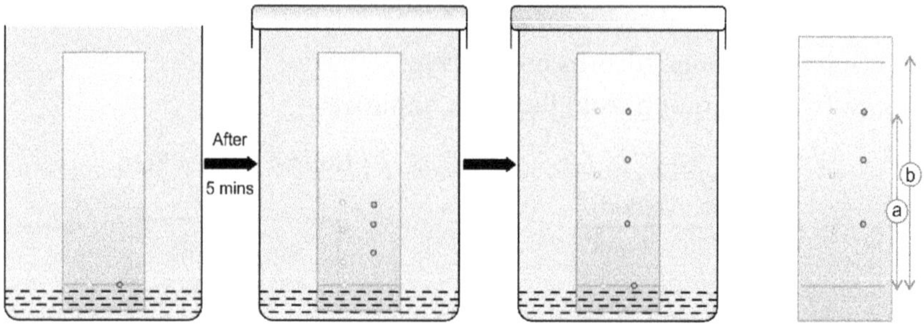

$$Rf = \frac{\text{distance travelled by the component}}{\text{distance travelled by the solvent}} = \frac{a}{b}$$

Fig. 10.7 Steps involved in TLC.

7. **Detection techniques:** After the development, the TLC plates are dried, and the analytes are detected. Detection of coloured samples can be done visually. The different types of detection techniques are
   1. Non-specific methods
   2. Specific methods
   1. **Non-specific methods:** These methods are used for the identification of compounds (qualitative analysis). The number of spots can be detected, but the nature of the compound cannot be detected.
      - **(i) Iodine chamber method:** Iodine crystals are added to the tank, and when the developed TLC plates are placed in the tank, the analyte spots appear as brown or amber-coloured spots.
      - **(ii) Sulphuric acid reagent:** The spraying reagent used is 70-80% of sulphuric acid with oxidizing agents like potassium dichromate, potassium permanganate or a few ml of nitric acid. After spraying this reagent, the plates are heated in an oven to give black spots, which are due to the charring of the compounds.
      - **(iii) Using a fluorescent adsorbent:** If the compounds are not fluorescent, they can be detected using a fluorescent adsorbent. The background is fluorescent and the compounds appear as dark spots when the plates are kept in the UV chamber. If the compounds are fluorescent in nature, they can be visualized as fluorescent spots in UV chamber, with a non-fluorescent adsorbent.

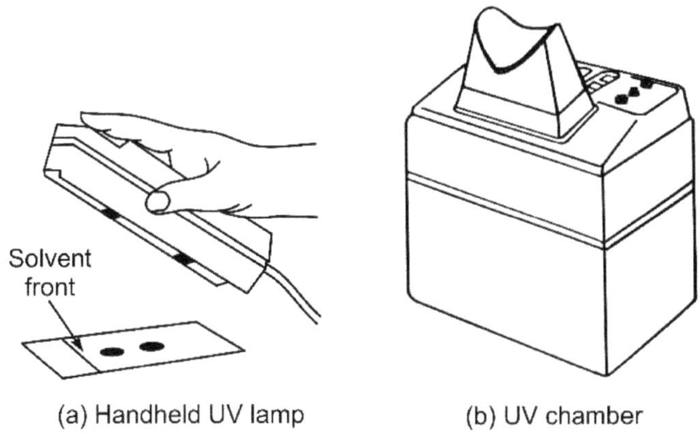

Fig. 10.8 UV detection methods.

2. **Specific methods:** Different detecting agents are used to identify the compounds. The agents used are specific for the given compound and are listed in table 10.1.

Table 10.1 Detecting agents with corresponding compounds.

Compounds	Reagent
Phenolic compounds and tannins	Ferric chloride
Amino acids	Ninhydrin in acetone
Alkaloids	Dragendroff's reagent
Cardiac glycosides	3,5-dinitrobenzoic acid
Aldehyde and ketone	2,4-dinitrophenyl hydrazine

The detecting techniques are further classified as

1. **Destructive techniques:** In these methods, the samples are destroyed by the reagent during detection. Hence sample recovery is not possible. E.g., Sulphuric acid reagent.
2. **Non-destructive techniques:** The sample is not destroyed during detection in these methods. Sample recovery is possible. E.g., UV chamber method, Iodine chamber method and densitometric method. In densitometry, the spot density is measured by a densitometer. This method is used for quantitative estimation. It is also called an *in-situ* method.

QUALITATIVE ANALYSIS

1. **R_f value:** To identify the compounds in TLC, a parameter called **R_f (retardation factor)** value is used. R_f value is the ratio of the

distance travelled by the solute to the distance travelled by the solvent front.

$$R_f = \frac{\text{Distance travelled by the solute}}{\text{Distance travelled by the solvent front}}$$

R_f values range from 0 to1. R_f value is characteristic for each compound for the given set of stationary and mobile phases. The compound can also be identified by comparison with the R_f value of the standard.

The factors affecting R_f values and reproducibility are

1. Increase in **layer thickness** decreases R_f value, because the mobile phase moves slower up the plate.
2. Moisture on the TLC plate
3. Vessel saturation
4. Temperature
5. Depth of mobile phase
6. Nature of the TLC plate
7. Sample size
8. Solvent parameters.

An increase in these parameters causes an increase in R_f values typically.

2. **R_x value:** In case the solvent front runs off the plate, the ratio of the distance travelled by the sample to the distance travelled by the standard is measured, and it is called as **R_x value**

$$R_x = \frac{\text{Distance travelled by the solute}}{\text{Distance travelled by the standard}}$$

The value is always closer to 1.

3. **R_m value:** To find out the compounds of a homologous series, **ΔR_m values are determined.**

$$\Delta R_m = \log \frac{1}{R_f} - 1$$

In a homologous series ΔR_m values are constant.

QUANTITATIVE ANALYSIS

Direct method: The quantity of the components can be determined by the densitometric analysis of individual spots.

Indirect method: The individual spots are eluted with a suitable solvent and determined by methods like UV visible, fluorescence, flame photometry and electrochemical methods.

8. **Development techniques:** The actual separation takes place in the plate development of thin-layer chromatography. A solvent system is introduced to the sample on the TLC layer to separate the mixture into individual substances. Separation can be achieved through various methods. The most common TLC development techniques are explained below.

   The different developmental techniques in TLC are

   1. One dimensional development

      Vertical and Horizontal, and multiple developments

   2. Two-dimensional development

1. **One dimensional development**

   Vertical Development: This is the most common TLC development method. The plate is placed in a suitable TLC developing chamber such that the solvent wets the adsorbent layer below the starting line. The solvent rises up the layer due to capillary forces transporting the sample mixture. Once the solvent front has reached the predetermined height (10-15 cm for TLC and 3-7 cm for HPTLC), the plate is removed from the chamber. The solvent front is marked with a pencil, and the plate is dried.

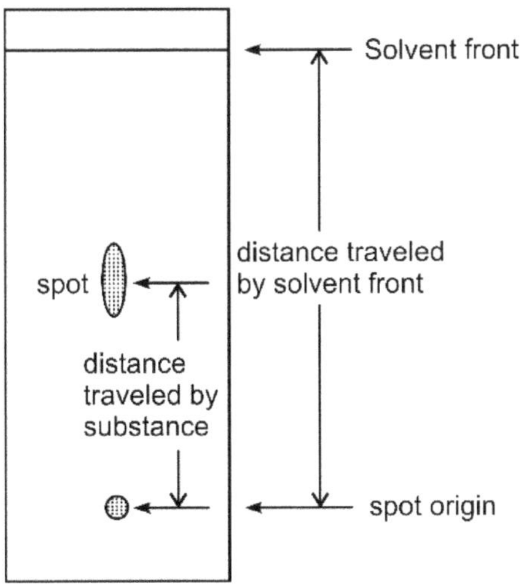

Fig. 10.9 Vertical development.

Horizontal Development: In this method, the plate is positioned horizontally inside the chamber, and the solvent is applied using a wick or capillary slit. Development can be performed on one or both sides of the TLC plate.

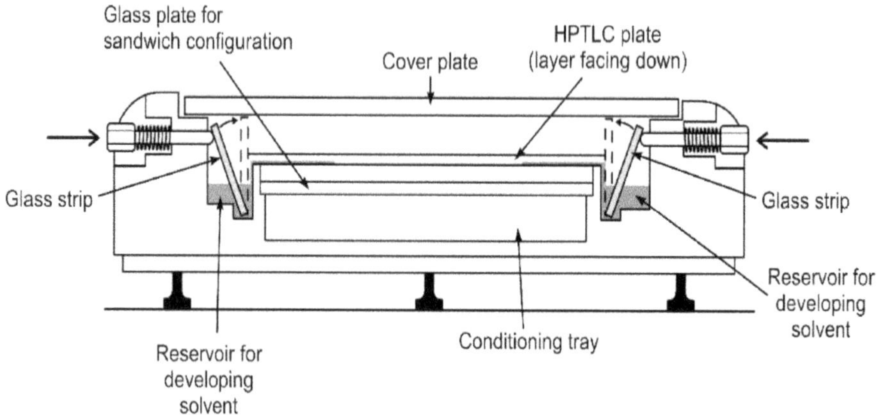

Fig. 10.10 Horizontal development.

Multiple Development: In this method, the TLC plate undergoes multiple developments with drying between each development. Re-concentration of the spots is caused by the repeated travelling of the solvent, producing elliptical shapes or narrow bands. The resolution is significantly improved for substances with R_f values below 0.5. Multiple developments can be performed over different separation distances, using the same solvent or different solvents of varying polarity. The different types are

Separate runs over the same migration distance

Stepwise, increasing

Stepwise, decreasing

Automated multiple developments, stepwise with a solvent gradient system

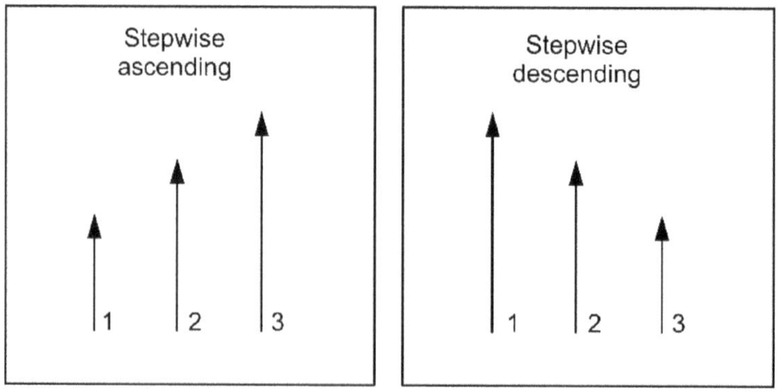

Fig. 10.11 Multiple developments.

Two-Dimensional Development

1. Two dimensions with one solvent system
2. Two dimensions with two solvent system

In two-dimensional TLC development, the sample is applied to a starting point in the corner of the TLC plate. The plate is placed in a normal chamber and developed from bottom to top. After drying, the plate is turned 90° and placed in another chamber with a different solvent and developed again. The end of chromatogram track from the first development is used as the starting line for the second development. The second development can be done with the same solvent or another solvent. Complex mixtures can be separated completely by two-dimensional chromatography.

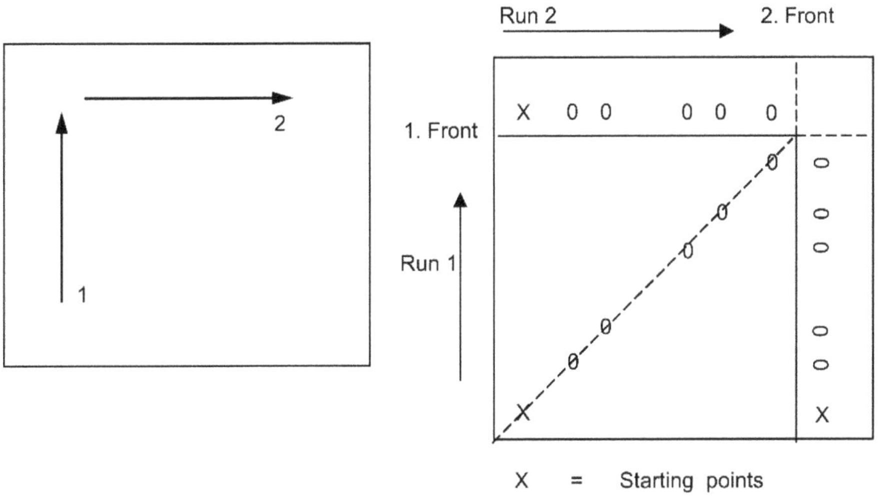

Fig. 10.12 Two-dimensional development.

APPLICATIONS OF TLC

1. Separation of a mixture of drugs of chemical, biological origin and plant extracts.
2. To check the purity of the samples and identification of drugs.
3. To purify the compounds
4. To check the completion of reactions
5. For identifying organic compounds. E.g., Acids, alcohols. Glycols, alkaloids, amines, proteins, peptides and antibiotics
6. Most widely used for identification tests, tests for purity and identification of related substances.
7. Separation of inorganic ions (cations and anions)
8. Separation of amino acids and vitamins

9. To detect decomposition products in drugs.
10. Quantitative analysis by TLC

It is done by two methods

1. Analysis of fractions on the plate - Photo densitometry.
2. Determination of fractions after elution from the supporting material.

After elution, the samples are quantified using methods like UV-Visible, Fluorimetry etc.

Advantages

1. Simple equipment and low cost
2. Rapid technique
3. Wide choice of stationary phases
4. Easy recovery of separated components
5. High efficiency of separation
6. Easy detection
7. More sensitivity
8. Both preparative and analytical scales are possible.
9. Allows the usage of corrosive spray reagents
10. Economical usage of solvents and stationary phases.

Disadvantages

1. The stationary phase needs activation.
2. Cannot differentiate isomeric and enantiomeric forms of a compound.
3. A large quantity of slurry is required to prepare a few TLC plates.
4. TLC is applicable only to nonvolatile compounds, thus limiting its use.

HIGH-PERFORMANCE THIN-LAYER CHROMATOGRAPHY

This is a sophisticated and automated form of TLC used to separate, identify, and quantify a mixture of components. It is also used as a micro preparation technique. The principle of separation is adsorption, as in TLC. In HPTLC, the particle size of the adsorbent is small and the layer thickness is thin, giving better resolution than TLC.

A comparison between TLC and HPTLC techniques is presented in Table 10.2.

Table 10.2 Comparison between TLC and HPTLC techniques.

Parameters	HPTLC	TLC
Adsorbent layer thickness	100μm	250μm
Mean Particle size	5-6	10-12
Plate height	12 μm	30 μm
Migration distance	3-6 cm	10-15 cm
Separation time	3-20 min	20-200 min
Number of samples per plate	< 36	< 10
Sample volume	0.1-0.5 μl	1-5μl
Mobile phase volume	Less consumption	More
Sampling	Autosampler	Manual
Scanning and detection	UV, Visible, Fluorimetric detection is possible for both qualitative and quantitative analysis. The densitometric scanner is used for the detection	Detection techniques are applicable. But scanners are not available for densitometric analysis.

CHAPTER 11

Paper Chromatography

Paper chromatography is a separation technique in which the mixture of components is separated on a chromatographic paper using a liquid mobile phase. The two types of paper chromatography are

1. Paper adsorption chromatography
2. Paper partition chromatography

In paper adsorption chromatography, the stationary phase paper is impregnated with silica or alumina, and the solvent is the mobile phase.

In paper **partition** chromatography, the **moisture** which is present in the **pores of the cellulose fibres** of the filter paper acts as the **stationary phase** and an immiscible **solvent** is used as the **mobile phase**.

Paper chromatography generally refers to paper partition chromatography because most of the separations are carried out by this method.

PRINCIPLE

The principle of separation in paper chromatography is partition. The moisture present in the cellulose layers of the filter paper acts as the stationary phase, and organic solvents/ buffers are used as mobile phases.

A small drop of the sample solution is applied as a small spot on the filter paper, and it is dried. The filter paper is kept inside the chamber containing the mobile phase, which rises by capillary action, and as it reaches the spots of the sample, the mobile phase carries the components along with it. The rate of movement of the components is dependent on their partition coefficients. When the mobile phase rises to ¾ th of the paper, the paper is removed from the chamber, dried and detected using suitable reagents. The movement of the components is expressed in terms of migration parameters like the R_f value.

MIGRATION PARAMETERS

The position of the migrated components is indicated by the terms such as R_f, R_x and R_m.

1. **R_f value:** To identify the compounds in paper chromatography, a parameter called **R_f (retardation factor)** value is used. R_f value is the ratio of the distance travelled by the solute to the distance travelled by the solvent front.

$$R_f = \frac{\text{Distance travelled by the solute}}{\text{Distance travelled by the solvent front}}$$

   R_f values range from 0 to 1. R_f value is characteristic for each compound for the given set of stationary and mobile phases. The compound can also be identified by comparison with the R_f value of the standard.

   The factors affecting R_f values and reproducibility are

   1. Nature of mobile phase.
   2. Vessel saturation
   3. Temperature
   4. Sample size and nature of the sample
   5. Nature of filter paper

   An increase in these parameters normally causes an increase in R_f values.

2. **R_x value:** In case the solvent front runs off the plate, the ratio of the distance travelled by the sample to the distance travelled by the standard is measured, and it is called as **R_x value**

$$R_x = \frac{\text{Distance travelled by the solute}}{\text{Distance travelled by the standard}}$$

   The value is always closer to 1.

3. **R_m value:** To find out the compounds of a homologous series, **ΔR_m values are determined.**

$$\Delta R_m = \log \frac{1}{R_f} - 1$$

   In a homologous series ΔR_m values are constant.

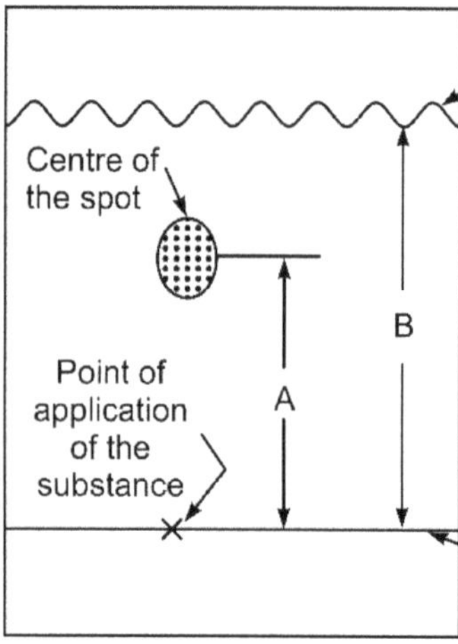

Fig. 11.1 Diagrammatic representation of R_f value.

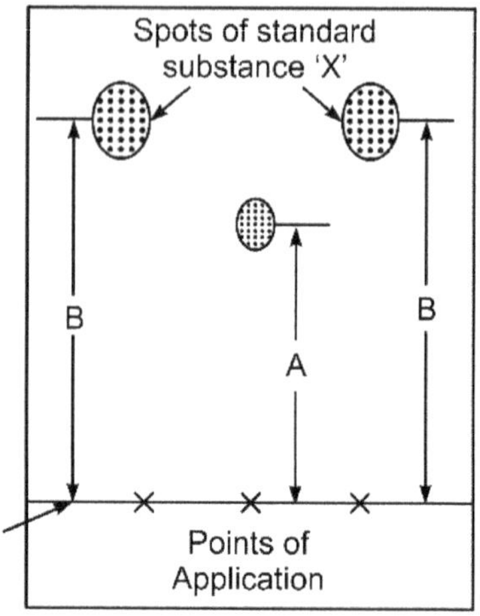

Fig. 11.2 Diagrammatic representation of R_x value.

EXPERIMENTAL DETAILS FOR QUALITATIVE ANALYSIS

CHOICE OF PAPER USED (STATIONARY PHASE)

The choice of the filter paper depends on

(a) Nature of the sample to be separated (hydrophilic, hydrophobic or neutral).

(b) Nature of separation, whether qualitative or quantitative

(c) Analytical or preparative separation

The different types of Whatman filter papers are grades like No.1, No.2, No.3, No.4, No.20, No.40 and No.42 etc. These papers have different sizes, shapes, porosities and thicknesses.

TYPES OF PAPERS

A. Pure cellulose papers (Whatman papers)

B. Modified cellulose papers

1. Chemically modified papers

   (a) Carboxyl papers (b) Acetylated papers (c) Hydrophilic papers

2. Impregnated papers

3. Loaded papers

   (a) Papers loaded with adsorbent powder

   (b) Papers loaded with Ion-Exchange celluloses

(c) Papers loaded with synthetic organic Ion-Exchange resins

(d) Papers loaded with inorganic Ion-Exchangers

C. **Glass fibretype papers**

A. **Pure cellulose papers (Whatman papers):** These types of papers are prepared from cotton linters low in organic and inorganic impurities and uniform in physical characteristics. Whatman papers have α Cellulose 98-99%and 1% of mineral content

B. **Modified cellulose papers:** Cellulose paper can be modified in several ways to alter its behaviour.

1. **Chemically modified papers (Hydrophobic papers)**

(a) **Carboxyl papers:** The exchange capacity of the paper is increased by increasing the carboxyl content (1.4%) by partial oxidation.

They are used for efficient separation of polar substances, Cationic separation of potential amines and amino acids.

(b) **Acetylated papers:** These papers are partially acetylated by treating with glacial acetic acid containing 5% acetic anhydride.

They are used in Reverse phase chromatographic separation of lipophilic substances like steroids, insecticides, pigments and also metal cations.

(c) **Hydrophilic papers:** e.g., Papers modified with methanol, formamide, glycol, glycerol etc.

2. **Impregnated papers:** Paper sheets are impregnated with oils to separate hydrophobic substances such as amines, lipids, steroids, vitamins, and pesticides (reverse phased chromatography)

3. **Loaded papers:** In these papers, powder, fibre, or resin are dispersed in a normal cellulose paper

(a) Paper loaded with adsorbent powder, E.g. Silica papers, alumina papers, zirconia papers, kieselguhr papers.

These papers are used to separate less polar and nonpolar substances (such as lipids, sterols, steryl esters, steroids, terpenes, dyes, insecticides, chloroplast pigments and inorganic ions).

(b) Papers loaded with Ion-Exchange celluloses

Chromatographic papers are coated with anionic or cationic exchangers

(c) Papers loaded with synthetic organic Ion-Exchange resins:

These papers are coated with micro pulverized ion-exchange resin, which is incorporated into α-cellulose pulp (reeve angle papers)

(d) Papers loaded with inorganic Ion exchangers: e.g. zirconium phosphate, hydrous oxide, and ammonium molybdophosphate

C. **Glass Fiber Type Papers:** These papers are manufactured from fine borosilicate glass fibres. Detection reagents that are too corrosive for cellulose-based papers (e.g. chromic-sulphuric acid charring solution) can be used on these papers. Glass fibre type papers can be used in extreme conditions of temperature and acidity where cellulose papers are unstable.

MOBILE PHASES

Pure solvents, buffer solutions or a mixture of solvents can be used as a mobile phase. The mobile phases can be classified as Hydrophilic and Hydrophobic mobile phases.

Hydrophilic mobile phases

Iso propanol: ammonia: water	9:1:2
n-butanol: glacial acetic acid: water	4:1:5
Methanol: water	3:1 or 4:1
t-butanol: water: formic acid	40:20:5

Hydrophobic mobile phase

Kerosene: 70% Isopropanol,

Dimethyl ether: cyclohexane

Single, two or three-phase solvent systems can be used.

APPLICATION OF SAMPLES

The sample is dissolved in the mobile phase and applied using a capillary tube or micropipettes. Sample in μg quantities like 10-20μl are used for spotting (low concentration). Spots are applied on the origin line, which is drawn by a pencil,5cm from the bottom of the filter paper. Each sample is spotted 2cm away from each other.

DEVELOPMENTAL TECHNIQUES

The different developmental techniques used in paper chromatography are

(i) Ascending development
(ii) Descending development
(iii) Ascending- descending development
(iv) Circular or radial paper chromatography
(v) Two-dimensional development

(i) Ascending development: It is otherwise called vertical development. The spotted (at the bottom) paper is kept vertically in the chamber containing the mobile phase. The solvent rises on the paper by capillary action against gravity.

(ii) Descending development: In this type of development, a special chamber holds the solvent at the top. The paper is spotted at the top, and the solvent is allowed to flow down the paper assisted by gravity. Hence the development is faster.

(iii) Ascending – Descending development: It is a hybrid of both ascending and descending techniques. First, the ascending technique is allowed to proceed. The filter paper is folded over a glass rod, allowing the ascending technique to be converted to descending. In this technique, the distance of travel of solute components increase leading to better separation.

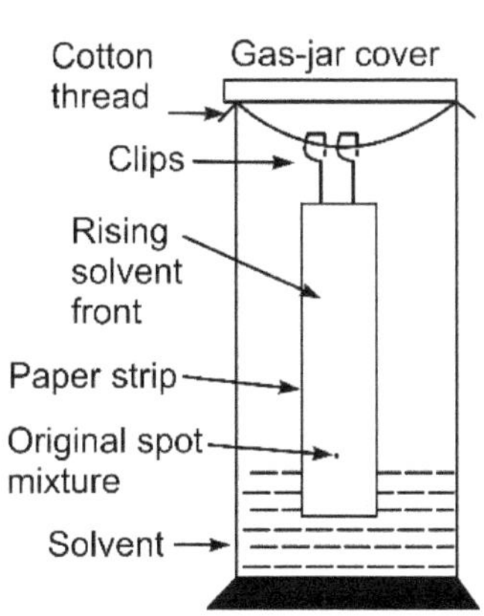

Fig. 11.3 Ascending development.

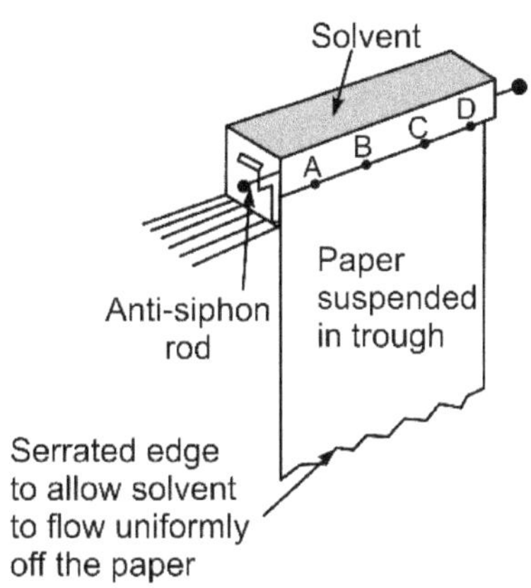

Fig. 11.4 Descending development.

(iv) Circular / radial paper chromatography: In this technique, the development takes place radially. A circular filter paper is used. The sample is spotted in the centre. After drying, the paper is placed on a petri dish with the mobile phase, and a wick from the filter paper is dipped into the mobile phase. As the solvent rises through the wick and moves through the paper, it uniformly carries the components in all directions.

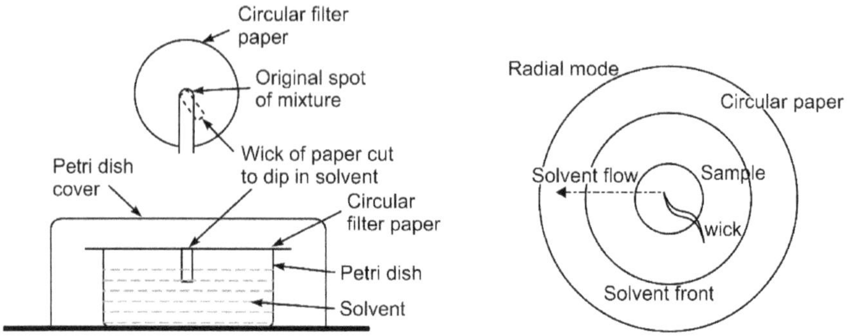

Fig. 11.5 Circular paper chromatography.

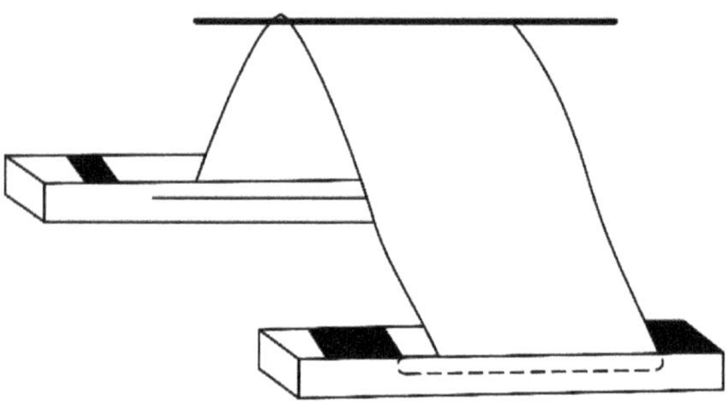

Fig. 11.6 Ascending – Descending development.

(v) Two-dimensional development

(a) Two dimensions with one solvent system

(b) Two dimensions with two solvent system

In two-dimensional paper development, the sample is applied to a starting point in the corner of the paper. The paper is placed in a normal chamber and developed once from bottom to top. After drying, the paper is turned 90° and placed in another chamber with a different solvent and developed again. The chromatogram track from the first development is used as the starting line for the second development. The second development can be done with the same solvent or another solvent. Complex mixtures can be separated completely by two-dimensional chromatography.

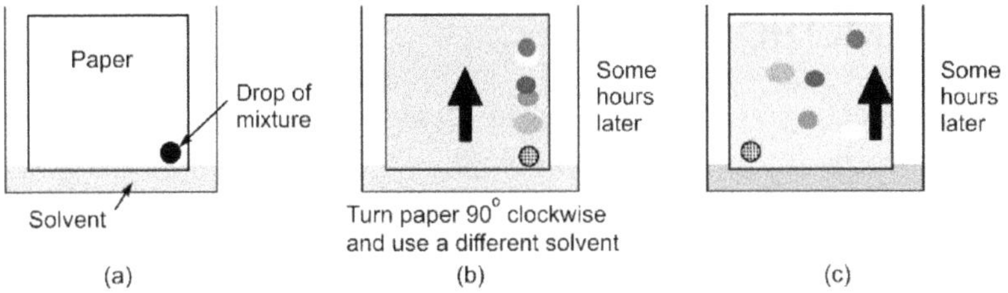

Fig. 11.7 Two-dimensional paper chromatography.

DETECTION TECHNIQUES

After the development, the chromatograms are dried and then detected. Detection of coloured samples can be done visually. The different types of detection techniques are

1. Non-specific methods
2. Specific methods

1. Non-specific methods: These methods are used for the identification of compounds (qualitative analysis).

The number of spots can be detected, but the nature of the compound cannot be detected.

(i) Iodine chamber method: Iodine crystals are added to the tank, and when the developed paper is placed in the tank, the analyte spots appear as brown or amber-coloured spots.

(ii) Using UV or Fluorescence: If the compounds absorb in the UV region they can be detected using UV chamber. E.g., Antibiotics. Fluoresent substances can be detected by fluorimetric methods. E.g., Quinine.

If the compounds are not fluorescent, they can be detected using a fluorescent adsorbent. The background is fluorescent and the compounds appear as dark spots when the plates are kept in UV chamber.

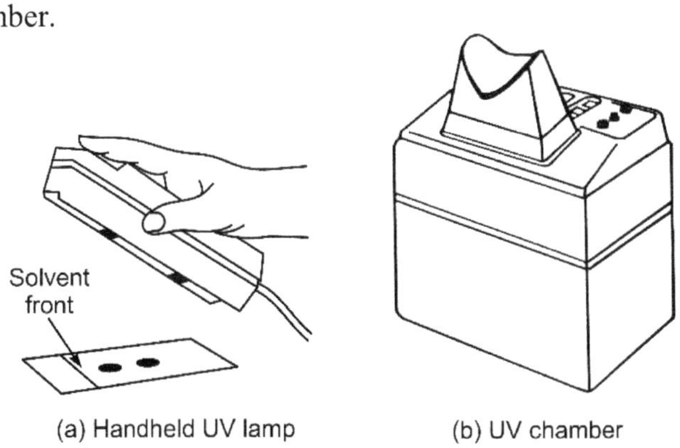

Fig. 11.8 UV chamber.

SPECIFIC METHODS

Different detecting agents are used to identify the compounds. The agents used are specific for the given compound.

Table 11.1 Some of the detecting agents for specific compounds.

Compounds	Reagent
Phenolic compounds and tannins	Ferric chloride
Amino acids	Ninhydrin in acetone
Alkaloids	Dragendroff's reagent
Cardiac glycosides	3,5-dinitrobenzoic acid
Aldehyde and ketone	2,4-dinitrophenyl hydrazine

The detecting techniques are further classified as

1. **Destructive techniques:** In these methods, during detection, the samples are destroyed by the reagent. Hence sample recovery is not possible. E.g., Sulphuric acid reagent.
2. **Non-destructive techniques:** The sample is not destroyed during detection in these methods. Sample recovery is possible E.g., UV chamber method, Iodine chamber method.

QUALITATIVE ANALYSIS

1. **R_f value:** To identify the compounds in TLC, a parameter called **R_f (retardation factor)** value is used. R_f value is the ratio of the distance travelled by the solute to the distance travelled by the solvent front.

$$R_f = \frac{\text{Distance travelled by the solute}}{\text{Distance travelled by the solvent front}}$$

   R_f values range from 0 to 1. R_f value is characteristic for each compound for the given set of stationary and mobile phases. The compound can also be identified by comparison with the R_f value of the standard.

2. **R_x value:** In case the solvent front runs off the plate, the ratio of the distance travelled by the sample to the distance travelled by the standard is measured, and it is called as R_x value

$$R_x = \frac{\text{Distance travelled by the solute}}{\text{Distance travelled by the standard}}$$

   The value is always closer to 1.

3. **R_m value:** To find out the compounds of a homologous series, **ΔR_m values are determined.**

$$\Delta R_m = \log \frac{1}{R_f} - 1$$

In a homologous series ΔR_m values are constant.

QUANTITATIVE ANALYSIS

The individual spots are eluted with a suitable solvent and determined by methods like UV visible, fluorescence, flame photometry and electrochemical methods.

Advantages of Paper chromatography

1. A simple and rapid technique
2. Inexpensive
3. Excellent resolving power.

Disadvantages of Paper chromatography

1. Only a minimum quantity of sample should be applied to avoid diffusion through paper leading to poor separation
2. Improper placement of paper leads to error in identification
3. If chamber saturation is not done, it will affect the resolution

Applications of Paper chromatography

1. Separation of organic and biochemical products
2. Separation of drugs and natural products
3. Separation of carbohydrates, vitamins, antibiotics, proteins, alkaloids, glycosides, and aminoacids.
4. Identification of drugs and related products.
5. Identification of decomposition products and drug metabolites in blood, urine etc.

CHAPTER 12

Ion Exchange Chromatography

Ion exchange is defined as a reversible reaction in which a mixture of similarly charged ions is exchanged using ion exchange resins. Cations or anions can be separated by this technique. The exchange of ions takes place based on the relative affinities of the ions for the ions in the ion exchanger. The ion-exchange chromatography is reported back from the 1850s.

PRINCIPLE

The basic principle is the attraction between oppositely charged particles. It is the reversible electrostatic interaction of charged species with the separation matrix. Ion exchange chromatography makes use of charge-charge interactions between the analyte in the sample solution and the functional groups which are present in the stationary phase (resin). The analytes are retained by the ionic interaction. The stationary phase surface presents ionic functional groups which interact with analytes of opposite charge.

The principle of separation is based on the reversible exchange of ions between the analyte ions in solution and ions in the ion exchange resin.

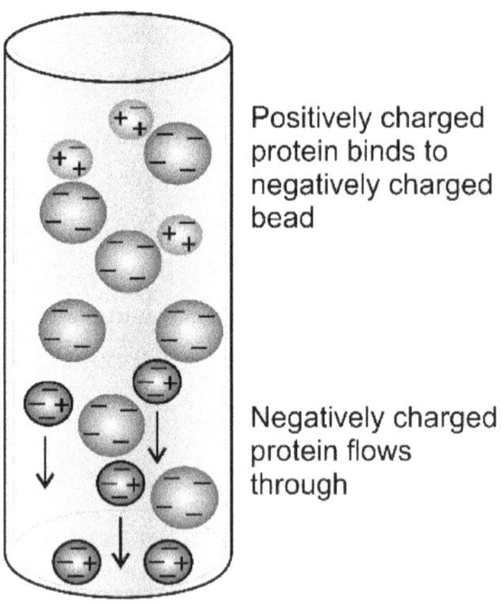

Fig. 12.1 Separation in Ion exchange chromatography.

TYPES OF ION EXCHANGE CHROMATOGRAPHY

(i) Anion exchange chromatography
(ii) Cation exchange chromatography

In Anion exchange chromatography, anion exchange resins are used (positively charged resin), which binds to the negatively charged analytes (anions). E.g., Q anion exchanger, DEAE (Diethylaminoethylcellulose) – anion exchanger.

$$\text{Stationary-OH}^- + A^- \rightarrow \text{Stationary-A}^- + OH^-$$

In cation exchange chromatography, the cation exchange resins are used (negatively charged) and bind to positively charged ions (cations). They are used for the separation of cations in solution. E.g., Sulfonic acid – S-cation exchanger,
Carboxymethyl – CM cation exchanger.

$$\text{Stationary-H}^+ + M^+ \rightarrow \text{Stationary-M}^+ + H^+$$

The bound analytes are then eluted by changing the pH of the buffer or by increasing ionic strength.

Ion exchange resin should have the following requirements

1. It must be chemically stable, rigid and inert
2. It should be insoluble in common solvents
3. It should have a sufficient degree of cross-linking
4. The swollen resin must be denser than water

CLASSIFICATION OF ION EXCHANGE RESINS

Classification of Ion exchange resins based on the chemical nature

1. Strong cation exchange resin
2. Weak cation exchange resin
3. Strong anion exchange resin
4. Weak anion exchange resin

Table 12.1 Types of ion exchangers with examples.

S. No.	Type of exchanger	Functional group	Commercially available media
1.	Strong cation exchange resin	Sulfonic acid (S)	RESOURCE™ S, Macro-Prep® High S, Macro-Prep® 25 S
2.	Weak cation exchange resin	Carboxymethyl (CM)	CM sephadex C-50, C-25, Macro-Prep® CM
3.	Strong anion exchange resin	Quaternary Ammonium (Q)	RESOURCE™ Q, Macro-Prep® High Q, Macro-Prep® 25 Q
4.	Weak anion exchange resin	Diethylaminoethyl (DEAE)	DEAE sephacel A-50, DEAE cellulose, Macro-Prep® DEAE

Classification Ion exchange resins based on the source

Natural:

Cation: Zeolytes,clay etc

Anion: Dolomite

Synthetic: Inorganic and organic resins

Organic resins are the commonly used resins. They are polymeric resin matrix with ion-exchange sites. The exchange sites are present in the polystyrene of the resin, and di-vinyl benzene is the cross-linking agent which offers mechanical strength to the resin.

Structure of Styrene and Di-vinyl benzene

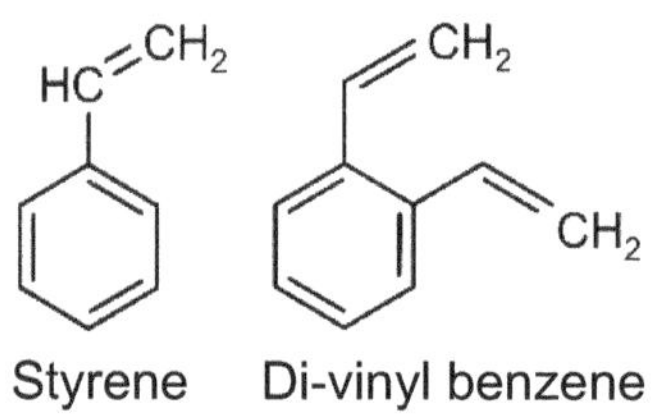

STRUCTURAL TYPES OF ION EXCHANGE RESINS

1. **Pellicular type:** The Particle size ranges from 30-40μ with an ion exchange film of 1-2μ thickness. **Their ion exchange capacity is very low.**
2. **Porous resin with coated exchanger beads:** Their particle size is 5-10 μ.They are porous in nature, and their efficiency is more
3. **Macro reticular resin bead:** A reticular network of the resin is present on the surface of the bead. It has low exchange capacity
4. **Bonded phase silica**: The surface of the support material is sulphonated and electro statically bonded to anion exchanger.

   It is **less efficient and has a low exchange capacity.**

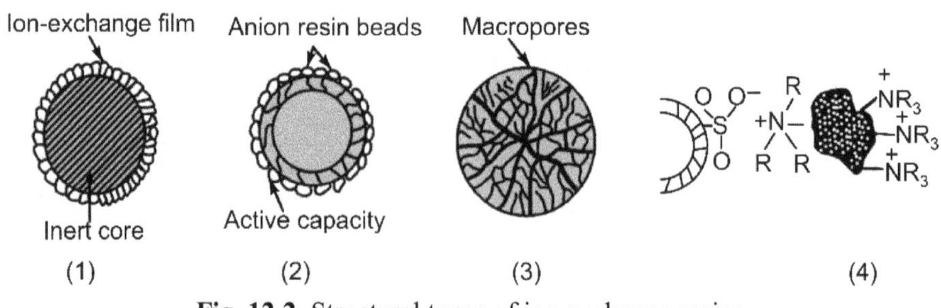

Fig. 12.2 Structural types of ion exchange resins.

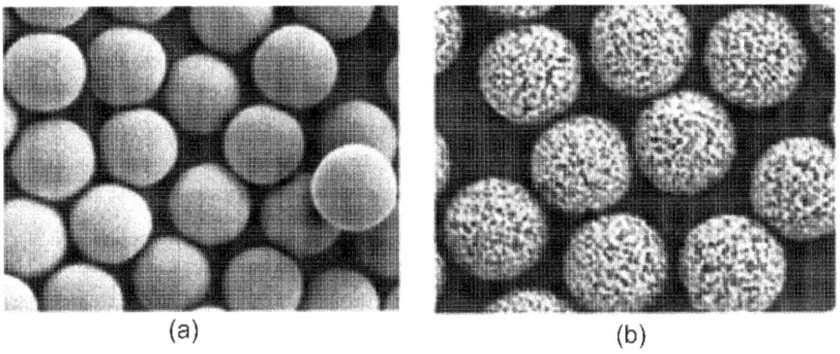

Fig. 12.3 Types of beads (a) Non-porous beads (b) Porous beads.

PROPERTIES OF RESINS

(i) **Particle size and porosity:** Decreased particle size offers more surface area, which in turn increases the rate of ion exchange. The range of particle size is 50-200mesh.

(ii) **Degree of cross-linking:** Increased concentration of cross-linking agents makes the resin rigid, leading to a decrease in swelling and decreased efficiency. On the other hand, the resin is soft, and swelling increases efficiency if the cross-linking agent concentration is less.

The quantity of cross-linking agents in the resin affects the separation.

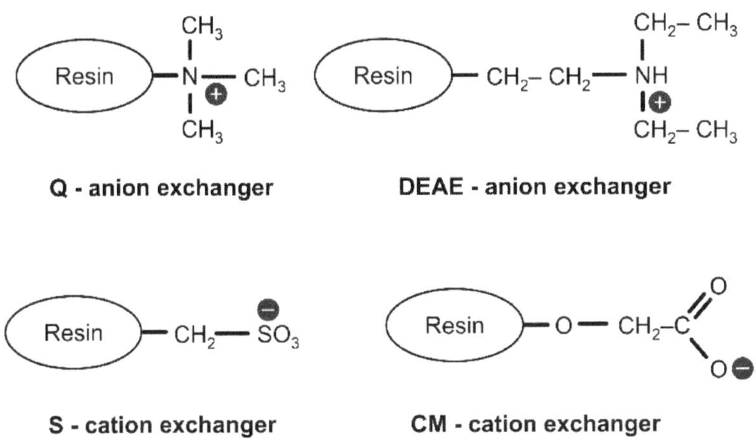

Fig. 12.4 Chemical structures of common ion-exchange media.

Mechanism of Ion exchange chromatography

The mechanism consists of 5 steps:

1. The ion diffuses to the exchanger surface. This occurs very quickly in homogeneous solutions.

2. The ion diffuses from the matrix surface to the exchange site, which is based on the degree of cross-linkage of resin and concentration of the solution. This step is considered to be the rate-determining step of the whole ion exchange process.
3. The exchange of ions occurs at the exchange site, which occurs instantaneously until equilibrium is attained.
4. The exchanged ion diffuses through the exchanger to the surface.
5. The molecules are separated by altering the pH or ionic concentrations or affinity elution, where there is greater affinity for the exchanger when the bound molecule is tightly bound to the stationary phase.

The ion exchange process is based on the affinity of the ions for the functional groups at the exchange site.

METHODOLOGY OF ION EXCHANGE CHROMATOGRAPHY

1. **Column and column packing:** Glass columns of 20:1,100:1 dimensions (length: diameter ratio) are used. Stainless steel columns are also used.
2. **Choice of ion exchange resin is based on**

   (a) Nature of ions to be separated-weak/strong

   (b) Charge on the ions to be separated –cation /anion.

   The efficiency of the ion is measured by ion exchange capacity. It is the total ion exchange capacity in terms of the exchangeable functional groups expressed as milli equivalents /gm of the resin. It is calculated for a cation exchanger as follows.

   A solution of sodium chloride of known concentration is passed through a column with the known weight of the resin. The acid eluting from the column is collected and titrated with a standard solution of alkali. The formula is

   $$\textbf{Capacity formula} = \frac{\mathbf{V \times N}}{\mathbf{W}}$$

   Where, V – volume of alkali solution,
   N – Strength of alkali solution in milli equivalents per litre,
   W – Weight of the resin in g.

   Similarly, anion exchanger capacity is determined by passing a solution of a definite concentration of sodium nitrate through the column. The concentration of eluted anions is determined by titration with a standard solution of silver nitrate.

3. **Column packing:** The wet packing method is used to pack the column. Resin is mixed with the mobile phase and packed uniformly in the column. The sample is dissolved in the mobile phase and introduced to the top of the column.
4. **Mobile phase:** The eluting solvents used are buffers, acids and alkalis of different strengths. E.g.,0.1N HC*l*, 0.1N NaOH, Phosphate buffer and acetate buffer, borate buffers, phthalate buffers etc.

   Organic solvents are not much useful. The pH should not be too low or too high to avoid interference with elution and high ionic strength is required for elution. pH should be 0.5-1 unit below pI (iso-electric point) in the cation exchanger and 0.5 -1 unit above pI in the anion exchanger.

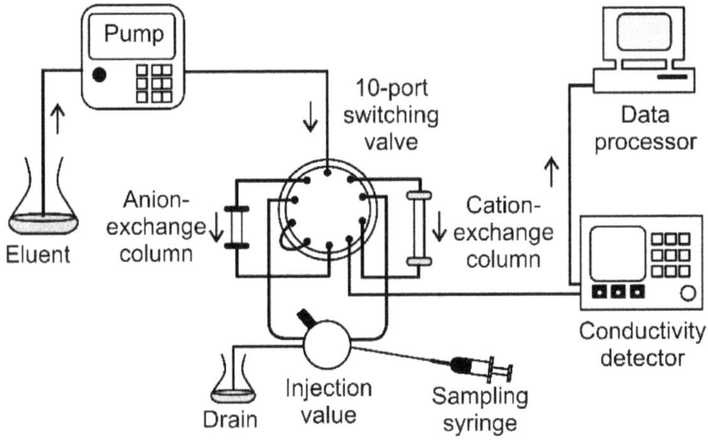

Fig. 12.5 Schematic diagram of Ion exchange chromatography.

5. **Sample preparation and loading:** The sample should be diluted, and it should be free of salt. It should be prepared with the same buffer which is used for the equilibration of the column. It should be filtered, and the sample size should not exceed the binding ability of the resin.
6. **Elution:** Components of the mixture separate and move down the column based on the affinity of the ion for the ion exchanger.

   There are two elution techniques **Isocratic** and **Gradient** elution

   Isocratic elution: The same composition of the solvent is used throughout the separation.

   Gradient elution: Increasing acidity or basicity of the mobile phase is used to separate complex mixtures.
7. **Detection:** Different fractions are collected based on time or volume and analysed by spectrophotometric, polarographic, conductometry or amperometric methods.

8. **Regeneration of ion exchange resin:** After separation, the ion exchange resin may not be useful for the next separation as exchangeable functional groups are lost.

But due to the cost of the ion exchange resins, they cannot be disposed off and hence reactivation is required.

REGENERATION

Regeneration makes the used ion exchange resin to be as efficient as a new resin. After the completion of the separation, the ion exchange resin should be regenerated by replacing the exchangeable cations or anions present in the original resin. Regeneration of ions is done as given below.

Cation exchange resin is regenerated by charging the column with a strong acid like HCl.

Anion exchange resin is regenerated by charging the column with a strong alkali like sodium hydroxide or potassium hydroxide.

FACTORS AFFECTING ION EXCHANGE CHROMATOGRAPHY

I. Cross-linking and swelling

II. Nature of ion exchange resin

I. Cross-linking and swelling: Increased quantity of cross-linking agent makes the resin rigid, which leads to a decrease in swelling and decreased efficiency. On the other hand, the resin is soft, and swelling is more with increased efficiency if the cross-linking agent quantity is less.

Thus the quantity of cross-linking agents in the resin affects the separation.

Table 12.2 Weak and strong types of anion and cation exchangers.

Exchange Type	Ion exchange group	Buffer counter ions	pH range	Commercial samples
Strong cation	Sulfonic acid (SP)	Na^+, H^+, Li^+	4-13	Capto*S
				SP Sepharose*
				SP Sephadex*
				TSKgel SP_5PW
Weak cation	Carboxylic acid	Na^+, H^+, Li^+	6-10	CM Cellulose
				CM Sepharose*
				CM Sephadex*
				CM Sepharose* CL6B
				TSKgel CM-5PW

Table 12.2 *Contd...*

Exchange Type	Ion exchange group	Buffer counter ions	pH range	Commercial samples
Strong anion	Quaternary amine (Q)	Cl^-, $HCOO_3$, CH_3COO^-, SO_4^{2-}	2-12	Q Sepharose*
				Capto*Q
				Dowex*1X2
				Amberlite*/Amberjet*
				QAE Sepharose*
Weak anion	Primary amine Secondary amine Tertiary amine (DEAE)	Cl^-, $HCOO_3$ CH_3COO^-, SO_4^{2-}	2-9	DEAE-Sepharose*
				Capto* DEAE
				DEAE Cellulose

II. Nature of ion exchange resin

(i) **Valency of the ions:** The ion exchange **rate increases** with an **increase in valency** at low concentration and room temperature.

$$Na^+ < Ca^{2+} < Al^{3+} < Th^{4+}$$

(ii) **Size of the ions:** Ion exchange rate **increases with a decrease in the size** of the hydrated ions

$$Li^+ < H^+ < Na^+ < NH_4^+ < K^+ < Rb^+ < Cs^+$$

(iii) **Polarizability: More polarisable** ions are preferred for ion exchange

$$I^- < Br^- < Cl^- < F^-$$

(iv) **Concentration: Dilute solutions favor** exchange of polyvalent anions

(v) **Charge on ions:** If the charge on the resin is higher than the charge on the solution, the exchange is favoured at a high concentration.

If the charge on the resin is lower than the charge on the solution, then the exchange is favoured at a low concentration

III. pH of the mobile phase (buffer): The pH should be one unit below pI for cation exchangers and one unit above for anion exchangers.

Cationic buffers are used in an anionic exchanger

E.g., Alkylamines, Tris, Aminoethyl alcohol

Anionic buffers are used in the cationic exchanger

E.g., Phosphate and acetate.

INSTRUMENTATION

General components of anion-exchange chromatography are given below

1. A high-pressure pump equipped with a pressure and flow indicator to deliver the eluent.
2. An injector for introducing the sample into the eluent stream and onto the column.
3. A column separates the sample mixture into individual components. The column can have an optional oven.
4. A detector to measure the analyte peaks as eluent emerges from the column
5. A data system for collecting and organising chromatograms and data.

APPLICATIONS

1. Water softening- Used for the removal of monovalent and divalent ions like potassium, calcium and magnesium
2. Demineralisation or deionisation of water - Removal of ions from water
3. Purification of solutions by removing ionic impurities
4. Separation of inorganic cations and anions
5. Used for the separation and purification of aminoacids, proteins, antibiotics, vitamins, fatty acids etc. in the pharmaceutical industry.
6. Isolation of dyes or metabolites from urine and blood
7. Used for the determination of the concentration of ionic solutions.
8. Used for the purification of proteins, nucleotides and small molecules
9. Separation of additives in food and drug samples.

CHAPTER 13

High Performance Liquid Chromatography (HPLC)

HPLC stands for High-performance liquid chromatography or High-pressure liquid chromatography. It is a type of column chromatography where the mobile phase is pumped with very high pressure into the column through the stationary phase. HPLC yields high performance and high speed compared to traditional column chromatography. It is a chromatographic technique that can be used for the separation and purification of the mixture of components and also for the quantification of the components.

The efficiency of separation in HPLC is very high because of the reduced particle size of the stationary phase (1 to 5μ).This reduction in particle size increases the surface area, which in turn increases the number of theoretical plates. In contrary to this, the decrease in particle size increases the resistance to the flow of the mobile phase. This generates more back pressure in the column, causing damage to the stationary phase, leading to decreased resolution. To overcome these difficulties, high pressure is used to force the mobile phase through the column and hence the name HPLC.

An HPLC chromatogram represents the separation of the components that occurs in the HPLC system. Peaks are rising from a baseline drawn on a time axis. Each peak represents the detector response for a different component. The chromatogram is a two-dimensional plot with the Y-axis (ordinate axis) giving concentration in terms of the detector response, and the X-axis (abscissa) represents the time. The chromatogram is plotted by the computer software. The area under the peak is proportional to the component concentration and is used for quantitative estimation.

TYPES OF HPLC

I. **Based on the principle of separation**

   (a) Adsorption chromatography

   (b) Partition chromatography

(c) Ion exchange chromatography
(d) Ion-pair chromatography
(e) Size exclusion/Gel permeation chromatography
(f) Affinity chromatography
(g) Chiral chromatography

(a) Adsorption chromatography: The separation of components in adsorption chromatography is based on the relative affinities of the components towards the stationary phase. The principle of separation is called adsorption, which is a surface phenomenon. The mixture (adsorbate), which is dissolved in the mobile phase, moves through the stationary phase (adsorbent) of the column. The component with more affinity for the stationary phase travels slower, and the component with less affinity for the stationary phase travels faster down the column. Thus, the components are separated based on their affinity difference for the stationary phase. No two components will have the same affinity for the given set of stationary, mobile phase and other conditions.

If the stationary phase is solid, the principle of separation is adsorption

E.g., GSC, TLC, Column adsorption chromatography, HPLC

(b) Partition chromatography: In this mode of chromatography, the separation of components is based on the partition coefficients of the individual components. The solute gets distributed between the two immiscible liquids based on its partition coefficient. The component which is more soluble in the stationary phase travels slower than the component soluble in the mobile phase. The components are separated based on their differences in partition coefficient since no two components will have the same partition coefficient for the given combination of stationary, mobile phase and other conditions.

The stationary phase is a liquid which is coated as a thin film over solid support.

If the stationary phase is a liquid, then the principle of separation is partition.

E.g., Gas-liquid chromatography, paper partition chromatography, column partition chromatography etc.

(c) Ion exchange chromatography: The principle involved is a reversible exchange of ions. The stationary phase used is ion exchange resin. For the separation of anions, anion exchange resin is used. For cation separation, cation exchange resin is used. Acids, alkalis and buffers are used as mobile phase.

(d) Ion-Pair Chromatography: In this technique, ion-pairing reagents like octane sulphonic acid, Tetraethyl ammonium hydroxide are used to convert an RP HPLC column into a temporary ion exchange column. Ion Pairing agents are ionic compounds that contain a hydrocarbon chain that imparts hydrophobicity to increase the retention of the ion pair. By adding pair ions with the opposite charge to the mobile phase, the pair ions form ion pairs with the ionic compounds, which neutralizes the charge, increasing hydrophobicity and thereby increasing retention.

If pair ions with a hydrophobic functional group (heptafluorobutyric acid in the example shown below) are added to the mobile phase, the hydrophobic functional groups are retained by the stationary phase. The mechanism is shown in figure 13.1.

(e) **Size exclusion/Gel permeation chromatography:** The separation in this chromato-graphy is based on the size of the solute particles. The mobile phase with the sample passes through the gel stationary phase. The gel acts as a molecular sieve and separates the solutes based on molecular size.

E.g., Soft gels: Dextran, Agarose and polysaccharide

Semi-rigid gels: Polystyrene, alkyl dextran.

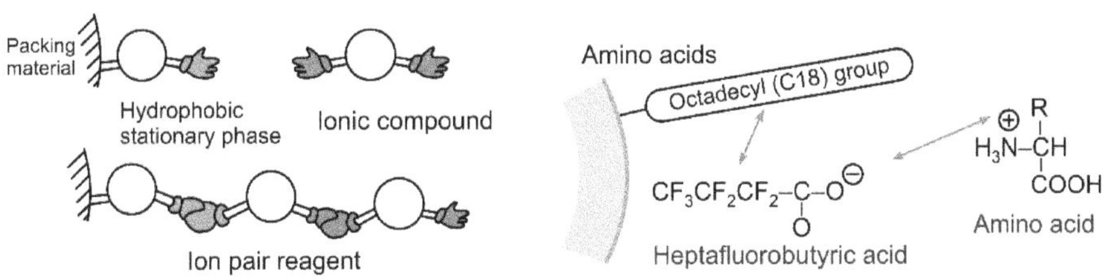

Fig. 13.1 Mechanism of Ion-Pair Chromatography.

(f) **Affinity chromatography:** This chromatography utilizes the specific interaction between the sample and a second molecule immobilized on a stationary phase. Affinity chromatography is mostly used in the field of Biotechnology, Microbiology, biochemistry etc.

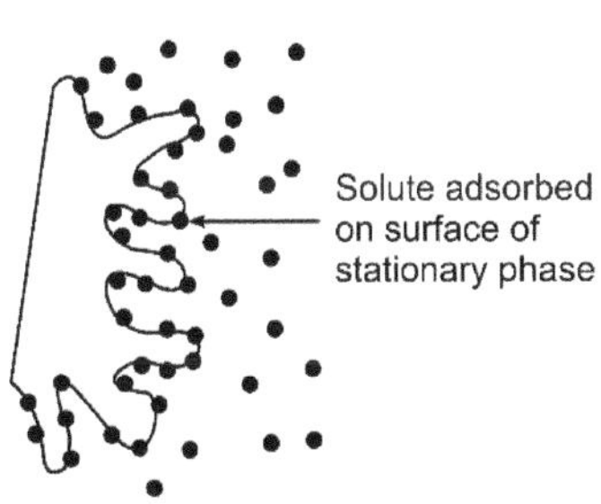

Fig. 13.2 Adsorption Chromatography.

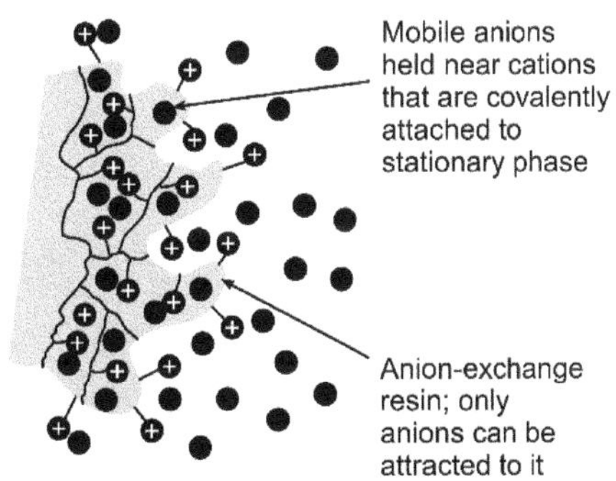

Fig 13.3 Ion-exchange Chromatography.

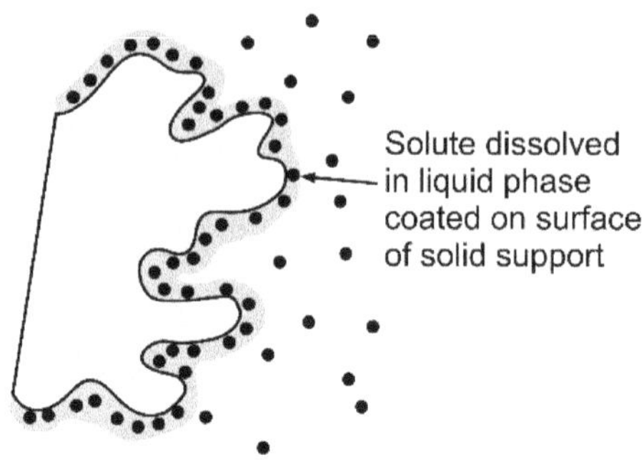

Fig 13.4 Partition Chromatography.

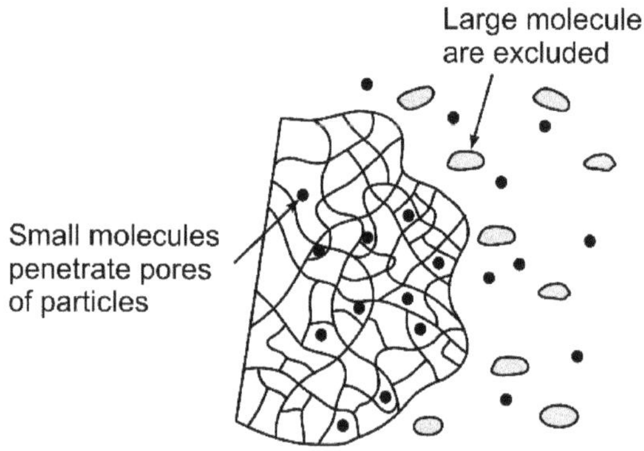

Fig. 13.5 Size exclusion Chromatography.

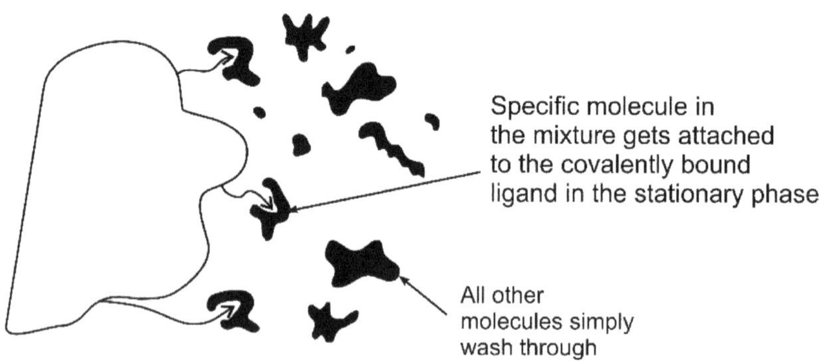

Fig 13.6 Affinity Chromatography.

(g) **Chiral chromatography:** Enantiomers have the same physical and chemical properties and can be separated only in a chiral environment. Separation of enantiomers (optical isomers) is done using either chiral stationary or mobile phase.

II. Based on elution technique

1. **Isocratic elution:** In this separation, the same mobile phase composition and hence the same polarity is maintained throughout the process.
2. **Gradient separation:** A technique in which the mobile phase composition or polarity is changed during the separation process. Linear gradients are the popular techniques for the efficient separation of components with a wide boiling range.

III. Based on the scale of operation

1. **Analytical HPLC:** The **sample size** is **low** in this technique. Qualitative and Quantitative analysis of the sample is carried out using this technique. Recovery of the sample is not possible.
2. **Preparative HPLC:** The **sample size** is **large**. Individual components can be recovered and reused.

IV. Based on the type of analysis

1. **Qualitative analysis:** Qualitative analysis is carried out for the identification of the compounds. It is also useful in finding out the presence of impurities and in finding the number of components.
2. **Quantitative analysis:** This analysis is useful in determining the quantity of the components in the sample mixture by comparing the peak areas of standard and sample.

V. Based on the mode of separation

1. Normal phase chromatography
2. Reversed phase chromatography

PRINCIPLE

The column consists of imaginary plates called as theoretical plates. A theoretical plate is the height of the column in which one equilibration of the solute particle happens with the stationary and mobile phases. When the number of theoretical plates in a column increases, the efficiency of separation also increases. The no of theoretical plates is related to the surface area of the stationary phase. The smaller the particle size more is the surface area. Thus smaller particles increase the efficiency of separation.

But smaller particles offer more resistance to the flow of the mobile phase, causing a back pressure in the column leading to the damage of the stationary phase. Hence the mobile phase is pumped through the column.

The principle of separation in HPLC by both normal phase and reverse phase mode is adsorption. When introduced into the column, the components of the sample mixture travel based on their relative affinities with the stationary phase. The component with more affinity towards the stationary phase (adsorbent) moves slowly, and the component with less affinity for the stationary phase travels faster with the mobile phase.

No two components can have the same affinity for the stationary phase under the given set of conditions, stationary and mobile phases. This forms the basis of separation in HPLC.

The principle of separation in HPLC varies with the type of HPLC. E.g., In partition HPLC, the principle is the partition, in ion exchange HPLC, ion exchange is the principle etc.

Working

1. The prepared mobile phase liquid is poured into the reservoirs after degassing.
2. The mobile phase is pumped into the column under high pressure to get the baseline.
3. The sample is injected through the injection port using injectors and swept into the high pressure liquid carrier stream between the pump and column.
4. As the mobile phase flows through the column, it carries the sample along with it, and the components are separated based on their affinities towards the stationary phase.
5. The detector detects the components as they emerge from the column.
6. The detector signals are amplified and recorded by the detector. The chromatogram contains detector response as a function of time.
7. The components are identified based on their retention time values compared to the standard, and the quantification is done using the peak area.

INSTRUMENTATION

COMPONENTS OF HPLC INSTRUMENT

1. Solvent delivery system
2. Sample injector system
3. Column
4. Detectors
5. Recorders and integrators

1. Solvent delivery system

The components are

(a) Solvent reservoir

(b) Pumps

(c) Mixing units

(d) Gradient controller
(e) Degasser
(f) Dampner

Table 13.1 Summary of HPLC components.

Solvent delivery system	Sample injector system	Columns	Detectors
Solvent reservoir Pumps 1. Reciprocating piston pump, 2. Syringe pump 3. Constant pressure pump Mixing units Gradient controller Degasser Dampner	(i) Septum injector (ii) Stop flow injector (iii) Rheodyne injector	1. Guard column 2. Analytical column 3. Capillary column 4. Fast column 5. Preparatory column 6. Chiral column	1. UV/Visible Detector – Fixed Wavelength – Variable Wavelength – Photo Diode Array (PDA) 2. Refractive index – Detector 3. Fluorescence Detector 4. Electrochemical Detector 5. Conductivity Detector 6. Evaporative light scattering (ELSD) detector 7. Mass detector (LC-MS) 8. Optical rotation detector (chiral detectors)

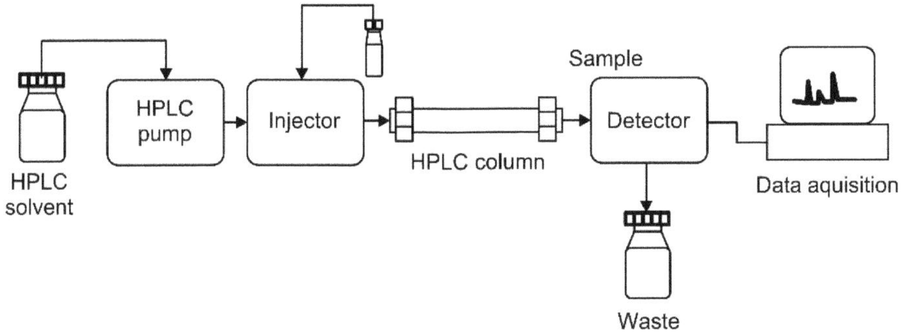

Fig. 13.7 Schematic diagram of HPLC instrument.

(a) **Solvent reservoir:** They are used for storing the mobile phase. They are usually made of glass and they should be kept above the level of the pump. Depending on the mobile phase composition (single solvent or mixture of two solvents), single or multiple solvent reservoirs are used.

(b) **Pumps:** The purpose of the pump is to maintain a constant flow of mobile phase through the HPLC system. This is accomplished regardless of the backpressure caused by the flow resistance of the HPLC column. The pump is used to force the mobile phase through the column at a specific flow rate, expressed in ml/min. Normal flow rates in HPLC are maintained in the range of 1 to 2 ml/min. Pumps can reach pressures up to the range of 6000-9000 psi (400- to 600-bar). The pumps can be used for both isocratic or gradient elution.

Types of HPLC pumps: The most commonly used pumps in HPLC are

1. Reciprocating piston pump
2. Syringe pump
3. Constant pressure pump

1. **Reciprocating piston pumps:** This pump consists of a piston driven by a small motor. The piston moves rapidly back and forth in a hydraulic chamber of volume 35-400ml.

   The piston pulls solvent from the mobile phase reservoir on the backstroke and the separation column valve is closed.

   The pump pushes solvent from the reservoir into the column on the forward stroke and the inlet valve is closed.

   Flow rates can be changed by altering the piston stroke volume or the stroke frequency during each cycle.

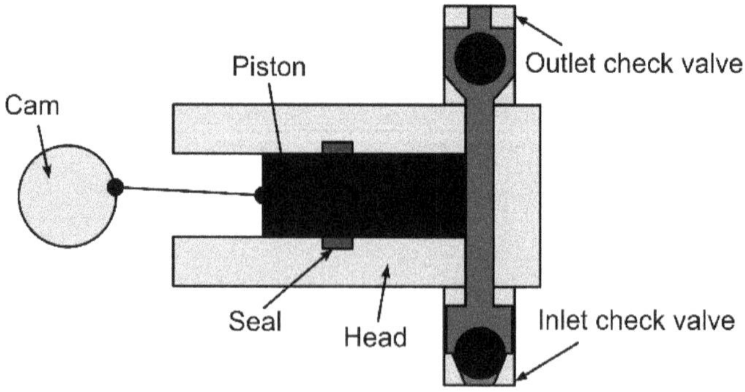

Fig. 13.8 Reciprocating Piston pumps.

An identical piston chamber unit with dual and triple head pump operates at 180 or 120 degrees out of phase (this system is significantly smoother because one pump is filling while the other is in the delivery cycle).

Disadvantages:

1. It produces a pulsed flow which is damped because pulses appear as baseline noise on the chromatograph.
2. Dual pump heads or elliptical cams are used to minimize such pulsations.

Advantages:

1. These pumps have a small internal volume of 35-400ml
2. It can give higher output pressures up to 10,000 psi.
3. Easily adapted to gradient elution.
4. It has got large solvent capacities & constant flow rates.
5. It is largely independent of column backpressure & solvent viscosity.

2. **Syringe type pump/Displacement pumps:** This pump delivers only a finite volume of the mobile phase. This pump has a volume between 250 to 500ml. These pumps are most suitable for small bore columns.

   A motorized screw delivers the mobile phase to the column at a constant rate in this pump. The rate of solvent delivery is controlled by changing the voltage on the motor.

   Advantages:

   The flow is independent of viscosity & backpressure.

   Disadvantages:

   It has a limited solvent capacity & poses a problem when solvents must be changed.

3. **Constant pressure pump:** In these types of pumps, the mobile phase is driven through the column with the use of pressure from the gas cylinder. A low-pressure gas source is needed to generate high liquid pressures. The rapid refill of the solvent chamber is achieved by the valve arrangement. These pumps provide continuous phase flow rates. It is not a constant flow pump. But it is a constant pressure pump. It can deliver high pressures. This pump provides a stable flow during the delivery stroke and stops flow on refill stroke. The cost is low.

   This type of pump provides pulse-less & continuous pumping with high flow rates. It is inconvenient for solvent gradient elution.

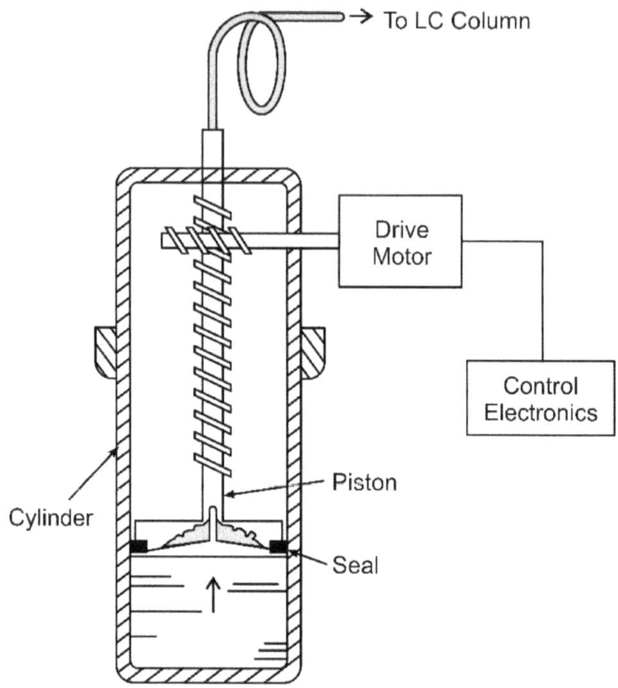

Fig. 13.9 Syringe pumps.

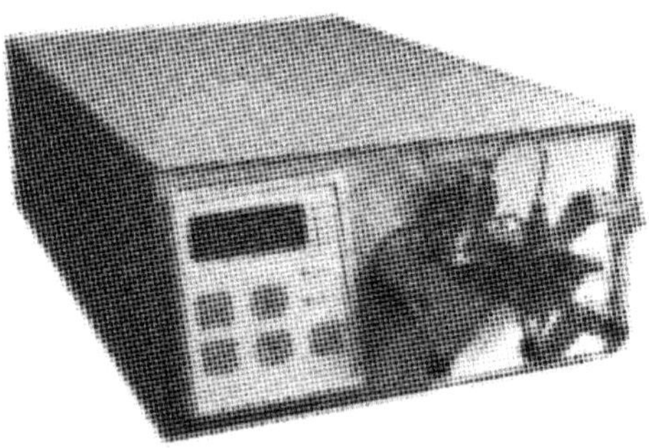

Fig. 13.10 Constant pressure pump.

(c) Mixing unit: The mixing unit is used for mixing the solvents in the required proportion and passing it through the column. The low-pressure mixing chamber uses helium for degassing solvents. In the high-pressure mixing chamber, there is no need of helium for degassing solvents.

The mixing unit can be a static mixer or a dynamic mixer.

(i) Static mixer: is packed with beads

(ii) Dynamic mixer: uses magnetic stirrer under pressure.

(d) **Gradient controller:** It is used in the gradient elution technique. The polarity of the solvent is increased gradually, and the solvent composition should be changed accordingly. This is achieved by two or more pumps.

(e) **Solvent degasser:** Organic solvents contain dissolved gases. When the solvents are pumped under high pressure, gas bubbles will be formed, and they interfere with the separation process, baseline steadiness and shape of the peak. Hence degassing of the solvent is necessary, and it is carried out by the following processes

1. **Vacuum filtration:** This method is accomplished by applying a partial vacuum to the solvent container. This method is not reliable.
2. **Purging with helium gas:** This method is carried out by passing helium gas through the solvent. It is an effective method. This is an expensive method.
3. **Ultrasonication:** This technique is carried out using an ultrasonicator. This converts the ultrahigh-frequency to mechanical vibration leading to the removal of air bubbles.

(f) **Dampeners:** Pumps cause a wavy baseline containing pulses. These pulses are dampened by pulse dampeners.

2. **Sample injector system:** The injector devices available are either for manual or auto-injection. The devices are
   (i) Septum injector
   (ii) Stop flow injector
   (iii) Rheodyne injector

   (i) Septum injector: These injectors are used to inject the sample through a rubber septum. They are not commonly used because the septum has to withstand high pressure.

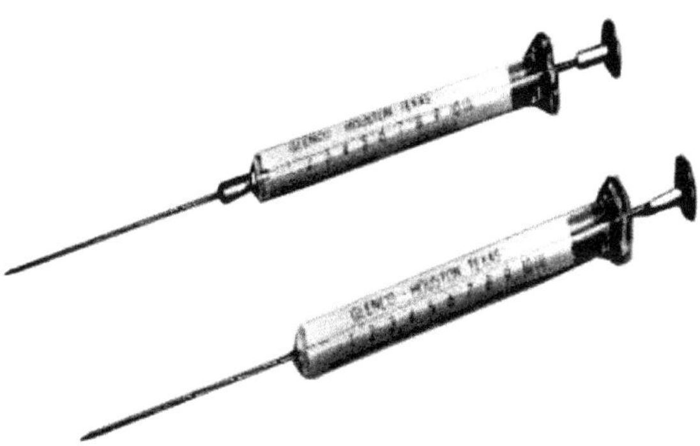

Fig. 13.11 Septum injector.

Disadvantage: The mobile phase leaches the septum, which results in ghost peaks.

(ii) Stop flow injector (on-line): In this type of injector, the mobile phase flow is stopped for some time, and the sample is injected through a valve.

Disadvantage: Formation of ghost peaks.

(iii) Rheodyne injector (loop valve): It is the most popular injector. The loop has a fixed volume of 20μl or 50μl. There are two modes in the injector.

(i) Load position

(ii) Inject position

The injector introduces the liquid sample into the flow stream of the mobile phase for analysis. It is equipped with six-port valves so that the sample can be injected into the flow path at continuous pressure. For a manual injector, the knob is manually operated to deliver the sample to the column.

The knob is set to LOAD position for sample injection using a syringe, the sample is injected into the sample loop, which is separated from the flow path

The knob is turned to INJECT position, and the eluent travels through the loop from the pump and delivers the sample to the column. Rheodyne injectors positions are shown in Figures 13.12(a) and 13.12(b).

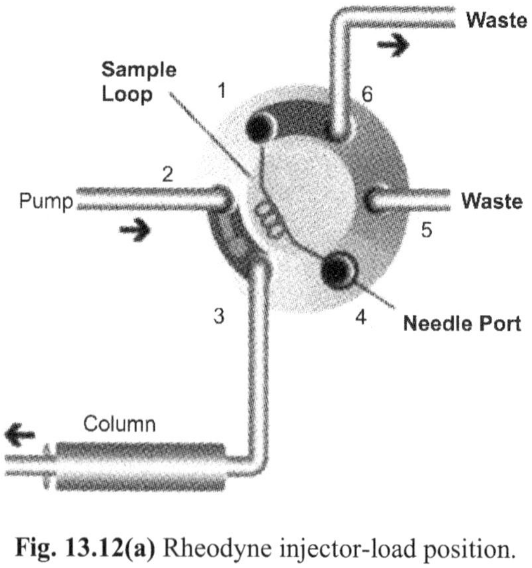

Fig. 13.12(a) Rheodyne injector-load position.

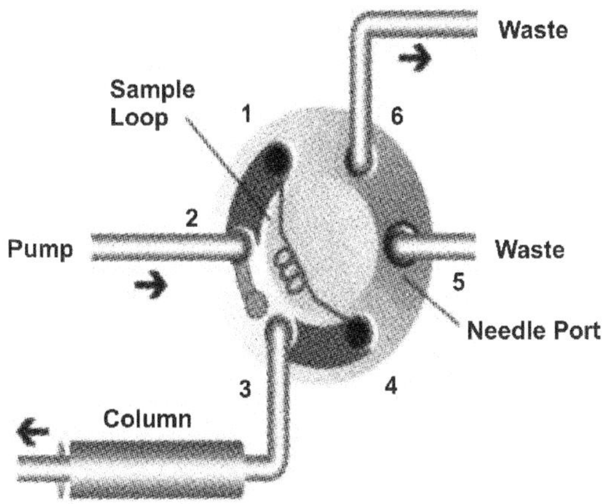

Fig. 13.12(b) Rheodyne injector-inject position.

Typical sample volumes for manual injectors are 5-to 20- μL. The injector must also be able to withstand the high pressures of the liquid system. An auto sampler is an automatic version for analysing many samples or when the manual injection is not practical. It can continuously inject a variable volume of 1 μL – 1 mL

3. **Columns:** Columns are the most important part of the instrument, and it is where the separation of components takes place. The columns are packed with the stationary phase through which the mobile phase is flowing through.

The various types of columns used in HPLC are

(i) Guard column
(ii) Analytical column
(iii) Capillary column
(iv) Fast column
(v) Preparatory column
(vi) Chiral column

(i) Guard column: This column is introduced before the analytical column, and it improves the life of the analytical column. Guard column packing is the same as that of the analytical column, but the particle size is larger. Guard column acts by

(a) By removing the particulate matter and contaminants from the solvents.
(b) By excluding the components that bind irreversibly to the stationary phase.
(c) It saturates the mobile phase with the stationary phase, so that loss of stationary phase in analytical column is minimized.

(ii) **Analytical column:** The analytical column is an important part of the HPLC instrument. This column decides the efficiency of separation. LC columns are usually constructed from smooth bore stainless steel tubing or glass. Glass columns are restricted to pressures lower than 600psi. Other materials used for column construction are polyethylene and PEEK (Polyether ether ketone). Column length is about 10 to 30 cm, and the internal diameter is about 4 to 10 mm.

Column packing is usually silica gel. Because of its particle shape, surface properties and pore structure, it gives a good separation. Other materials used are alumina, polystyrene divinyl benzene or an ion exchange resin

Mainly, there are three types of column packing particles; microporous particles, Pellicular particles and bonded phase particles.

Pellicular particle: These are also called superficially porous particles with a particle size of 40 μm in diameter. The pores are coated on an inert core. The inert core is made up of glass or some other hard material. The porous material is made up of polymethacrylates or polystyrene-divinylbenzene. These particles have high mechanical stability and excellent pH stability (pH 2-12).

Porous particle: Porous particles are of 5-10μm in diameter. They are made of silica or aluminium and contain microscopic pores running through the particle to increase the surface area for more interaction with analytes and the mobile phase. E.g., Porous polyvinyl chloride.

Bonded phase particles: These particles also contain an inert core made up of silica. The stationary phase is chemically bonded on that inert core by different linkages like silicate ester, silicate carbon and siloxanes.

E.g., Silica C-18 for reverse phase chromatography of peptides/proteins.

The common columns used in RP-HPLC are C_{18} – Octadecyl silane (ODS) column, C_8- Octyl column, C_4 – Butyl column, CN- Nitrile, NH_2 – Amino column.

(iii) **Capillary column:** Three types of capillary columns are available. Open tubular, wall coated and SCOT columns. These columns are discussed in GC. The advantages of these columns are decreased sample size(nl), decreased flow rate, decreased solvent volume usage with efficient separation.

(iv) **Fast column:** These are shorter columns packed with particles of 3µm in diameter. Their advantages are increased sensitivity, decreased analysis time and increased reproducibility.

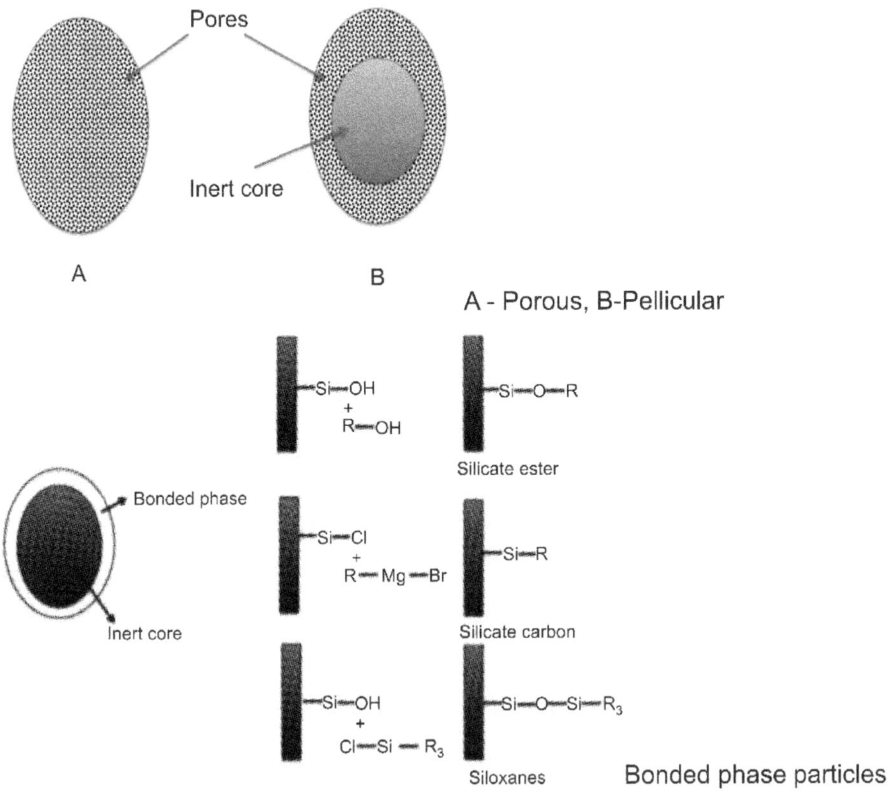

Fig. 13.13 Types of column packing material.

(v) **Preparatory column:** The length of these types of columns is 10-15 cm and the internal diameter is 25 mm. The particle size used is 15-100µm. They are bigger in dimensions and can handle more sample quantities. They are used in preparatory applications.

(vi) **Chiral column:** These columns are used in the separation of enantiomers. Chiral columns contain chiral stationary phases.

4. **Detectors:** Detectors are used to detect components eluting from the column by producing an electrical signal. The output of the detector is connected to a recorder or computer.
The selection of the detector is based on the property of the compounds to be separated.

Commonly used detectors in HPLC

There are two types of detectors used in HPLC

1. **Selective detectors (solute property):** These detectors respond to a particular physical or chemical property of the solute and are independent of the mobile phase.

   E.g., Absorbance detectors, Fluorescence detectors, electrochemical detectors, Mass spectrometric detectors.

2. **Universal detectors (bulk property):** These detectors measure the difference in the physical property of the mobile phase due to the presence of solute particles compared to the mobile phase alone. They are universal in application. They have poor sensitivity and limited range. Such detectors are usually affected by even small changes in the mobile-phase composition. Hence they cannot be used in gradient elution. E.g., Refractive index detectors, Evaporating light scattering detectors.

   The various detectors used in HPLC are

   1. UV/Visible Detector
   2. Refractive index - Detector
   3. Fluorescence Detector
   4. Electrochemical Detector
   5. Conductivity Detector
   6. Evaporative light scattering detector (ELSD)
   7. Mass detector (LC-MS)
   8. Optical rotation detector (chiral detectors)

   1. **UV–VISIBLE DETECTORS:** It is a photometric detector. Substances that absorb UV light can be detected by this solute property detector. These are versatile detectors with the best sensitivity and linearity. They are cost-effective, popular and widely used. There are three types of UV detector

      (a) Fixed wavelength detectors

      (b) Variable wavelength detectors

      (c) Photodiode array detectors

      (a) Fixed Wavelength detector: Detector operates at 254 nm only because most of the compounds absorb at this wavelength

      Simplest and cheapest of the UV/VIS detectors

      Limited in flexibility

      Limited in types of compounds that can be monitored

      (b) Variable Wavelength detector: In this detector, a single wavelength is monitored at any given time but operates in the wavelength range 190-900 nm.

      More expensive requires more advanced optics

More sensitive due to photomultiplier tube

(c) **Photo Diode Array Detector:** In this detector, the absorbance of solutes is measured simultaneously at several different wavelengths. Light from the emission source, such as a deuterium lamp, is collimated by an achromatic lens system. The total light passes through the sample cell and then to a holographic grating. In this way, all wavelengths of light emitted by the source pass through the sample. The dispersed light from the grating is allowed to fall onto a diode array. The array contains many hundreds of diodes, and the output from each diode is processed by a computer and stored. The working of the PDA detector is shown in Figure 13.14.

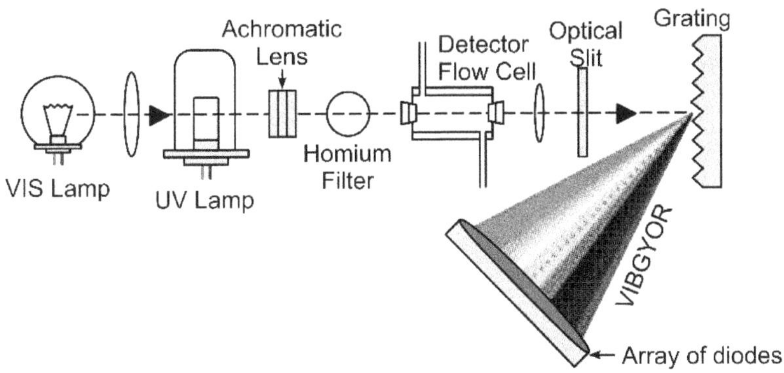

Fig. 13.14 Photo Diode array Detector.

2. **Refractive index detector:** A Refractive index detector measures the molecule's ability to deflect light in a flowing mobile phase in a flow cell relative to a static mobile phase contained in a reference cell. The amount of deflection is proportional to the concentration of the solute in the mobile phase. The refractive index (RI) detector is one of the least sensitive LC detectors. This detector is extremely useful for detecting the compounds that are non-ionic, not showing ultraviolet light absorption and substances that do not exhibit fluorescence. E.g. sugar, alcohol, fatty acid and polymers.
3. **Fluorescence Detector:** These detectors are used for the substances that give fluorescence when subjected to radiation from a source. The excitation light is usually a low-pressure mercury lamp providing relatively high-intensity UV light at 253.7 nm. Many substances that fluoresce will be excited at this wavelength. The excitation light is focused by a quartz lens through the cell. A second lens, set normal to the incident light, focuses the fluorescent light onto a photocell.

As it is very sensitive, its response is only linear over a relatively limited concentration range.

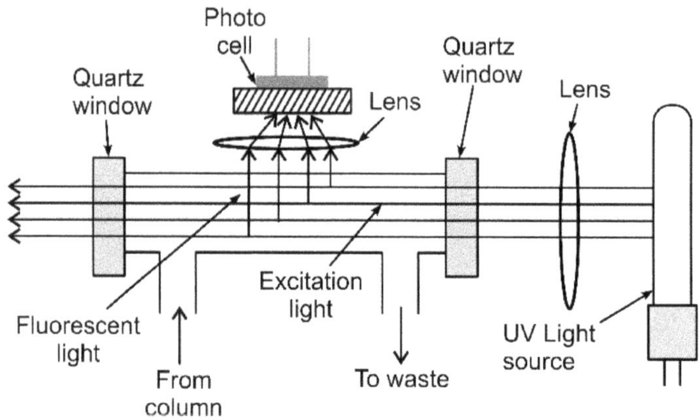

Fig. 13.15 Fluorescence detector.

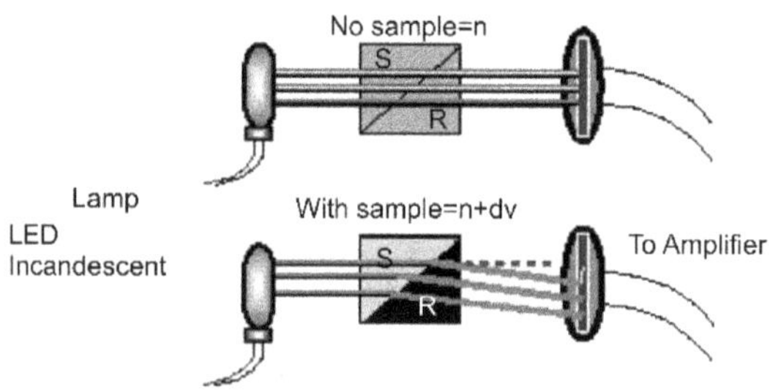

Fig. 13.16 Refractive index detector.

4. **Electrochemical detectors:** The current resulting from an oxidation/reduction reaction of the analyte at a suitable electrode is measured in this detector. The current produced is directly proportional to the analyte concentration. The eluent should be electrically conductive.

   E.g. of drugs detected using this detector are phenol, catecholamines, nitrosamines, and organic acids in the ng range
5. **Conductivity detectors:** This detector is used in ion-exchange chromatography for the detection of ionic compounds. The ability of the mobile phase to conduct current when placed in a flowcell between two electrodes is measured. Conductivity detectors measure the resistance, which is directly proportional to the concentration of ions present in the solution. Two electrodes placed in the mobile phase form each corresponding to one arm of a Wheatstone Bridge.
6. **Evaporative light scattering detector (ELSD):** Detection is based on the scattering of a beam of light by particles of the compound.

The three steps involved in detection are

- Nebulisation
- Desolvation
- Detection

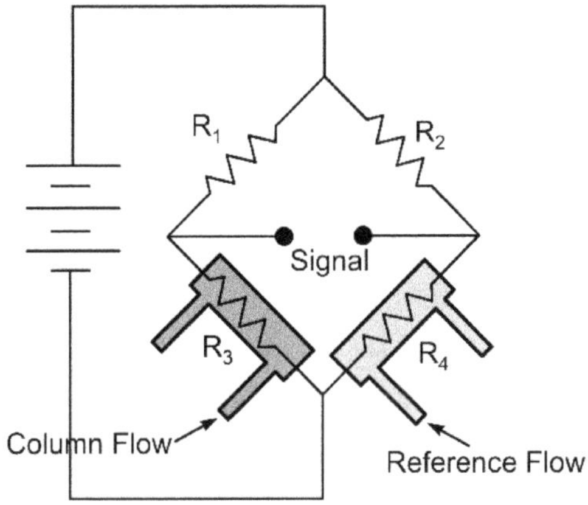

Fig. 13.17 Wheatstone Bridge arrangement in conductivity detectors.

A stream of inert gas nebulises the flow from the column. (Nebulizing is to convert a liquid into a fine spray or mist). The volatile mobile phase is evaporated, leaving tiny particles of the analytes. The particles, when passed through a laser beam, they scatter the laser light. The scattered light is measured at right angles to the laser beam by a photodiode detector. It is a universal detector. The compound does not require a chromophore for detection by this detector.

7. **Mass detector:** The HPLC system in which the Mass spectrophotometer is used as the detector is called LC-MS. In this method, the separation power of HPLC is combined with the detection power of Mass spectrometry. Mass spectrometry (MS) is a powerful analytical tool that can supply both structural information about compounds and quantitative data relating to mass.
8. **Chiral detectors:** Optically active compounds such as amino acids, sugars, terpenes and other compounds containing asymmetric carbon are detected by chiral detectors. There are two types of chiral detection techniques,
   1. Polarimetry or optical rotary dispersion (ORD)
   2. Circular dichroism (CD).

   ORD detectors are based on differences in refractive index

   CD detectors identify the enantiomers by measuring the differential absorption of right and left-handed circularly polarized light.

5. **Recorders and integrators:** Recorders record the responses from the detector. They record the baseline and all the peaks with respect to time. Integrators are the data processors. They record all the data related to every peak like R_t, peak area, peak width and height etc. Computers are used for data processing.

   Advantages of HPLC:
   1. Speed
   2. Efficiency
   3. Accuracy
   4. Versatile and extremely precise when it comes to identifying and quantifying chemical components.

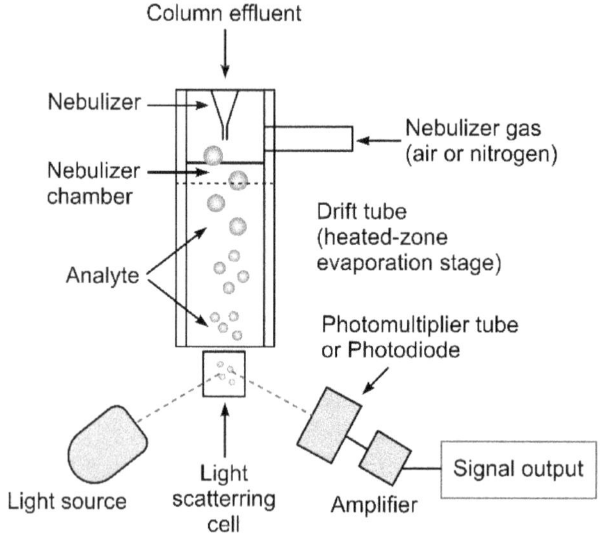

Fig. 13.18 Evaporative light scattering detector (ELSD).

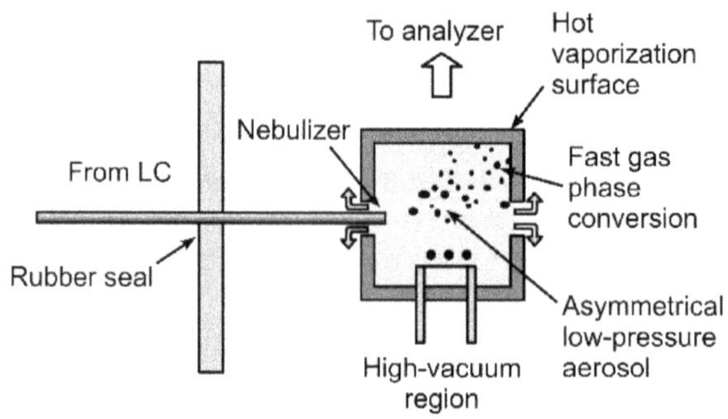

Fig. 13.19 Mass detector.

Disadvantages of HPLC:

1. **Cost:** Costly, requiring large quantities of expensive organic solvents.
2. **Complex to operate:** The compounds that are irreversibly adsorbed onto the stationary phase of the column cannot be detected.
3. Volatile substances are better separated by gas chromatography.

APPLICATIONS

1. **Qualitative analysis (identification):** It is carried out by comparing the retention time of the sample with the retention time of the standard. If the operating conditions are the same, the retention time also remains the same. It is used in fields like environmental, Pharmaceutical, food, forensic, nutraceuticals and cosmetic industries
2. **To check the purity of the compound:** The presence of additional peaks in the chromatogram shows the presence of impurities when compared with the standard chromatogram. The peak areas can be used to calculate the percentage purity of the sample.
3. **Detection of impurities:** The presence of additional peaks, when compared with reference material, identifies the impurities. The peak areas can be used to calculate the percentage of impurities.
4. **Quantitative analysis**
   (a) **Direct comparison method:** From the peak areas of the standard and the sample, the quantity of the sample can be calculated.

   Peak area = Peak height X width at ½ height

   $A_1/A_2 = \alpha(w_1/w_2)$ where,

   A_1 & A_2 are the peak area of the sample and standard.

   α- Response factor

   w_1/w_2 is the weight or concentration of sample and standard.

   (b) **Calibration curve method:** Serial dilutions of standard solutions are prepared and injected in HPLC. A calibration graph is constructed by plotting peak area vs concentration. The concentration of the unknown sample is determined from the calibration graph.

   (c) **Internal standard method:** A known concentration of the internal standard (a compound with similar retention characteristics) is added to the standard solution and sample solution. The unknown solution concentration is determined using the ratios of the sample with internal standard and standard and internal standard. This method avoids the extraction steps when the sample matrix is complex in nature.

5. **Multi component analysis:** HPLC is also used for the determination of multiple components in a formulation simultaneously.
6. Isolation and identification of drugs and metabolites in biological fluids
7. Used in analyzing the mixture of components in natural products.
8. Useful in Biopharmaceutical and pharmacokinetic studies.
9. **Stability studies of drugs are performed using HPLC.**
10. Purification on the preparative scale can be carried out with HPLC.

CHAPTER 14

High-Performance Thin Layer Chromatography

HPTLC

High-Performance Thin layer chromatography (HPTLC) is an instrumental technique that is a sophisticated, automated, and improved form of TLC. This powerful analytical tool in combination with an automated sample application and **densitometric scanning** is suitable both for qualitative and quantitative analysis. It is otherwise called planar chromatography or flatbed chromatography. It involves the same theoretical principle as that of TLC. This technique provides efficient separation in a shorter period of time.

PRINCIPLE

The principle of separation in HPTLC is adsorption as in thin-layer chromatography. There are two phases, the stationary phase, and the mobile phase. Sample is loaded onto the stationary phase and is moved along by the mobile phase. The mobile phase moves up the plate by capillary action. The components of sample mixture undergo repeated interactions with the stationary phase and mobile phase and this leads to the gradual separation of the sample components into bands or zones

The components move in the stationary phase based on their affinity towards the stationary phase (adsobent). The component with more affinity for the stationary phase moves slowly and component with lesser affinity for the stationary phase travels faster. Thus the sample components are separated based on their affinity towards the stationary phase and their solubility in the mobile phase. The main applications of HPTLC are identification, quantification and micro preparation.

Steps involved in the separation of components in HPTLC

1. Selection of chromatographic Layer (stationary phase)
2. Layer prewashing
3. Layer Pre-conditioning
4. Mobile phase-optimization

5. Activation of pre-coated plates
6. Sample and Standard preparation & application
7. Preconditioning (chamber saturation)
8. Chromatographic development and drying
9. Scanning and documentation of the chromatoplate
10. Detection of spots

1. **Selection of chromatographic Layer (stationary phase)**

   Smaller plates (10x10 or 10x20 cm) with shorter development distance (6 cm) are used in HPTLC leading to shorter anslysis time (7-20 min). Both hand made plates and pre-coated plates can be used. Hand made plates are made of cellulose, cellulose with starch as binder, silica gel with starch and acetylated cellulose with binder ($CaSO_4$ (1/2) H_20). These handmade plates are not used much now a days.

   Procoated plates are available with different support materials and different adsobent layers with varying thickness.

   The various support materials used in TLC plates are glass, polyester/polyethylene and aluminium. The various adsorbents used in plates are silicagel, silicagel 60F, aluminium oxide magnesium silicate, magnesium oxide, polyamide, cellulose, kieselguhr, ion exchangers and modified polar silicagel layers containing bonded amino, cyano, diol and thiol groups. The particle size of the adsobent is in the range of 5-6 μm and the thickness of the layer is about 100μ. The reduced particle size increases the surface area which helps in greater resolution, increased efficiency, decreased analysis time and sensitivity.

2. **Layer prewashing**

   Plates should be handled only at the top upper edge to avoid contamination. The significance of pre-washing is to remove impurities including water vapour and other volatile impurities from atmosphere which are adhered to the stationary phase. Prewashing improves the reproducibility and useful in quantitative analysis.

   The common prewash solvents are methanol or methanol: water (9:1), Chloroform: methanol (1:1) chloroform: methanol: ammonia (90:10:1). The different methods used for layer prewashing are ascending, dipping and continuous techniques. After developing the plate using any one of these techniques in a twin-trough chamber, the plate is dried and then used.

3. **Layer Pre conditioning**

   The dried plates are equlibrated with the laboratory atmosphere like temperature and humidity. Then they are stored in a suitable container to protect from dust and fumes.

4. **Mobile Phase - optimization**

   The mobile phase solution is done based on the nature of stationary phase and the physico chemical properties of the analyte. The mobile phase can be a pure solvent or a mixture of solvents. The mobile phase systems that are used commonly are diethyl ether, methylene choride, choroform and hexane for normal phase development. For reversed phase, the solvent systems include methanol, acetonitrile and THF mixed with water.

5. **Activation of pre-coated plates**

   Activation of pre coated plates is required for removing moisture from plates. Activation of plates is done by heating the plates in an oven at 110-120° C for 30 minutes. This removes water molecules that are absorbed on the surface of adorbent layer.

6. **Sample and standard preparation and application**

   The solvent used for dissolving sample should be non-polar and volatile. Sample and standard are dissolved in the same solvent. As a little quantity of sample is spotted the sample solution should be a concentrated solution. After this the plates are dried. Mobile phase can also be used as solvent for sample and standard.

   Sample application

   The concentration of the sample is usually in the range of 0.1-1μg and volume used for spotting the sample and standard is 0.5-5μl. The sample spot size should not exceed 1mm in diameter. The different types of sample applicators used are

   (i) Capillary tubes
   (ii) Microbulb pipettes
   (iii) Microsyringes
   (iv) Automatic sample applicators

   Application of sample in the form of narrow bands leads to maximum resolution and sensitivity.

7. **Preconditioning (Chamber saturation)**

   Chamber saturation influences the separation profile of the mixture components. Unsaturation of the chamber leads to higher R_f values. Reproducibility is also increased with chamber saturation

   Saturation of the chamber is done by lining the inner wall of the developing chamber with filter paper and closing the chamber with lid. The equilibration is allowed to continue for 20 minutes. This allows uniform distribution of solvent vapors.

8. **Chromatographic development and drying**

   After spotting the plates with sample and standard, the plates are air dried and placed in the developing chambers vertically. The mobile phase is allowed to rise over the stationary phase which is called development

   The various developmental techniques are;-

   1. Ascending
   2. Descending
   3. Horizontal
   4. Circular
   5. Automatic multiple development
   6. Gradient

After the development of the plate, the plates are removed and air dried.

9. **Scanning and documentation of the chromatoplate**

The detector spectrophotometer used in HPTLC is called densitometer or scanner. It consists of a sample light beam in the form of rectangular slit. The bands or zones are converted into peak and peak height/area by the scanner. The peak height/area is related to the concentration of substance in the band. The instrument measures and records the peak height and area. The plates of HPTLC after development will be evaluated for the following parameters

(a) R_f Value of the spot
(b) Area of each spot
(c) Height of each spot
(d) Spectra of each spot
(e) Purity of each spot

10. **Detection of spots**

(i) Non destructive techniques

After drying the plate to make it free from mobile phase, zones are detected. UV detection is the first choice because it is a nondestructive technique. Other detection technique used is fluorescence, in which the spots can be visualized at 254 nm (short wavelength) or at 366nm (Long wave length). For non fluorescent compounds, fluorescent stationary phase (silica gel GF) can be used.

(ii) Derivatization

Destructive techniques

Derivatization is carried out by spraying or immersing the plates in suitable reagent. These techniques are used when the compound cannot be detected directly. A reagent specific for the separated components is sprayed on the plate to develop colors.

Eg: Ninhydrin reagent is used for amino acids.

Uses of Derivatization techniques

1. Detection of components in a mixture
2. Non detectable substances are converted to detectable substances
3. Detection limits are increased.
4. For selective detection of few components.
5. To convert non fluorescent compounds to fluorescent compounds.

(iii) Iodine chamber method

The plates can also be detected by placing in chambers saturated with iodine vapour

Non-UV absorbing compounds like ethambutol, dicyclomine can be detected by dipping the plates in 0.1% iodine solution

DOCUMENTATION

Each developed plate in HPTLC is documented in digital format. The type of plate, chamber system, mobile phase composition, running time and detection method are the important parameters that are documented.

EVALUATION OF HPTLC PLATE

Factors affecting HPTLC

1. Type of stationary phase
2. Mobile Phase
3. Layer thickness
4. Temperature
5. Mode of development
6. Sample quantity
7. Detection methods

The validation parameters performed for a method in HPTLC are precision, accuracy, limit of detection, limit of quantitation, ruggedness and robustness.

Advantages of HPTLC

1. Simple, robust, efficient and rapid_
2. Better resolution with low limit of detection
3. Both quantitative and qualitative analysis can be performed.
4. Used in fingerprint determination of herbal products.

Applications of HPTLC

(i) Pharmaceutical Industry
Used in a quality control, identification and purity testing etc,

(ii) Food Industry.
HPLTC is used in QC, testing of additives, pesticides and also in stability testing.

(iii) Clinical application
HPTLC is also applicable in drug screening metabolism studies and stability testing etc.

(iv) Process development and optimization in industries.

(v) Used in poison investigations of forensic studies.

(vi) Pesticides analysis in drinking water can be done using HPTLC.

(vii) Used in Biomedical Analysis.

(viii) Fingerprint profiling of natural products, Plant ingredients is done using HPTLC.

(ix) Cosmetic analysis can also be performed with HPTLC.

(x) Analysis of Drug in biological fluids can be carried out using HPTLC

CHAPTER 15

Gas Chromatography

Gas chromatography is a most widely used powerful technique in separation chemistry to analyze volatile substances in the gaseous phase. In gas chromatography, gas is used as the mobile phase. If the stationary phase is a solid adsorbent, the technique is termed as gas-solid chromatography (GSC). A liquid on an inert support is used as stationary phasc in gas-liquid chromatography (GLC). Thus, based on the stationary phase, the gas chromatography is classified as GSC or GLC. Gas-liquid chromatography is the most commonly used method to separate volatile organic compounds. In identification of molecules, the combination of gas chromatography and mass spectrometry is an invaluable tool.

A GC chromatogram is a representation of the separation of the components that occurs in the GC column. Each of the peaks in the chromatogram represent the signal corresponding to a component eluting from the GC column into the detector. The x-axis shows the Retention time (R_t), and the y-axis shows the intensity of the signal. The chromatogram is plotted by the software in the computer. The area under the peak is proportional to the component concentration and is used for quantitative estimation.

THEORY

When a gas comes into contact with the adsorbent, some quantity of gas gets adsorbed on its surface. Adsorption isotherm is a graph or a relation between the amounts of adsorbate adsorbed on the surface of adsorbent and pressure at a constant temperature. The two important equations in adsorption are Freundlich and Langmuir adsorption isotherms. The **Freundlich equation** or **Freundlich adsorption isotherm** gives the observed experimental relation between quantity of a gas adsorbed onto a solid surface and the gas pressure. The same relationship can be applied to the solute concentration adsorbed onto the surface of a solid and the concentration of the solute in the liquid phase. It is mathematically expressed as

$$x/m = Kp^{1/n} \text{or } x/m = Kc^{1/n}$$

where

x = mass of adsorbate

m = mass of adsorbent

p = Equilibrium pressure of adsorbate if gas is used as mobile phase.

C = Equilibrium concentration of adsorbate in solution if the mobile phase is a liquid.

K and n are constants for a given set of adsorbate and adsorbent.

At high pressure 1/n = 0, hence extent of adsorption becomes independent of pressure.

Thus, the Freundlich adsorption isotherm fails at higher pressure.

The **Langmuir adsorption model** explains adsorption by assuming an adsorbate behaves as an ideal gas at isothermal conditions. According to the model, adsorption and desorption are reversible processes.

The mass of solute adsorbed per unit weight of adsorbent (m) depends on the concentration (c) of the solute. Langmuir equation is based on the assumption that only a monolayer is adsorbed and there is only one binding site on the adsorbent surface. The mathematical expression is given as

$$m = \frac{K_1 K_2 c}{1 + K_2 c}$$

where

K_1 – No of active adsorption sites /unit wt of adsorbent

K_2 – Affinity of the solute for the adsorbent.

c – Concentration of adsorbate

Langmuir assumed only one binding site but actually there are number of sites on the adsorbent surface and multiple layers of adsorption also take place against his monolayer adsorption assumption.

The law governing the separation in GLC, where the stationary phase is a liquid is Henry's law of partition which states that

x/m = Kc where K is the constant and c is concentration. K values differ with different pairs of vapor adsorbent combinations.

PRINCIPLE

In **GSC,** where the stationary phase is a solid, the principle of separation is **adsorption**. This technique has got limited applications like separation of low molecular weight gases like H_2S, CS_2, CO_2, Rare gases, CO and nitrogen oxides.

Principle of separation in **GLC is partition**. The stationary phase is a liquid which is coated as a thin film over a solid support. The mobile phase used is a gas. The components of the mixture to be separated are converted to vapors. These vapors are carried into the column after mixing with the mobile phase gas. The solubility of the component in the stationary or mobile phase (partition coefficient) determines the rate of elution of the component. The component which is more soluble in the mobile phase travels faster and gets eluted first. Thus the separation is based on the partition coefficient of the component for the given set of stationary and mobile phase combination. Under the given conditions, partition coefficient is unique for each component and no two components can have same partition coefficient.

$$\text{Paritition coefficient} = \frac{\text{Concentration of the sample in stationary phase}}{\text{Concentration of sample in mobile phase (gas)}}$$

Criteria for the compounds to be analyzed by GLC

1. **Volatility of the sample:** The mixture to be separated must be volatile in nature so that it can be mixed with the mobile phase.
2. **Thermo stability of the sample:** The sample should be vaporized by heating before entering into the column. If the sample is decomposed while heating, (thermo labile), then the sample cannot be separated and detected. Thus thermostability becomes an important criterion for the compound to be detected by GLC.

INSTRUMENTATION

Components of gas chromatography are

1. Carrier gas
2. Flow regulators /Flow meters
3. Injection devices
4. Columns
5. Temperature control devices
6. Detector
7. Recorders and integrators.

1. **Carrier Gas:** The carrier gas acts as the mobile phase and it carries the sample mixture through the column for separation into its components. The commonly used carrier gases are Helium (He), nitrogen (N_2), hydrogen (H_2), and argon (Ar). The choice of carrier gas is often dependent on the type of detector which is used. The carrier gas system also contains a molecular sieve to remove water and other impurities. **Helium and nitrogen are the most commonly used gases**.

Table 15.1 Components of gas chromatography.

Carrier gas	Flow regulators /Flow meters	Injection devices	Columns	Temperature control devices	Detector
Hydrogen Helium Nitrogen Argon	Rota meter Soap bubble meter	Split injectors Splitless injectors On-column injectors Automatic injectors	Analytical Preparative Packed Capillary WCOT SCOT PLOT	Preheaters Thermostatically controlled oven	**Concentration dependent detectors** Thermal conductivity detector, electron capture detector **Mass flow dependent detectors** FID, FPD, MS, AES and nitrogen phosphorous detectors.

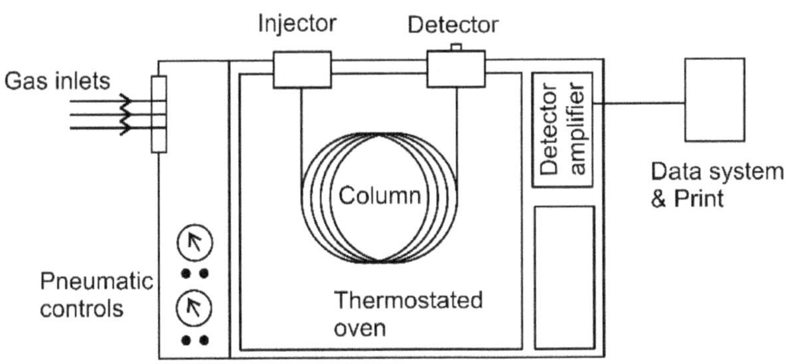

Fig. 15.1 Schematic diagram of gas chromatography.

Criteria for the carrier gas

1. It should be cheap, inert and readily available.
2. It should be of high quality and should not have fire hazard.
3. It should be suitable for the analyte and the detector.
4. It should give good column performance with speed of analysis.

Hydrogen: Hydrogen gas has good thermal conductivity and low density. It can be used with thermal conductivity detector and flame ionization detector.

Disadvantages:

1. It reacts with unsaturated compounds
2. Inflammable

Helium: Helium gas has got excellent thermal conductivity. It is the most commonly used carrier gas. It is inert in nature. It has low density and it allows greater flow rates. It is a safe gas. It has relatively wide optimum linear velocity range.

Disadvantage: Expensive

Nitrogen: It is an inexpensive and safe gas. Its sensitivity is less.

As the carrier gases are compressible, they are stored under high pressure in cylinders.

2. **Flow Regulators and Flow Meters:** The high pressure of the carrier gas cylinders necessitates the use of flow regulators so that gas can be delivered with uniform pressure or flow rate.

   Flow meters are used for measuring the flow rate of carrier gas. There are two types of flow meters.

   (a) Rota meter

   (b) Soap bubble meter

   (a) Rota meter: It is a calibrated glass tube which has a float held on a spring. The level of the float indicates the flow rate of the carrier gas. It is placed before the inlet of the column.

   (b) Soap bubble meter: It has a graduated pre calibrated glass tube attached with a inlet tube at the bottom for the carrier gas. The soap solution is stored in a rubber bulb. When this bulb is pressed, a drop of the soap solution gets converted to a bubble as the pressurized carrier gas comes in through the gas inlet. As the gas travels up, it takes the bubble along with it. The distance travelled upwards gives the measure of carrier gas flow rate.

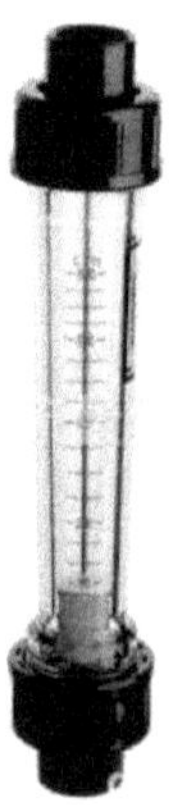

Fig. 15.2 Rota meter.

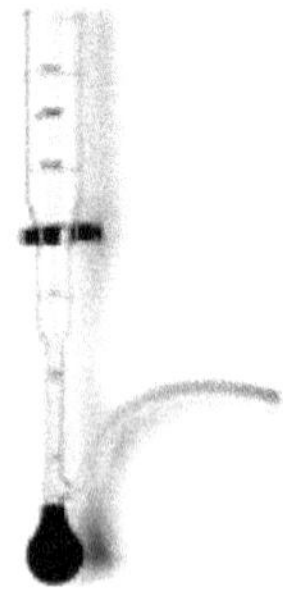

Fig. 15.3 Soap bubble meter.

3. **Injection Devices:** The sample is introduced into the column head through the injection device. The injection port is included in a oven that helps to maintain the temperature 20-50°C above the boiling point of the sample, so that the sample can be converted into vapor.

   Gaseous samples are introduced into the column using air tight **hypodermic needle** of 0.5 ml-10 ml capacity through gas sampling valves.

   For **Liquid** samples, **Hypodermic syringes** are used to inject through self sealing rubber septum. (0.1 -100μl capacity)

   Solid samples are **dissolved in volatile solvent** and then **injected** through a septum

   Types of injectors

   (a) Split injectors
   (b) Split less injectors
   (c) On-column injectors
   (d) Automatic injectors

   (a) Split injectors: Split injection is the most popular and versatile method in capillary GC analysis. The sample is introduced into the inlet and is vaporized as it moves downstream. Large portions of the vaporized sample have to be exhausted before the sample is separated in the column and detected. The split line has a role to protect the column from any sample overload and increase the moving velocity of the component in the injector port. The sensitivity of the injectors are low but the resolution is not affected.

   (b) Split less injectors: The split less injector is suitable for relatively high boiling point compounds with a low analyte concentration. The entire sample reaches the column in these injectors. They are used in high capacity columns such as Support-Coated Open Tubular (SCOT)/heavily coated Wall-Coated Open Tubular (WCOT) columns.

   (c) On-column injectors: Inlet temperature is kept below the boiling point of the sample solvent and the tip of the micro syringe is inserted directly into the tip of the capillary column for sample injection. Thereafter, by raising the temperature of the inlet and column, the sample is gradually vaporized directly inside the capillary column.

   (d) Automatic injectors: These injectors are used when large number of samples are analyzed and also for improving reproducibility.

4. **Columns:** Columns are the most important part of the instrument. They are made up of glass, stainless steel, copper, aluminium, nylon and other synthetic plastics. Glass columns are inert but they are fragile in nature.

   Classification of columns: columns can be broadly classified into two types

   (i) Analytical columns: These are packed columns made up of glass or stainless steel. They are about 1-1.5 m length and 3-6 mm in outer diameter. These columns can handle only a small quantity of samples.

   (ii) Preparative column: They can handle large quantity of sample. They are larger in size with about 3-6 m in length and diameter of 6-9 mm.

   Analytical columns are further subdivided into

   (a) Packed columns

   (b) Capillary columns /Open tubular column/ Golay column

   (a) Packed columns: These columns are prepared by packing granular stationary phase in metal, aluminium, stainless steel, copper, poly tetra fluoro ethylene or glass tubing. In GSC, the column packing is adsorbents which are size graded or porous polymers. The commonly used adsorbents are Kieselguhr, silica or alumina, hydrated amorphous silica with metal oxides like Fe, Al, Mg, Ca, Na, K and synthetic polymers like squalene, Teflon etc.

   In GLC, a liquid is coated over the size graded solid inert support. The inert supports are mostly diatomaceous earths like silica, hydrated amorphous silica with metal oxides or synthetic polymers like squalene and Teflon used in the form of small spherical beads. The stationary phase liquid may be non-polar (e.g. silicone oils-methylsilicone type), polar (polyethylene glycol, silicone oils with cyanopropyl groups) or of intermediate polarity (e.g. phenyl methyl silicone phase, dinonyl phthalate) depending on the type of the separation. The inner diameter of the column ranges from 1.5 mm to 6 mm.

   Advantages

   1. The porous polymers are stable upto 250°C with no column bleed and no base line drift.
   2. Polar compounds are not adsorbed.
   3. Higher sample capacity and used for preparative work
   4. Porous polymer beads are easily packed in the column and they are mechanically strong.
   5. Highly reproducible retention data is obtained.

Micro-packed columns have inner diameter ranging from 0.3-1mm and at lengths from 1-15 m. Particle size ranges from 0.007-0.3 mm in diameter.

The stationary phase is chosen based on the mode of separation and the nature of the analyte.

(b) Capillary columns: These are open tubular columns or Golay columns. They are made of long capillary tubing (30-90m) and the internal diameter is 0.10-0.2 mm. The material of construction is stainless steel, copper, nylon or glass etc.

Capillary columns are classified into

(i) WCOT column (Wall coated open tubular column)

(ii) SCOT column (Support coated open tubular column)

(iii) PLOT column (Porous layer open tubular column)

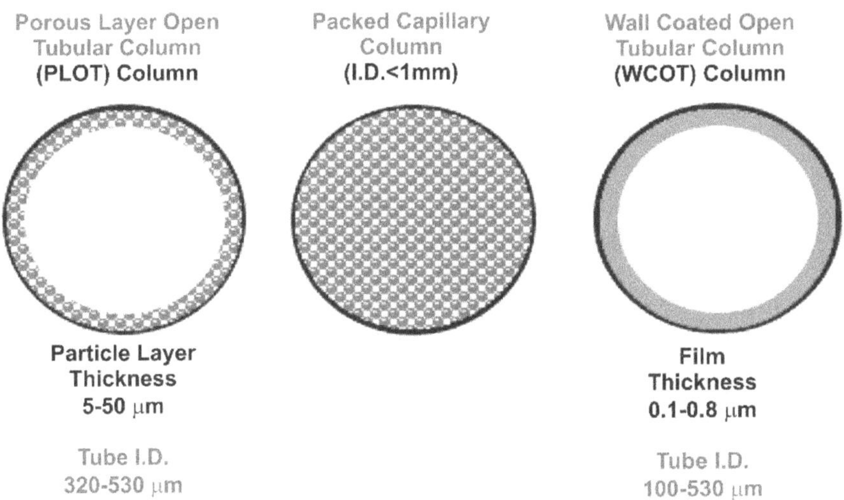

Fig. 15.4 Types of capillary columns.

WCOT column: The inner wall of the capillary column is coated with thin, uniform layer of stationary phase (0.5-1 μ). A very efficient, popular WCOT column is fused silica wall coated open tubular column (FSWC). It is used for the separation of small sample size and it is very inert. There is no resistance offered for the flow of the carrier gas in these columns, because there is no packing in the column.

SCOT column: These columns have a thin layer of (30μm) of supporting material coated on the inner wall of the capillary column and these support material are coated with thin layer of liquid phase. SCOT has more quantity of stationary phase than WCOT and hence can handle more quantity of sample.

PLOT column: This column is similar to SCOT column. The only difference is that the PLOT column does not have liquid stationary phase. They are used for GSC. The stationary phase coating is 5-50 microns thick.

SCOT columns are less efficient than WCOT columns.

Capillary columns are more efficient than packed column.

If the stationary phase is a solid adsorbent (GSC), the principle of separation is adsorption.

If the stationary phase is a liquid coated on a porous material (GLC),the separation principle is partition.

Equilibration of the column: Equilibration of the column is done before the introduction of sample in packed columns. Equilibration is done by passing the heated carrier gas continuously through the column for a specified period of time (24 hrs) at a particular temperature.

This equilibration helps in getting zero base line when the carrier gas alone is passed through the column.

5. **Temperature controlling devices:** The column temperature can be controlled by jackets containing vapors of boiling liquid, electrically heated metal blocks or circulating air baths. Compounds of low boiling point are eluted at lower temperature. Compounds of high boiling point require temperature programming to avoid broader and shallow peaks.

   The devices used in temperature programming are

   1. Pre heaters
   2. Thermostatically controlled oven

   1. **Pre heaters** are used to vaporize the sample and mix it with the mobile phase or carrier gas. They are present along with the injecting devices.
   2. **Thermostatically controlled oven:** The principle of separation in GLC is partition. The partition coefficient of the sample varies with temperature. Hence the maintenance of temperature in the column and the injection devices is very important for the resolution of the components. Since the columns are very long they are used in the coiled form and enclosed in the thermostatically controlled oven. The oven can maintain temperature difference up to 0.1°C.

6. **Detectors:** Detectors are the important part of gas chromatography. The solute particles get eluted along with the carrier gas from the column and enter the detector. The detector produces electrical signals proportional to the concentration of the solute components. These signals are amplified and recorded as chromatographic peaks.

In GC, the area under the peak is proportional to the concentration of the analyte.

Properties of ideal detector

1. Sensitivity should be high even in small concentrations.
2. It should be able to detect wide range of samples.
3. It should give linear and rapid response even at high temperatures
4. It should be non destructive, simple, easy to maintain and inexpensive
5. It should be stable and reproducible.

The Detectors used in Gas chromatography are classified as

1. Concentration dependent detectors
2. Mass flow dependent detector

Concentration dependent detectors: The signal produced is directly proportional to the concentration of solute in the carrier gas. These detectors are **non destructive** detectors.

Dilution with detector gas lowers the detector response

E.g., **Thermal conductivity detector and electron capture detector**

Mass flow dependent detector: These detectors are **Destructive in nature** i.e. the sample cannot be recovered. Signal produced is proportional to the rate at which the solute particles enter the detector. The detector is unaffected by the dilution of carrier gas.

e.g., **FID, FPD, MS, AES** and **nitrogen phosphorous** detectors.

1. **Thermal Conductivity detector/Katharometer:** It is a nondestructive detector. The principle of Katharometer is that **the thermal conductivity of the pure gas changes in presence of the sample component**. (Organic compound)

   Thermal conductivity detector has two platinum wires made of uniform dimensions and they form the two arms of Wheatstone bridge as shown in figure 11.5 b. Through one of the platinum wires, always pure carrier gas flows through and the effluent from the column passes through the other platinum wire. The two platinum wires are electrically heated and they have uniform temperature and electrical resistance.

   When only pure carrier gas is passed through both wires, there is no temperature or resistance change which is recorded as base line. When the compound emerges from the column, the wire through which column effluent passes experiences a change in thermal conductivity of the gas leading to change in temperature and resistance of the wire. The difference in the resistance is amplified and recorded as signal.

   Hydrogen and helium gas have high thermal conductivity and they are very much suited as carrier gas for TCD.

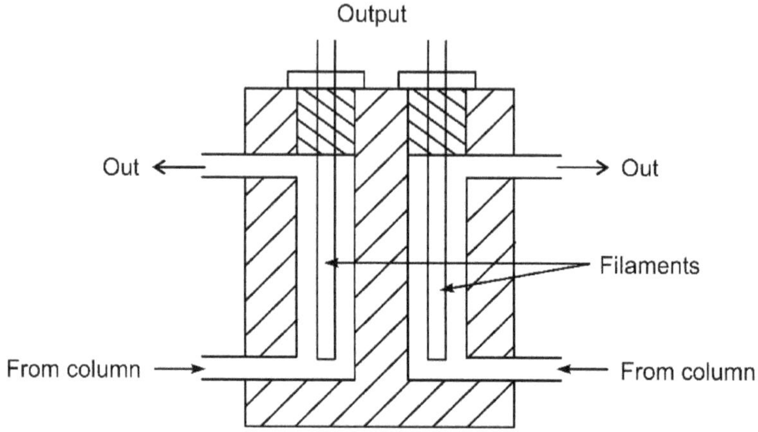

Fig. 15.5(a) Thermal conductivity detector.

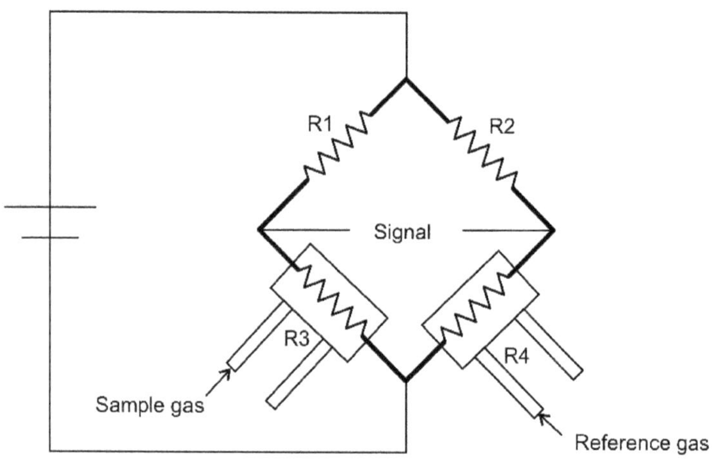

Fig. 15.5(b) Wheatstone bridge.

Advantages

1. Simple and inexpensive
2. Accurate, linear and rugged
3. Applicable to most compounds. Hence called as universal detectors
4. **Non–destructive** type. It can be used for preparative chromatography.

Disadvantages

1. Sensitivity is low
2. Biological samples cannot be analyzed.
3. Fluctuations in flow rate and temperature affect the outcome.
4. The response obtained is relative response only. Absolute response is not obtained.

2. **Electron capture detector (ECD): The difference in the electron affinity of the substances is used as the principle of ECD.**

   ECD has two electrodes, the anode and the cathode. The column effluent passes between the electrodes. The cathode is treated with a radioactive isotope like ^{65}Ni or ^{3}H emitting electrons as it undergoes decay. When a potential of 20 eV is applied, the secondary electrons are produced by these isotopes. The emitted electrons are collected by the anode producing a constant current.

   If helium is preferred as carrier gas for the column, a make-up gas such as nitrogen or argon/methane is used to increase detector sensitivity. The function of the make-up gas is to improve the detector ionization yield. In other words: make-up gas does not play a role in the chromatographic process in the column. It is only added the moment the carrier gas leaves the column.

   When only carrier gas is flowing between the electrodes, all the secondary electrons are collected by the positive electrode and constant current is recorded as base line. When the carrier gas with the effluent molecules is flowing between the electrodes, the effluent molecules having affinity for the electrons (electronegative components) capture the electrons. This causes a reduction in the constant current. The difference in current is recorded as signal. A schematic diagram of electron capture detector is given in figure 11.6. Choice of the carrier gas depends on the electron affinity of the analyte in these detectors. For analytes of high electron affinity, argon gas is used and for low electron affinity analytes nitrogen, helium, hydrogen or carbon di oxide is used.

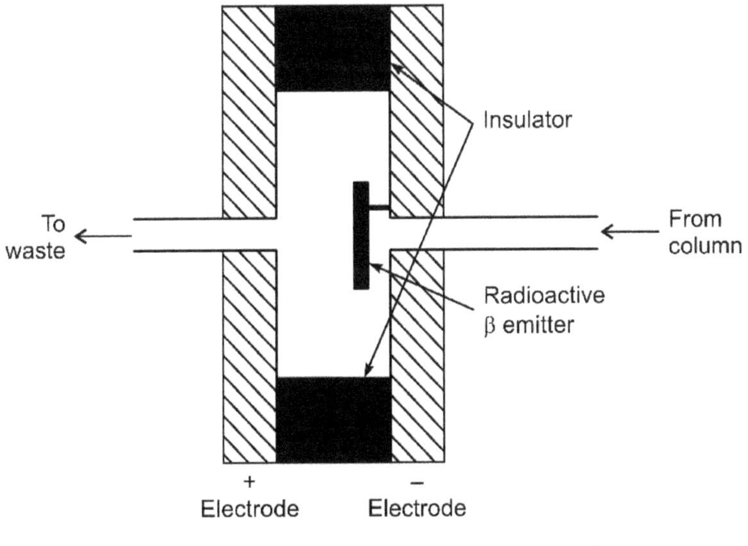

Fig. 15.6 Schematic diagram of electron capture detector.

Advantages:

1. Highly sensitive. Even nanogram quantity of substances can be detected for halogens, nitriles etc.
2. Highly selective
3. Non-Destructive
4. More sensitive than TCD and FID

Disadvantages:

1. Can be used **only for components with electron affinity** eg: Halogenated compounds, Pesticides etc.
2. Carrier gas should be pure
3. Insensitive to amines, alcohols and hydrocarbons.

3. **Flame ionization detector (FID):** These detectors are based on the **principle of change in electrical conductivity of carrier gases due to the ions of the components.** At standard temperature and pressure, gases are insulators, but the presence of ions makes them as conductors. In the given conditions if the gas molecules are not ionized, the conductivity of the gas is due to the solute ions present in it.

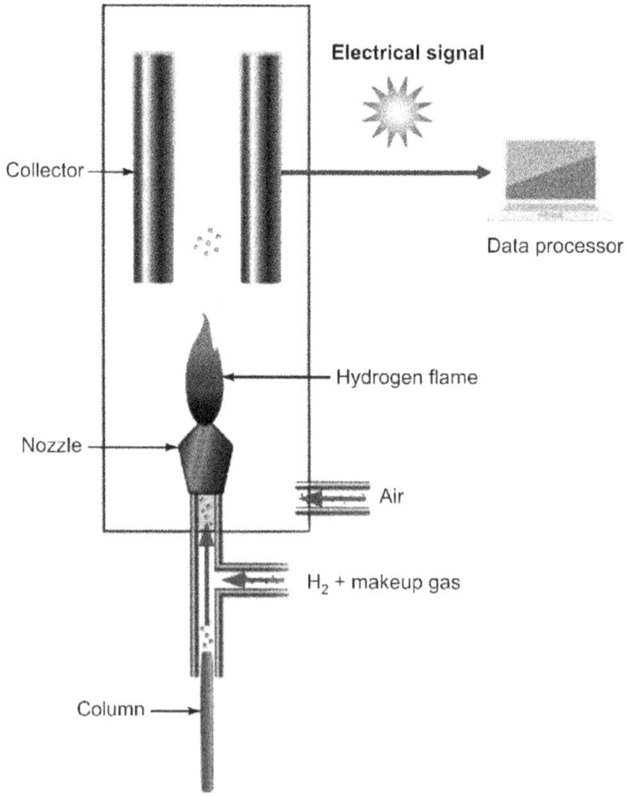

Fig. 15.7 Flame ionization detector (FID).

If a carrier gas other than hydrogen, like nitrogen or argon is used, then they are mixed with hydrogen and they reach the platinum tip of the burner acting as cathode. Silver gauze placed above the burner tip acts as anode. The sample in carrier gas is burnt in air in the detector.

When the carrier gas alone passes through the cathode, there is no ionization taking place and as a result no current is flowing through the system. When a sample component emerges from the column effluent with the carrier gas, the sample gets ionized by the thermal energy from the flame. The collection of these ions by the anode causes a potential difference and current is flowing. This current is amplified and recorded as signal.

Advantages

1. Rugged and sensitive. Background noise is low. Hence μg quantities of solute can be detected.
2. Presence of water vapor is not affecting the performance.
3. Responds to most organic analytes except formic acid.
4. Excellent linearity.

Disadvantages

1. Destructive detector. Sample recovery is not possible
2. Weakly sensitive to carbonyl, amine and alcohol.
3. Not sensitive to non-combustibles like H_2O, CO_2, SO_2 and these cannot be detected.

4. **Flame photometric detector (FPD):** The thermal energy of the flame in this detector excites the solute particle atoms and the excited atoms emit characteristic radiation which is detected by the detector. The amount of emitted radiation is directly proportional to the solute concentration in the carrier gas.

   This detector is used for the detection of heavy metals like chromium, selenium, tin etc in organo metallic compounds and sulphur and phosphorous containing compounds. Analysis of pesticides, coal, air and water pollutants are also carried out with this detector.

5. **Argon ionization detector:** Carrier gas used in this detector is argon gas. The argon atoms are excited to a meta stable state using radioactive energy and these argon meta stable molecules collide with solute molecules in the effluent carrier gas and ionize them. These ions are detected by the increase in current

   Excitation of argon atoms is carried out with α or β particles. α particles obtained from radium –D, β particles obtained from ^{90}Sr or tritium. These high energy particles are used for the ionization of argon atoms.

Advantages:

1. Most of the organic compounds can be detected.
2. High sensitivity

Disadvantages:

1. Response is relative response not absolute. Response varies with temperature of detector.
2. Poor linearity
3. Less sensitive for halogenated compounds and sensitivity is affected by water vapor.

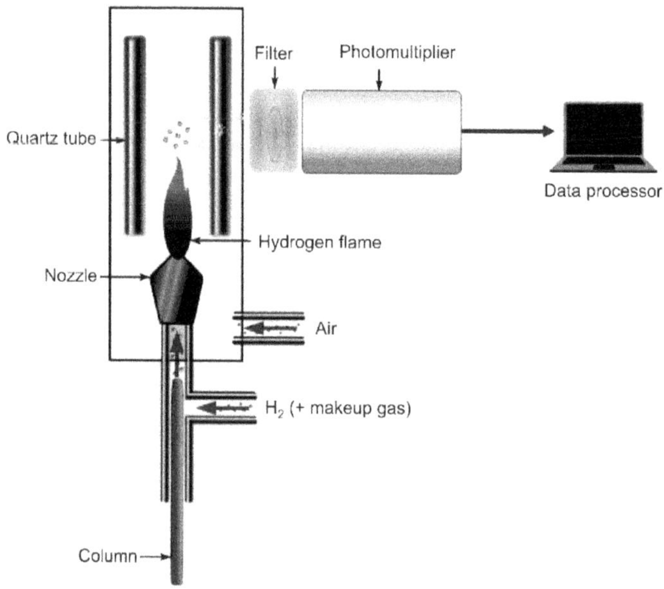

Fig. 15.8 Flame photometric detector.

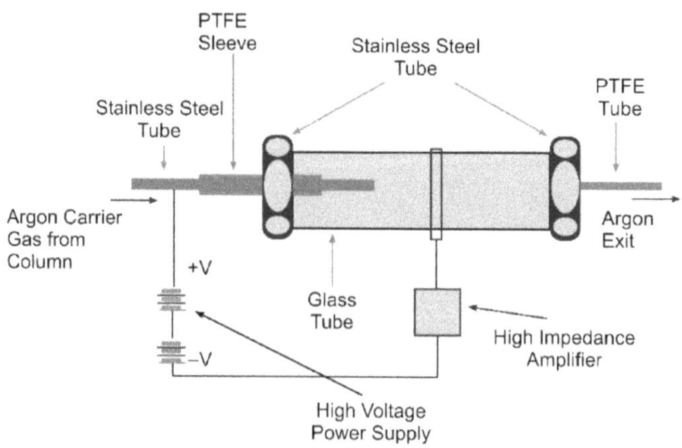

Fig. 15.9 Argon ionization detector.

6. **Thermionic Detector/Nitrogen-Phosphorous Detector (NPD):** A NPD is based on the same basic principles as an FID. A special bead of rubidium is mounted in a silica lattice between the jet and the polarization electrode. This bead is fused to a platinum wire. The bead is heated either electrically or by the flame. Compounds are burned in plasma supplied with hydrogen and air surrounding the rubidium bead. Nitrogen and phosphorous containing compounds produce ions that are attracted to the collector. The number of ions hitting the collector is measured and a signal is recorded. A small amount of alkali metal vapor in the flame greatly enhances the formation of ions from nitrogen and phosphorus-containing compounds.

   The NPD is about 500 times more sensitive in detecting phosphorous-containing compounds, and 50 times more sensitive to nitrogen-containing compounds when compared to FID.

   Applications: Organophosphate in pesticides and in drug analysis for determination of amino drugs or basic drugs

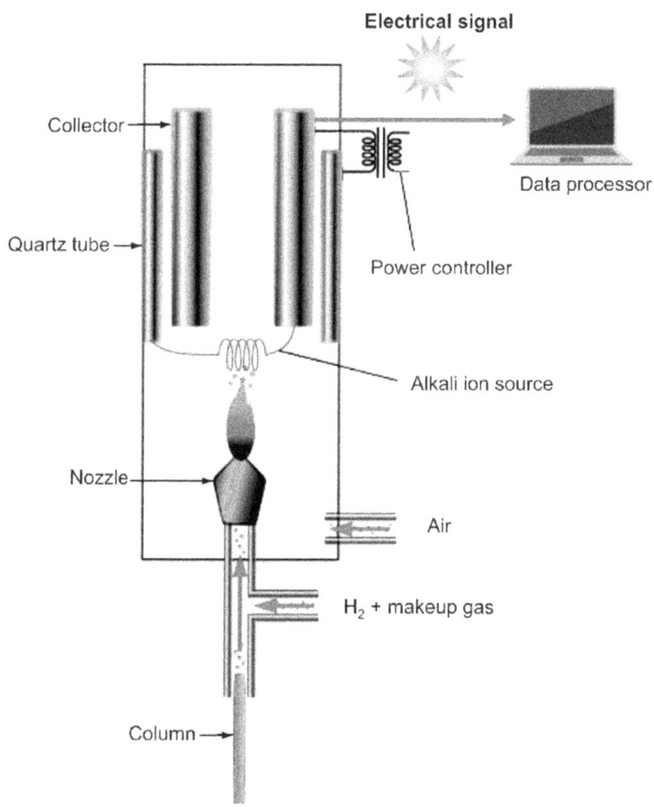

Fig. 15.10 Thermionic Detector/Nitrogen-Phosphorous Detector (NPD).

7. **Electrolytic Conductivity Detector:** It is an element-selective detector for halogen, sulfur and nitrogen containing compounds.

   Halogens, sulfur or nitrogen containing compounds are mixed with a reaction gas in a small reactor tube made of Ni. The products from the reaction tube are then dissolved in a liquid, which produces a conductive solution. The conductivity changes due to the ionic species is measured.

   Each detector requires gas, called the detector gas, based on its principle of detection. For example, the flame ionization detector (FID) uses a hydrogen flame so it requires hydrogen and air.

   Analysis using a capillary column requires a makeup gas added just before the detector to act as an auxiliary gas and ensure the detector receives a rapid supply of compounds. Makeup gas reduces the effects of increasing and decreasing column flow rates on detector sensitivity by increasing the sample transfer speed inside the detector and preventing peak broadening. A summary of the detectors in given in the table 15.2.

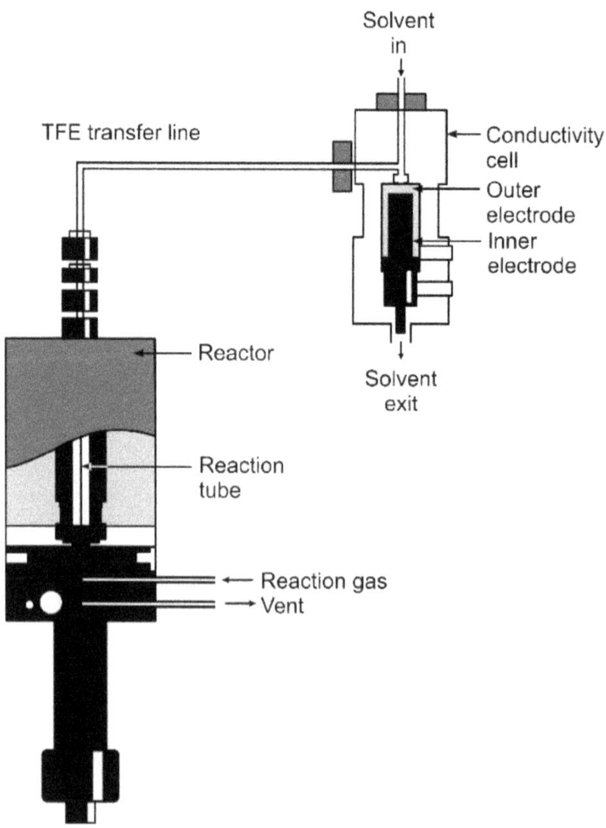

Fig. 15.11 Electrolytic conductivity detector.

8. **Recorders and integrators:** Recorders record the responses from the detector. They record the base line and all the peaks with respect to time.

   Integrators: They are the data processors. They record all the data related to every peak like R_t, peak area, peak width and height etc.

   Temperature Programming: Temperature programming is controlled increase of temperature during an analysis. In a mixture containing compounds with a wide boiling range, efficient separation within a short analysis time is not possible. In temperature programming, the components with wide boiling range are resolved efficiently in a shorter analysis time and they can be eluted fast with improved peak shapes.

   Two types of temperature programming are used

   (a) **Isothermal programming:** In this type of temperature programming, the same temperature is maintained throughout the process of isolation. This type of programming is used in separation of components with closely similar boiling points. Adequate separation in short analysis time is obtained at a particular temperature.

Table 15.2 Summary of Gas chromatography detectors.

Detectors	Type	Carrier gas	Make up gas (capillary column)	Selectivity	Sensitivity	Detection limit
Thermal conductivity detector (TCD)	Concentration	He	He or Ar or N_2 or H_2 ,etc.	Universal	Low	10ppm (10 ng)
Flame ionisation	Mass flow	H_2 and Air	He or N_2	Organic compounds (other than formaldehyde and formic acid)	Highly sensitive	0.1 ppm (0.1 ng)
Electron capture detector (ECD)	Concentration	Mainly N_2	Mainly N_2	Halides, nitrates, nitriles, peroxides, anhydrides and organo metallics	Sensitive to electronegative groups	0.1 ppb (0.1 pg)
Flame photo-metric	Mass flow	H_2 and Air	–	Sulphur, phosphorous, tin, boron, arsenic, Germanium, selenium, chromium.	Highly sensitive	10 ppb (10 pg)
Argon ionization detector	Concentration	Argon	–	Organic compounds	Highly sensitive	0.1 ppm

(b) Linear programming: There are three types of linear programming

1. Temperature increasing linearly with time
2. Linear increase followed by a period of Isothermal programming
3. Multi linear programming

1. Temperature increasing linearly with time: In this method the oven temperature is increased linearly over a period of time. The rate of change of temperature is maintained constant throughout separation. eg: Initial temperature followed by 5°C /minute increase up to the required temperature till the end of separation.

This linear programming is used for the separation of complex mixtures containing low and high boiling point compounds.

2. Linear increase followed by a period of Isothermal programming: This linear programming is used for the separation of complex mixtures and the temperature is maintained constant till all the components are resolved.

3. Multi linear programming: This programming changes the oven temperature from an initial value to final temperature with various rates, times and temperatures. An example of multilinear programming is shown in figure 15.12.

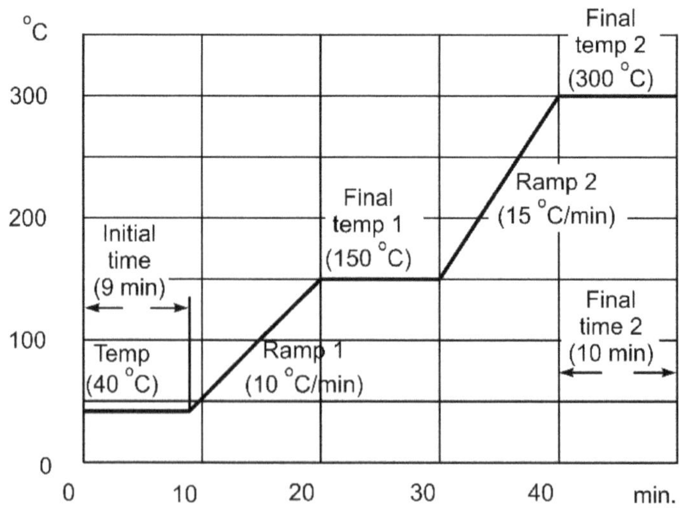

Fig. 15.12 Example of multi linear programming.

Three variables play important role in temperature programming

(i) **The initial temperature:** The temperature where most of the volatile components are well separated is kept as the initial temperature. It is generally well below the boiling point of the lowest boiling component.

(ii) **The Final temperature**: It is the temperature at which highest boiling component leave the column after separation. The temperature is near the boiling point of highest boiling component in the sample mixture.

(iii) **Rate of rise of temperature:** It can be linear, multi linear, convex or concave.

Derivatization of sample: It is the technique used to improve the process of separation of the sample by column or detection by detector. **Derivatization is the process of chemically modifying the compound to produce a new compound, so that it can be analyzed by GC.**

There are two types of Derivatization

(a) Pre column derivatization

(b) Post column derivatization

Pre column derivatization: The components are converted to volatile and thermo stable derivatives. Derivatization is performed offline.

Pre column derivatization is done for the following reasons

1. Substance is less volatile or less stable.
2. Components to be separated are thermo labile
3. To reduce tailing and improve the separation factor

Eg: Carboxylic acids, sugars are converted to less polar compounds by treating with reagents like BSA reagent. (Bis tri methyl silyl acetamide reagent)

Post column derivatization: Post column derivatization is performed only for enhancing the detectability of the analytes. This derivatization is done.

1. To improve detector response.
2. The ionization or electron affinity of the components is increased.
3. This is an on-line detection technique. The flow rate is neither stopped nor altered.

Pretreatment of solid support: Pretreatment of solid support is carried out.

1. To overcome tailing.
2. For the separation of non-polar components like esters, ethers etc.

The different methods used in derivatization are

1. Silylation
2. Acylation
3. Per fluoroacylation
4. Alkylation
5. Esterification
6. Condensation
7. Cyclisation

1. **Silylation:** Silylation is a chemical reaction in which a reactive hydrogen atom in OH, COOH, SH, NH, CONH, POH, SOH or enolisable carbonyl is replaced with a silyl group, using Trimethyl silyl (TMS).

   The silylation helps in the reduction of the polarity of the analyte, increases its stability, and improve the GC behavior of the solute.

   Eg. of silylating agents: Hexa methyl disilane(HMDS), Trimethyl chlorosilane (TMCS), Trimethyl silyl imidazole (TMSI), Bis Trimethyl silyl acetamide (BSA).

   The functional groups that can be silylated are alcohol, phenol, carboxyl, amine and amide.

2. **Acylation:** Acylation is replacing the active hydrogens from an analyte with functional groups like OH, SH, NH CONH, etc with acyl group(R-C=O).

   The acylation is also used for reducing polarity and improving the behavior of the analytes in the chromatographic column. Acylation is used to enhance the detectability in GC with ECD and FID detectors.

   Common acylating agents are formic acid, acetyl chloride, acetic anhydride, N-Methyl-bis trifluoro acetamide (MBTFA), bis (trifluoro acetamide), trifluoroacetic acid (TFA), propionic anhydride and butyric anhydride.

   Alcohols, amines and phenol are derivatized by acylation.

4. **Alkylation:** Replacement of the active hydrogens in an analyte with an alkyl (R) group is alkylation and this results in the reduction of polarity of the sample. The functional groups which can undergo alkylation are OH, COOH, SH, NH, or CONH. Alkylation enhances the detectability of the analytes by ECD.

   Eg of alkylating agents are Dimethyl formamide, Tetra butyl ammonium hydroxide, Diazomethane.

   Carboxylic acids and Phenols are derivatized by alkylation.

5. **Esterification:** The esterification reaction is the alkylation of carboxylic acid or the acylation of the alcohol.

6. **Condensation:** Ketones and aldehydes present in the sample are derivatized to prevent hydrogen bonding. The agent used is methoxylamine.
7. **Cyclization:** Compounds containing two functional groups in close proximity undergo cyclization to form heterocyclic rings.

PARAMETERS USED IN GC

Retention Time (R_t)

It is the difference in time from the point of injection to the peak maxima. Retention time is the time required for the elution of 50% of the component from the column. The unit for R_t is minutes or seconds. The solutes which are not retained by the column travel straight to the detector and t_m is the time taken for the unretained solute to travel through the column. It is shown in figure 15.13

Retention volume (V_r): Retention volume is the volume of carrier gas required to elute 50% of the component from the column. It is a product of retention time and flow rate.

Retention volume = retention time × flow rate

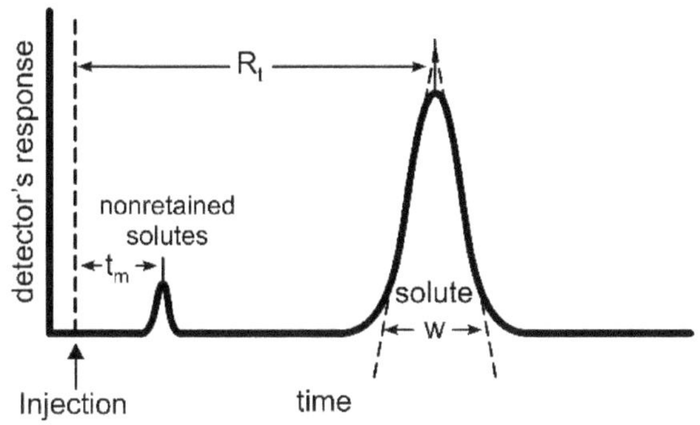

Fig. 15.13 Retention time.

Separation factors(S): It is the ratio of partition coefficient of the two components to be separated. It is expressed as

$$S = K_a / K_b = \left(\frac{t_b - t_0}{(t_a - t_0)} \right)$$

Where

t_0 = Retention time of unretained substance

K_b, K_a= Partition coefficients of b and a

t_b, t_a= retention time of substance b and a

S = depends on liquid phase and column temperature

If the difference in partition coefficients of two compounds are more, the separation factor is more and the peaks are far apart. If the difference in partition coefficients is less, then the peaks are closer and the separation factor is less.

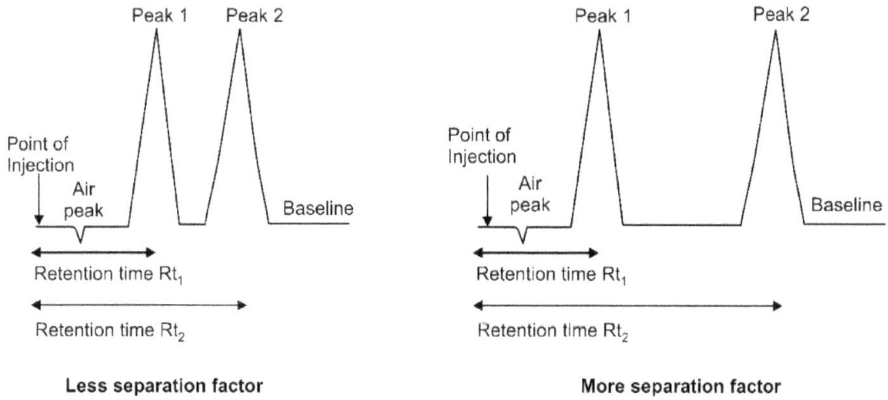

Fig. 15.14 Separation factor.

Resolution: It is a quantitative measure of separation of two components. It is defined as the difference in retention times between the two peaks, divided by the combined widths of the elution peaks. Resolution should be greater than one.

$$R_S = \frac{2(R_{t2} - R_{t1})}{w_1 + w_2}$$

Theoretical plates (Plate theory): This theory was developed by Martin and Synge in 1941. In plate theory the column is viewed as divided into a number of adjacent imaginary segments called as theoretical plates. In each theoretical plate, a complete equilibration of the solute occurs between stationary and mobile phase.

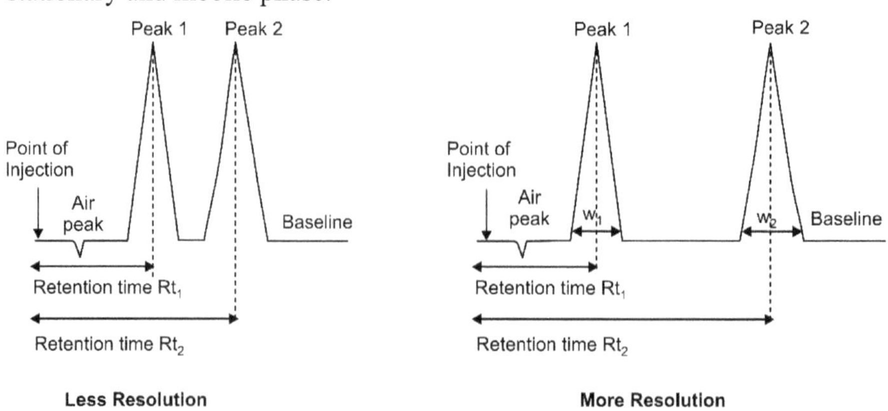

Fig. 15.15 Resolution.

The **(HETP)** Height Equivalent to Theoretical Plates is defined as a unit of column length sufficient to establish equilibrium between the solute in the mobile phase and that in the stationary phase throughout the unit.

The equal interaction of the solute components of the mixture with the mobile phase and stationary phase leads to the retention of the molecules (slow rate of movement).

If each solute molecule is interacting with the mobile phase and stationary phase in a different manner, then they will have different rates of migration leading to separation of the components.

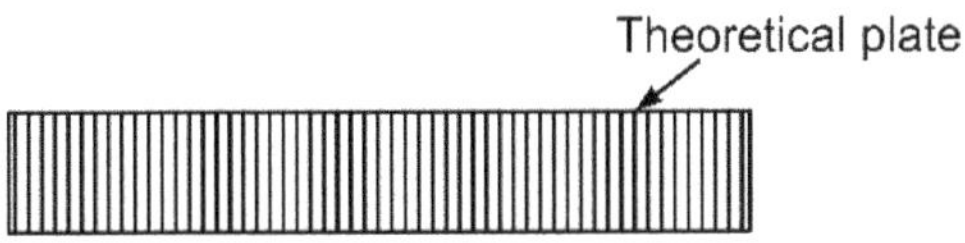

Fig. 15.16 Column showing imaginary theoretical plates.

SIGNIFICANCE OF THEORETICAL PLATES

Efficiency (good separation of the components) of the column increases with

1. Increase in number of theoretical plates. (N)
2. Decrease in HETP (Height equivalent to theoretical plates)

$$H = L/N$$

where
L- Length of the column
N- Number of plates
H – HETP or Height of the theoretical plates.

Van Deemter equation gives the HETP

$$\mathbf{HETP = A + (B/u) + Cu}$$

where
A = is the Eddy diffusion
B = Longitudinal diffusion
C = Mass transfer
U - Average mobile phase velocity

Eddy diffusion - (A term) - is caused by the different paths taken by the solute particles in the column resulting in peak broadening. It is independent of flow rate.

Longitudinal diffusion – (B term) – is caused by less analyte concentration in the edges of the column than in the centre leading to peak broadening.

Increased flow rate can control B term and peak broadening can be avoided.

Mass transfer – (C term) – is the movement of the analyte or mass transfer between mobile and stationary phases.

Increased flow rate increases the resistance to mass transfer leading to band broadening.

The Van Deemter plot is shown below in figure 15.17, indicating the desired plate height (H or HETP) and flow rate as optimum efficiency and optimum flow rate respectively.

A column is efficient when the HETP is minimum. Therefore, the flow rate corresponding to minimum value of HETP is used.

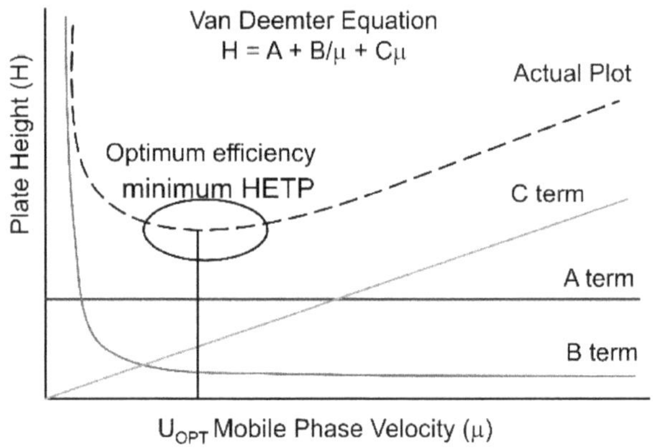

Fig. 15.17 Composite curve of Van Deemter.

Efficiency of the column (No of theoretical plates): The number of theoretical plates in a column represent the efficiency of the column. It is determined using the formula

$$N = 16\frac{(R_t^2)}{(W^2)}$$

Where N – no of theoretical plates

R_t - retention time

W – peak width at base.

More number of theoretical plates indicate the high efficiency of the column. Gas chromatographic columns normally have 600 - 1000 plates/meter where as in HPLC it varies between 8000- 12000 plates/meter.

Asymmetry factor: A chromatographic peak follows gaussian distribution and it should be symmetrical about its centre. But in actual practice, The peak may not be symmetrical due to some factors, and it shows tailing or fronting.

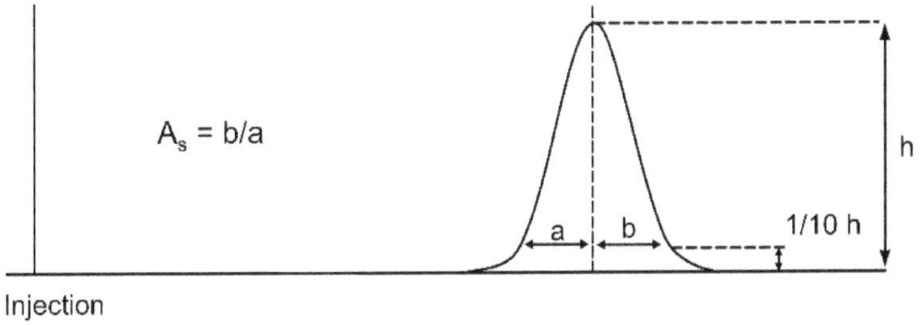

Fig. 15.18 Asymmetry factor.

b - distance from the peak midpoint (perpendicular from the peak highest point) to the trailing edge of the peak measured at 10% of peak height.

a - is the distance from the leading edge of the peak to the peak midpoint (perpendicular from the peak highest point) measured at 10% of peak height.

Asymmetry factor(A_S) should be between 0.95 to 1.05.

If A_S > 1 the peak is showing tailing and if A_S < 1 fronting is observed in the peak.

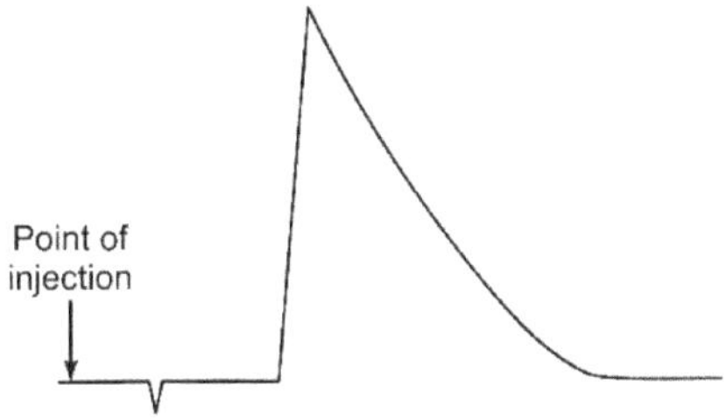

Fig. 15.19 Tailing in a peak.

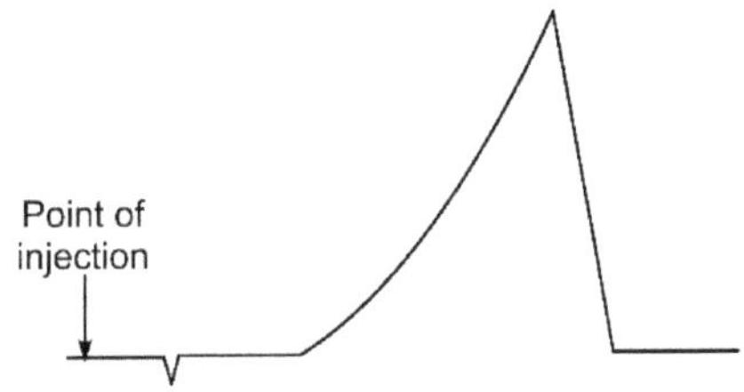

Fig. 15.20 Fronting in a peak.

Tailing Factor: Tailing Factor (T_f) is the USP coefficient of the peak symmetry. The formula for tailing factor is given as

$$T_f = (a + b)/2a$$

where a is the distance from the leading edge of the peak to the peak midpoint (perpendicular from the peak highest point) measured at 5% of peak height and b is the distance from the peak midpoint (perpendicular from the peak highest point) to the trailing edge of the peak measured at 5% of peak height.

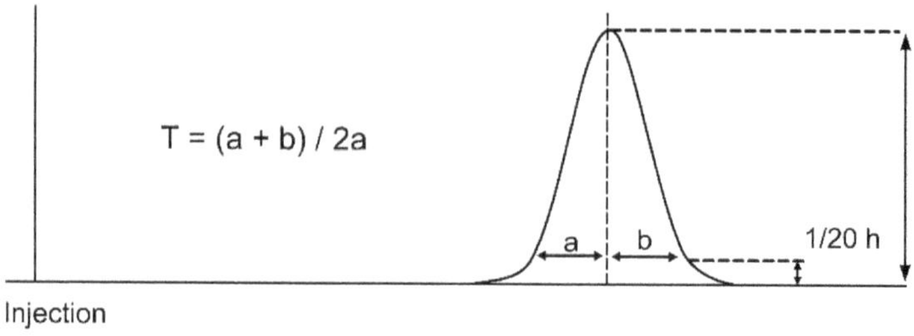

Fig. 15.21 Tailing factor in a peak.

APPLICATIONS

1. **Qualitative analysis:** It is carried out by comparing the retention time of sample with the retention time of the standard. If the operating conditions are same, the retention time also remains the same.
2. **To check the purity of the compound:** Presence of additional peaks in the chromatogram shows the presence of impurities when compared with the standard chromatogram. The peak areas can be used to calculate the percentage purity of the sample.
3. **Detection of impurities:** Presence of additional peaks when compared with a reference material identifies the impurities. The peak areas can be used to calculate the percentage of impurities.
4. **Quantitative analysis**
   (a) **Direct comparison method:** From the peak areas of the standard and the sample, the quantity of sample can be calculated.

      Peak area = Peak height × width at ½ height

      $A_1/A_2 = \alpha(w_1/w_2)$ where,

      A_1 & A_2 are the peak area of sample and standard.

      α- Response factor

      w_1/w_2 is the weight or concentration of sample and standard.

   (b) **Calibration curve method:** Serial dilutions of standard solutions are prepared and injected in GC. A calibration graph is constructed by plotting peak area vs. concentration. The concentration of the unknown sample is determined from the calibration graph.

   (c) **Internal standard method:** Known concentration of the internal standard (compound with similar retention characteristics) is added to the standard solution and sample solution. The unknown solution concentration is determined using the ratios of sample with internal standard and standard with internal standard. This method is used to avoid the extraction steps when the sample matrix is complex in nature.

5. **Multi component analysis:** GC is also used for the determination of multiple components in a formulation
6. **Isolation** and identification of drugs in urine, plasma and serum
7. **Analysis** of mixture of components like amino acid, plant extracts, volatile oils etc.
8. **Pharmaceutical applications:**
   (a) Quality control and analysis of antibiotics (penicillin), antiviral (amantidine), General anesthetics (chloroform, ether), sedative /hypnotics (barbiturates) etc.
   (b) Assay of drugs like Atropine sulphate etc.
   (c) Presence of related compounds

CHAPTER 16

Electrophoresis

Electrophoresis is a physical method of analysis in which the compounds that acquire charge in the presence of an electric field are separated. Electrophoresis is defined as the **movement of charged particles in an electric field**, leading to their separation. It is a separation technique that is based on the differences in the mobility of charged particles in an electric field. The technique was pioneered in 1937 by the Swedish chemist Arne Tiselius to separate proteins. It is one of the widely used techniques in molecular biochemistry, microbiology and biochemical research. It is an efficient technique for the separation of proteins in a mixture.

In practice, a positive (anode) and negative (cathode) electrode are placed in a solution containing ions. When a voltage is applied across the electrodes, solutes of different charges, *i.e.*, anions (negative) and cations (positive) move through the solution towards the electrode of opposite charge.

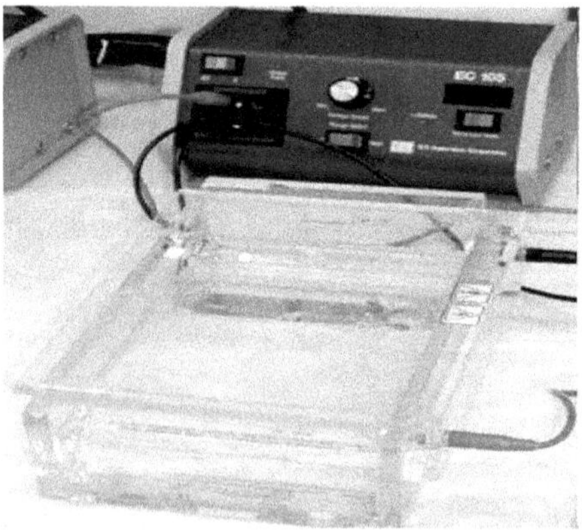

Fig. 16.1 Electrophoresis Apparatus.

PRINCIPLE

The basic principle is that the rate of migration (separation) of ions depends upon the e/m (charge to mass) ratio. Molecules having different molecular weights will have different charge/mass ratios. This fact is responsible for the differential migration of charged particles.

When a voltage is applied across the electrodes, a potential gradient (E) develops and is given as

$$E = V/d$$

where V – Voltage and d- the distance between electrodes.

The charged molecules migrate towards oppositely charged electrodes under the influence of an electric field. The positively charged molecules move towards the cathode and the negatively charged molecules move towards the anode.

The migration of molecules under the influence of current, experiences a frictional force. If the charge on the molecule is Q coulombs, then the velocity v of the charged molecule is given as

$$\mathbf{v = EQ/f}$$

where

f is the frictional force which retards the mobility of the molecule.

The frictional force is dependent on size, shape, hydrodynamic volume of the molecule, matrix pore size and viscosity of the medium.

The **electrophoretic mobility, μ** of an ion is defined as the ratio of velocity to the potential gradient

$$\mu = v/E = Q/f$$

where

$$f = 6\pi r\eta \text{ (Stokes law)}$$

i.e. $$\mu = Q/ 6\pi r\eta$$

where

Q – Charge on the molecule (esu)

μ - Electrophoretic mobility

r – Radius of the molecule (cm)

η - Viscosity of the medium (poise)

Thus in electrophoresis, molecules with identical or similar charges can also be separated if the molecules have different frictional forces.

Working Principle

Biological molecules exist in a solution as electrically charged particles at a given pH. They will exist as anionic (negatively charged/basic), Zwitterions and cationic (positively charged / acidic) ions. Zwitterions are amphoteric molecules having no charge on them.

The total charge of molecules depends on the pH. When electricity is applied to the medium containing biological molecules, they migrate differentially depending on their net charge & molecular size and thus, different proteins/DNA can be separated.

Depending on the kind of charge the molecules carry, they move towards the cathode or anode. An ampholyte becomes positively charged in acidic condition and migrate to the cathode. In alkaline conditions, they become negatively charged and migrate to anode. The electrophoresis mechanism is illustrated in figure 16.2.

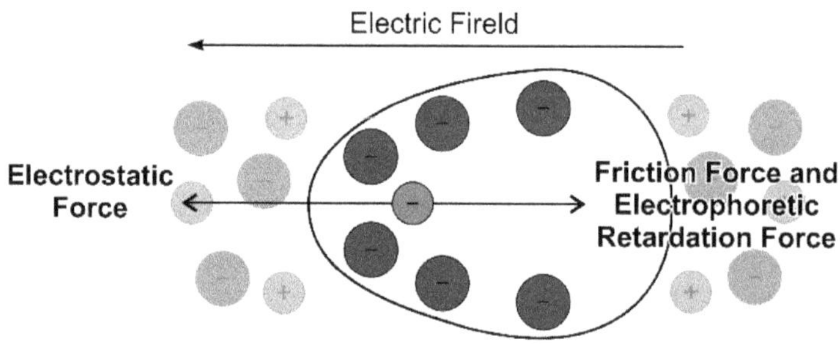

Fig. 16.2 Electrophoresis mechanism.

FACTORS AFFECTING ELECTROPHORETIC MOBILITY

1. Factors related to the electric field
2. Factors related to sample
3. Factors related to the buffer
4. Factors related to supporting medium
5. Viscosity of the medium

1. **Factors related to the electric field**
   (a) **Voltage:** The rate of migration is proportional to VQ/d where V is Voltage, Q is the charge on the ion, and d is the distance between electrodes. Therefore, an increase in voltage causes a proportional increase in the rate of mobility.
   (b) **Current:** The migration distance of the ion is proportional to the current in the electrophoretic system.
   (c) **Resistance:** The current and rate of migration are inversely proportional to the resistance, which in turn depends on the nature of the medium, the buffer and its concentration. Resistance is directly proportional to the length of the supporting medium. It is inversely proportional to cross-sectional area and ion concentration of the buffer.

(d) **Temperature:** Resistance decreases with an increase in temperature. An increase in temperature causes a decrease in viscosity of the liquid leading to decreased resistance and hence increased mobility. A decrease in resistance causes an increase in current and more heat will be produced. This heat evaporates the solvent and decreases the resistance.

2. **Factors related to sample**

(a) **Charge on the ion:** Migration rate increase with an increase in the charge on the ion

$$\mu = Q/\ 6\pi r\eta$$

Q – Charge on the molecule (esu)

μ - Electrophoretic mobility

E.g., Ca^{2+} will move faster than Na^+

(b) **Size and shape of the molecule:** The size of the molecule is inversely related to migration. Smaller molecules exhibit faster migration rates when compared to larger molecules. Molecules with different shapes but similar sizes show different migration rates. The frictional resistance for the mobility depends on the shape of the molecule.

(c) **pK_a:** The mobility of molecules increases with a decrease in ionic strength. The degree of ionization is dependent on the pH of the buffer. Thus, the pH of the mobile phase is chosen based on the pK_a of the analyte.

(d) **Diffusion:** Is based on Fick's law of diffusion, which states that the movement of ions occurs from the region of their higher concentration to the region of lower concentration

3. **Factors related to the buffer**

(a) **Composition of buffer:** The commonly used buffers are formate, acetate, citrate, borate, phosphate, EDTA and pyridine. The buffer should not interact with the sample and the support medium.

(b) **pH and ionic strength:** Mobility increases with decreased ionic strength. The pH of the buffer greatly affects the electrophoretic mobility, particularly when the sample is a weak acid/ weak base because the degree of ionization is dependent on pH.

4. **Factors related to the supporting medium**

(a) **Adsorption:** Adsorption of solute molecules on the supporting medium causes the tailing of the sample. It decreases the migration rate and separation efficiency.

(b) **Electro osmosis:** It is caused by the relative charge produced between water molecules and the surface of the supporting medium. The charge may be caused by the interaction of the ionic molecules (sample) with the ionic side chain in the supporting medium.

E.g., sulphonate group in agar and carboxyl group on paper

5. **Viscosity of the medium:** The mobility of ions is inversely proportional to the viscosity of the medium.

TYPES OF ELECTROPHORESIS

Electrophoretic techniques can be broadly divided into two types

(i) **Zone electrophoresis**
  (a) Paper electrophoresis
  (b) Gel electrophoresis
  (c) Thin layer electrophoresis
  (d) Cellulose acetate electrophoresis

(ii) **Moving boundary electrophoresis**
  (a) Capillary electrophoresis
  (b) Iso-tachophoresis
  (c) Isoelectric focusing
  (d) Immunoelectrophoresis

MOVING BOUNDARY ELECTROPHORESIS

This method allows the movement of charged particles in a free moving solution in the absence of a supporting medium.

Disadvantages:

1. Complete separation is not possible.
2. Only the fastest and slowest components can be separated in pure form.
3. Preparative and quantitative analysis cannot be performed
4. Stabilisation of ion boundaries is complicated, and there is a need for specialized equipment

ZONE ELECTROPHORESIS

The disadvantages of moving boundary electrophoresis are eliminated by the use of a stabilizing medium in Zone electrophoresis. It involves the migration of charged particles which are supported on a relatively inert and homogenous solid or gel framework. Separated components are distributed into different zones in the support media.

E.g. of supporting media are paper, agar, cellulose, starch, gels, polyacrylamide gels.

PAPER ELECTROPHORESIS

It is one of the simplest electrophoretic techniques which makes use of special filter papers as the supporting medium. This technique is mostly used for the separation of proteins and amino acids. It is a simple and economical method. Paper electrophoresis is adapted well to routine laboratory use.

PRINCIPLE

The principle is the same for all electrophoretic techniques as given above. The charge carried by the molecule depends on the pH of the medium. The mobility of the ion depends on the voltage applied and the charge on the ion.

WORKING PRINCIPLE

In this technique, Whatman filter paper No.1 or No.3 in a 3 or 5 cm wide strip is used as the supporting medium. The filter paper is moistened with the buffer, and the ends of the paper strip are immersed in beakers of electrolytes. The sample is applied as spots in the centre of the paper. A potential of 5V/cm of paper length is applied. The separation is carried out for several hours. After separation, the paper is dried and stained to get coloured bands.

INSTRUMENTATION

The instrumentation of electrophoresis consists of two parts.

1. Power pack
2. Electrophoretic cell

1. **Power pack:** The power pack provides DC and can control both voltage (0-500 V) and current output (0-150 amp).
2. **Electrophoretic cell:** The electrophoretic cell consists of
   1. Electrodes
   2. Buffer reservoirs
   3. Support for paper
   4. Transparent insulating cover

TYPES OF PAPER ELECTROPHORESIS

1. **Vertical paper electrophoresis** – Filter paper is mounted vertically. The sample is applied in the centre, and movement of the separated sample occurs in both directions depending on the charge.

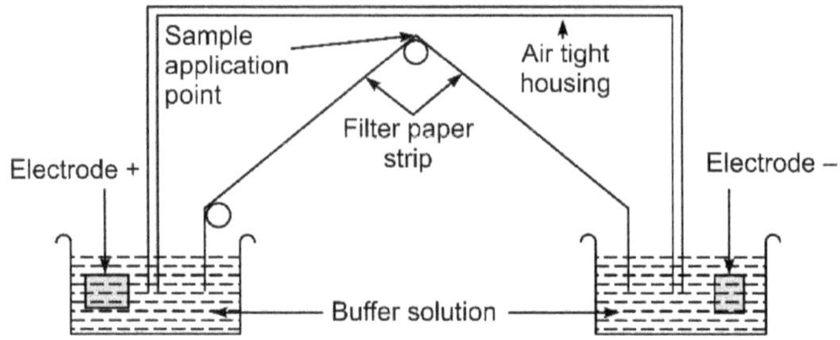

Fig. 16.3 Vertical Electrophoresis.

2. **Horizontal paper electrophoresis-** Filter paper is mounted horizontally. The sample is applied in the centre, and movement of the separated sample occurs depending on the charge.

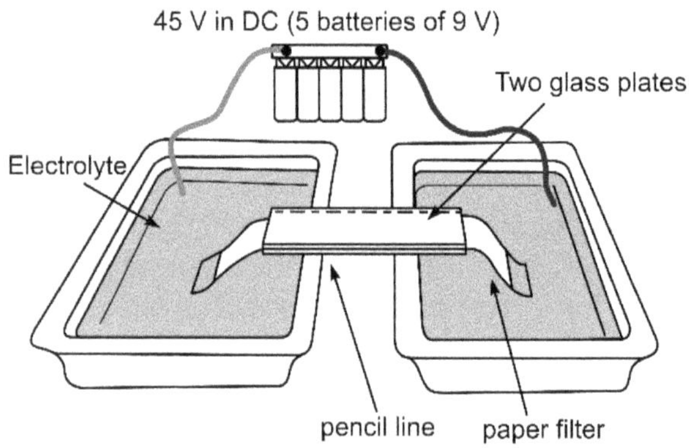

Fig. 16.4 Horizontal Electrophoresis.

3. **Continuous paper electrophoresis** – Predetermined sample volume is applied continuously on the centre of the paper. The suitable voltage causes migration and separation of samples.

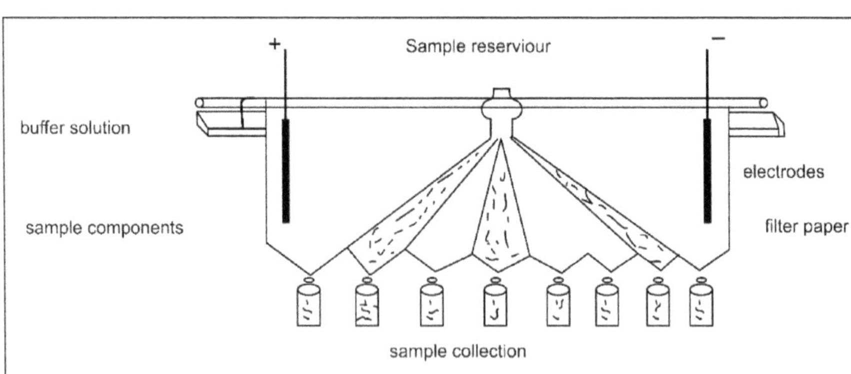

Fig. 16.5 Continuous paper electrophoresis.

Components

(i) **Paper:** Filter paper of good quality contains 95% α-cellulose. It has less adsorption capacity, and Grade No 1 or No 3 paper is used. The filter paper is moistened with buffer and both ends are dipped in buffer solutions in the electrode chambers.

(ii) **Electrodes:** Platinum electrodes are used. DC volt of about 8-15 V is applied

Based on the voltage applied, the electrophoresis can be classified as

Low voltage electrophoresis: Provides a voltage gradient of 5V/cm and a current of 0-150mA. Used for the separation of amino acids, proteins and sugars.

High voltage electrophoresis: Provides voltage gradient up to 100 V/cm. Rapid analysis consumes less time and bands are sharp. Useful for the separation of small ions derived from small peptides and amino acids.

(iii) **Buffers**: Buffers of different pH and ionic strength are used in separation. The buffer (pH) selection depends on the nature of the substance to be separated. The buffer is kept in the electrode chamber on both sides, and the ends of the filter paper are dipped in the buffer after moistening the paper with buffer.

The ionic strength of the buffer affects migration velocity. Mobility decreases with increasing ionic strength. Low ionic strengths lead to diffused bands. Usually, 0.05-0.5 ionic strength is used in separation.

E.g., Veronica buffer (baritone buffer) pH 8.6

Tris-acetate buffer –pH 7.6

Citrate buffer pH 3 or 6.8

Detection: The graph obtained for the unknown sample is compared with the graph of the standard sample for qualitative analysis.

The different techniques used for the detection are

1. **Fluorescence:** The staining reagents used are
   1. Ethidium bromide – used for the detection of DNA and RNA. It gives fluorescence under UV light.
   2. Fluorescamine – used to detect amino acids, peptides and proteins.
   3. Dansyl chloride - used in the detection of amino acids, peptides and proteins
2. **UV absorption:** Detection is carried out between 260-280nm. Used for the detection of amino acids, peptides and proteins.
3. **Staining**
   1. Proteins are stained with Dansyl chloride, Fluorescamine, Bromophenol blue in acetic acid.

2. Nucleic acids are stained with Ethidium bromide
3. For polysaccharides, iodine is used as the staining agent.

   After staining, different biomolecules appear as distinct bands within the gel.

Advantages:

1. Simple technique
2. Economical
3. More number of samples can be analysed simultaneously.

Disadvantages:

1. Time-consuming
2. Certain compounds like proteins, hydrophilic molecules cannot be resolved due to the adsorptive properties of paper leading to tailing and distortion of component bands.
3. Low field strength of 20V/ cm only can be used. It requires a very efficient cooling system.
4. Electro osmosis

Applications:

1. Serum analysis for diagnostic purposes.
2. Analysis of muscle proteins, egg white proteins, milk protein, snake and insect venom can be carried out
3. Alkaloids identification
4. Environmental studies.

GEL ELECTROPHORESIS

The supporting material used in this technique is a gel. The gel is polymerized in the shape of thin slabs and it has wells to load the sample.

Gel electrophoresis is carried out by two methods

1. Vertical gel electrophoresis
2. Horizontal gel electrophoresis

1. **Vertical gel electrophoresis:** Vertical gel electrophoresis contains a stacking gel and a resolving gel. The stacking gel concentrates proteins that are loaded into the well so that the proteins can start to migrate simultaneously. After stacking, the resolution gel separates the proteins based on the molecular size. The top chamber of this system contains the cathode, while the bottom chamber contains the anode. The negatively charged linear strands of proteins migrate toward the anode (top to bottom) upon separation. Vertical gel electrophoresis is usually chosen for separating protein due to the ease of preparation of polyacrylamide gel vertically.

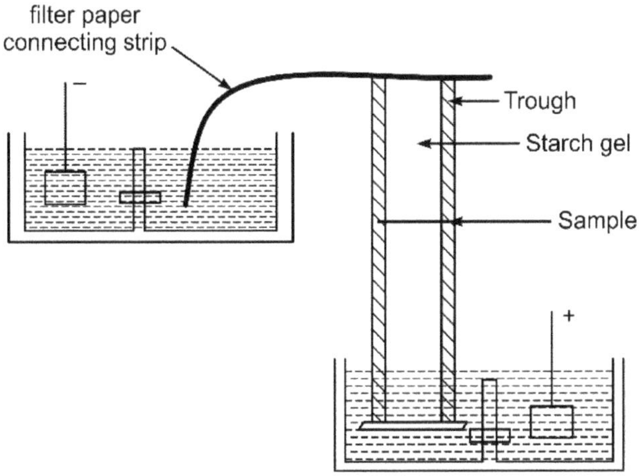

Fig. 16.6 Vertical Gel Electrophoresis.

2. **Horizontal gel electrophoresis:** Horizontal gel electrophoresis is used to separate DNA and RNA. Prior to separation, the DNA and RNA are loaded into the wells of agarose gel in the electrophoresis chamber. The chamber is connected to a cathode and anode, through which an electric field is created by an external power supply. DNA and RNA are negatively charged, they migrate from a negative end to a positive end.

   The various types of the gel used in gel electrophoresis are

   1. **Agarose gel electrophoresis**
   2. **Polyacrylamide gel electrophoresis**
   3. **Starch gel electrophoresis**

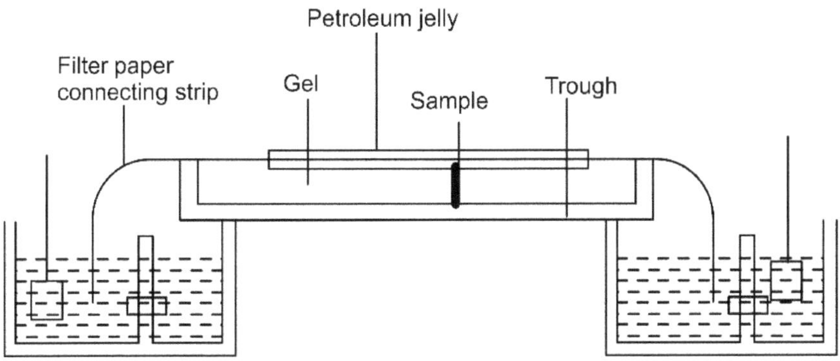

Fig. 16.7 Horizontal starch gel electrophoresis.

1. **Agarose gel electrophoresis:** Agarose gel is a polysaccharide obtained from seaweeds. It is a linear polymer composed of repeating units of D and L – galactose. Agarose melts at 90° and forms a gel at

40°C. Gel formation results in the formation of a mesh of channels with a diameter of 50-200nm.The agarose gel formation is shown in figure 10.8.

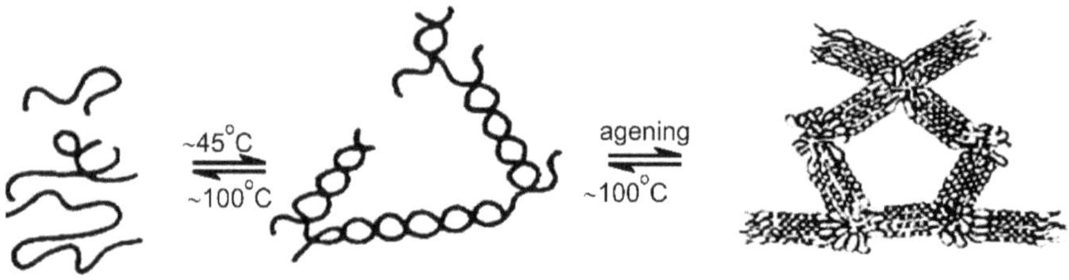

Fig. 16.8 Formation of Agarose gel.

Sample (DNA) is pipetted into the sample wells. The application of an electric current causes the negatively-charged DNA to migrate towards the cathode, positive end. The rate of migration is proportional to size. Small fragments move more quickly. DNA is visualized by including a dye in the gel. E.g., Ethidium bromide. DNA fragments take up the dye as they migrate through the gel. Examination under ultraviolet light causes the DNA to fluoresce. The various steps involved in Agarose gel electrophoresis is shown in figure 10.10

Applications of Agarose Gel Electrophoresis

1. Estimation of the size of DNA molecules
2. Analysis of PCR products, e.g. in molecular genetic diagnosis or genetic fingerprinting
3. Separation of DNA and RNA.
4. Agarose gels are used for the purification of DNA fragments.

Advantages

1. Agarose gels are simple and rapid to prepare.
2. The gel is easily poured and does not denature the samples.
3. The samples can be recovered.

Disadvantages

1. Sometimes gels can melt during electrophoresis.
2. The buffer can become exhausted.
3. Occasional unpredictability in the running of DNA and RNA material

2. **Polyacrylamide gel electrophoresis:** Polyacrylamide gels are chemically cross linked gels formed by the polymerization of acrylamide with a cross linking agent, usually N, N'-methylenebisacrylamide. Polyacrylamide gel electrophoresis **(PAGE)**

is a technique widely used in biochemistry, forensic chemistry, genetics, molecular biology and biotechnology to separate biological macromolecules, usually proteins or nucleic acids according to their electrophoretic mobility. The process of ion migration in PAGE is shown in figure 16.9.

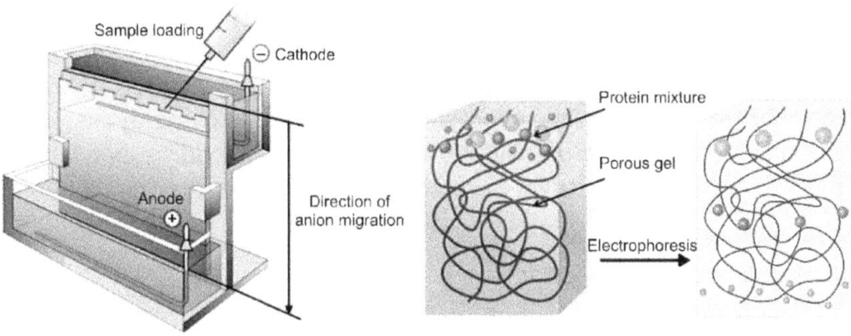

Fig. 16.9 Polyacrylamide gel electrophoresis (PAGE).

The most commonly used form of polyacrylamide gel electrophoresis is the Sodium dodecyl sulphate Polyacrylamide gel electrophoresis **(SDS- PAGE)**.It is used mostly for the separation of proteins.

The mobility of a substance in the gel depends on both charge and size. Hence the general electrophoresis techniques cannot be used to determine the molecular weight of biological molecules. To overcome this difficulty, different protein molecules with different shapes and sizes are denatured with SDS so that the proteins lose their secondary, tertiary or quaternary structure.

The proteins are covered by SDS and are negatively charged. When these denatured protein molecules are loaded onto the gel and placed in an electric field, they migrate towards the anode (positively charged electrode).They have acquired uniform charge by treatment with SDS, and hence the electrophoretic mobility depends primarily on size. The protein molecules are separated by a molecular sieving effect based on size. After staining (protein-specific), the size of a protein can be calculated by comparing its migration distance with that of a known molecular weight ladder (marker).

Buffer: Buffers allow the current to be carried through the sample, and they resist pH changes in the overall solution. The choice of the buffer depends upon the isoelectric point of the analyte. In DNA electrophoresis, buffers like TAE (Tris-acetate-EDTA) and TBE (Tris-borate-EDTA) are used. In protein electrophoresis, SDS (sodium dodecyl sulfate) is commonly used. These buffers facilitate the separation of the samples into readable gels.

Dye: A dye is used to monitor the migration of DNA into a gel or during gel electrophoresis. It is known as DNA gel loading dye. Eg: bromophenol blue, Ficoll 400, Xylene cyanol and glycerol. It is utilized as a colour indicator to monitor the migration of DNA in gel electrophoresis. The loading dye contains Ficoll or glycerol that gives density to the DNA sample. Henceforth, DNA cannot come out and diffuse in the buffer. DNA migration can be strictly monitored. The loading dye is the dye that is used for making the DNA markers, whereas the **tracking dye** is used to stain the DNA. The loading dye is used in the agarose and polyacrylamide gels, whereas the tracking dye is used in the agarose gel. The bromophenol blue is used as a loading dye, whereas the SYBR, an asymmetrical cyanine dye, is used as a tracking dye.

Applications:

1. Measuring molecular weight.
2. Peptide mapping and estimation of protein size.
3. Determination of protein subunits or aggregation structures.
4. Estimation of protein purity.
5. Analysis of the number and size of polypeptide subunits.

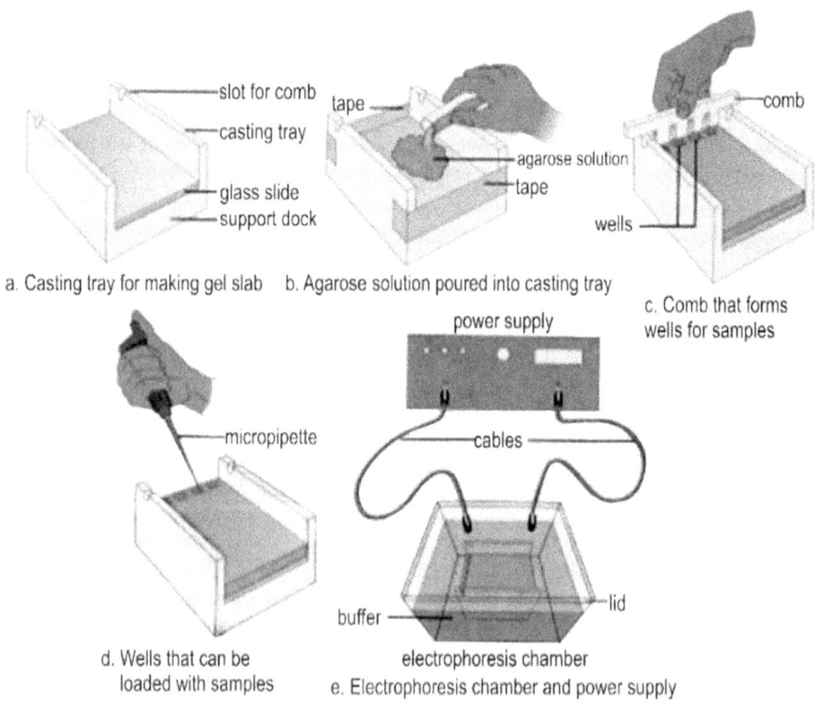

Fig. 16.10 Steps involved in Agarose gel electrophoresis.

Advantages of PAGE

1. Stable chemically cross linked gel with greater resolving power (Sharp bands)
2. Large quantities of DNA can be separated without significant loss in resolution
3. The purity of DNA recovered is extremely high.
4. The pore size of the polyacrylamide gels can be changed easily by changing the concentrations of the two monomers.
5. Low molecular weight fragments can be separated

Disadvantages of PAGE

1. Gels are tedious to prepare and handle.
2. Requires a longer time for preparation than agarose gels.
3. Monomers are toxic
4. Gels often leak, and a new gel is needed for each experiment

3. **Starch gel electrophoresis:** Starch gels are slightly more opaque than agarose or polyacrylamide types and are used for protein electrophoresis. They are formed from partially hydrolysed potato starch. A suspension of granular starch is boiled in a buffer to get a clear colloidal suspension. The semisolid gel is formed on cooling due to the intertwining of the branched chains of amylopectin. Petroleum jelly is used to avoid swelling and shrinking.

Advantages:

1. High resolving power and sharp zones are obtained.
2. Reasonable yield is obtained in the case of proteins
3. Can be used for analytical as well as preparative electrophoresis.

Disadvantages:

1. Electroosmotic effect.
2. Variation in pore size from batch to batch.

TWO-DIMENSIONAL GEL ELECTROPHORESIS (2-D ELECTROPHORESIS)

In the first dimension, proteins are resolved according to their isoelectric points (PI) using immobilized pH gradient electrophoresis (IPGE), isoelectric focusing (IEF), or non-equilibrium pH gradient electrophoresis. (Horizontal separation)

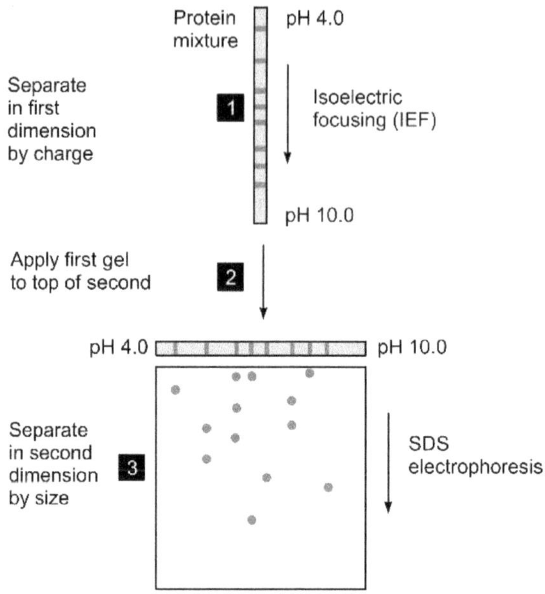

Fig. 16.11 Steps involved in 2D electrophoresis.

In the second dimension, proteins are separated according to their approximate molecular weight using SDS-PAGE. (Vertical separation).

CAPILLARY ELECTROPHORESIS

Capillary electrophoresis (CE) is an analytical technique used to separate ions based on their electrophoretic mobility under the applied voltage. The separation medium used is a capillary tube.

In capillary electrophoresis, the conducting buffer is filled in a capillary tube whose inner diameter is 25–75 μm. Samples are introduced in one end of the capillary tube. As the sample migrates through the capillary, the components separate and elute from the column at different rates. A component with a lower migration rate will be retained and have a longer retention time.

PRINCIPLE

The basic principle is that the rate of migration (separation) depends upon the e/m (charge to mass) ratio. Molecules having different molecular weights will have different charge/mass ratios. This fact is responsible for the differential migration of charged particles.

When a voltage is applied across the electrodes, a potential gradient (E) develops and is given as

$$E = V/d$$

where

V – Voltage and d- the distance between electrodes.

The charged molecules migrate towards oppositely charged electrodes under the influence of an electric field. The positively charged molecules move towards the cathode, and the negatively charged molecules move towards the anode.

The migration of molecules under the influence of current experiences a frictional force. If the charge on the molecule is Q coulombs, then the velocity v of the charged molecule is given as

$$v = EQ/f$$

where

f is the frictional force which retards the mobility of the molecule.

The frictional force is dependent on size, shape, hydrodynamic volume of the molecule, matrix pore size and viscosity of the medium.

The **electrophoretic mobility, μ** of an ion is defined as the ratio of velocity to the potential gradient

$$\mu = v/E = Q/f$$

where

$$f = 6\pi r\eta \textbf{ (Stokes law)}$$

i.e. $$\boldsymbol{\mu = Q/\, 6\pi r\eta}$$

where

Q – Charge on the molecule (esu)

μ - Electrophoretic mobility

r – Radius of the molecule (cm)

η - Viscosity of the medium (poise)

Thus in electrophoresis, molecules with identical or similar charges can also be separated if the molecules have different frictional forces.

The capillary is filled with the buffer of specific pH for the separation of the analyte. The sample is introduced into the capillary by pressure injection or by electrokinetic injection. When a high voltage is generated (> 300V/cm), the sample components move through the capillary at different speeds. Positive components migrate to the negative electrode, and the negative components migrate towards the positive electrode and are detected by the detector.

WORKING

The size and charge on the ion determine its mobility in electrophoresis. The charge is dependent on pH. The pH can be changed to alter the migration of components to get the best separation. The pH is decided based on the pK_a values of the components.

Capillary is made up of fused silica-containing surface silanol groups (Si-O-H), which is slightly acidic in nature. In higher pH values, lots of negative charges are present on capillary walls ($Si-O^-$) due to the loss of proton (H^+). The capillary wall, which has a negative charge, develops a second layer of cations attracted to it. The inner cation layer is stationary, while the outer layer is free to move along the capillary. The applied electric field causes the free cations(+ve) to move towards the cathode(-ve), creating a powerful bulk flow. When the cations are travelling, they drag the buffer fluid with them. This is called **Electro Osmotic Flow** (EOF).

The EOF is flowing towards the cathode, negative electrode. During a separation, uncharged molecules move at the same velocity as the electroosmotic flow (with very little separation). Positively-charged ions move faster, and negatively-charged ions move slower.Thus +ve, -ve and neutral components all can be detected and separated. The diagrammatic representation of electroosmotic flow is given in figure 16.12

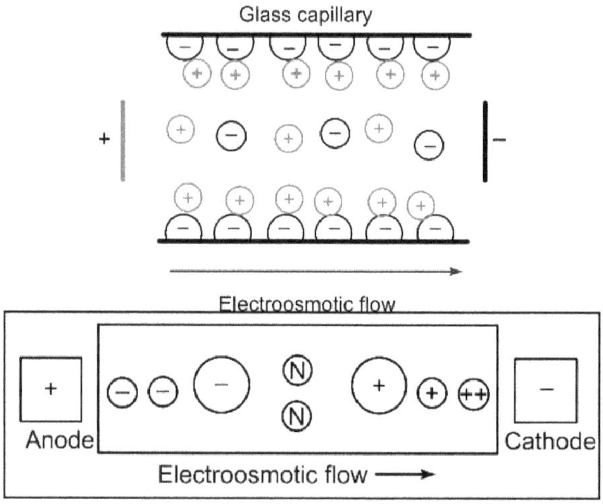

Fig. 16.12 Electroosmotic flow.

DIFFERENT MODES OF CAPILLARY ELECTROPHORESIS

The different modes of capillary electrophoresis are

1. Capillary zone electrophoresis (CZE)
2. Capillary gel electrophoresis (CGE)
3. Micellar electrokinetic capillary chromatography (MEKC)
4. Capillary electrochromatography (CEC)
5. Capillary isoelectric focusing (CIEF)

6. Capillary isotachophoresis (CITP).
7. Electro chromatography (EKC)

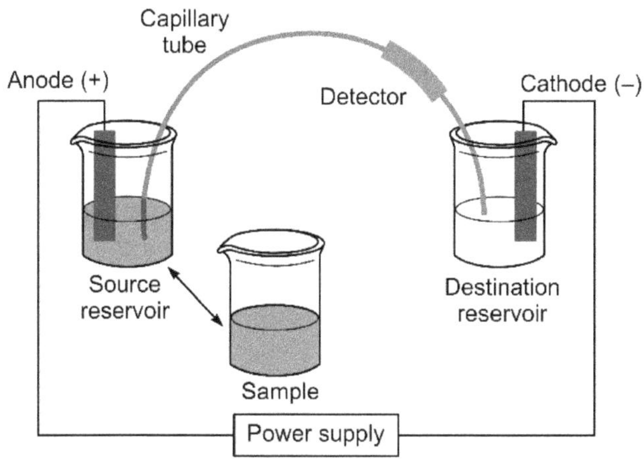

Fig. 16.13 Schematic diagram of instrumentation of Capillary electrophoresis.

The capillary electrophoresis can be classified into continuous and discontinuous systems, as shown in flow chart 16.14.

A continuous system has a background electrolyte acting throughout the capillary as a buffer. The continuous system is further classified into kinetic (constant electrolyte composition) and steady-state (varying electrolyte composition) processes.

A discontinuous system keeps the sample in distinct zones separated by two different electrolytes.

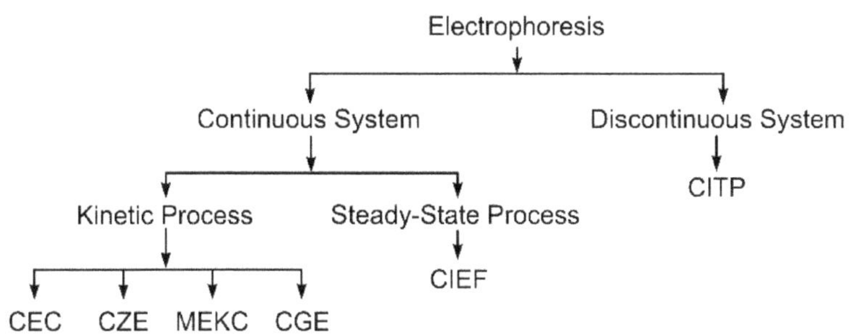

Fig. 16.14 Flow chart showing the types Capillary of electrophoresis.

1. **Capillary Zone Electrophoresis (CZE):** Capillary Zone Electrophoresis (CZE) is the most commonly used technique. It is also known as **free solution capillary electrophoresis**. The separation is based on the differences in electrophoretic mobility. The velocity of the ion is directly proportional to the electrophoretic mobility and the

magnitude of the electric field. The electrophoretic mobility is directly proportional to the charge on the molecule and inversely proportional to the viscosity of the solvent and radius of the atom.

2. **Capillary Gel Electrophoresis (CGE):** A gel matrix is used in the capillary. Separation is based on the size of the components. Different sized but same mobility components are separated by this technique. CGE is used for protein and DNA separation. Smaller molecules move faster and the bigger molecules move slowly in CGE.
3. **Micellar Electrokinetic Capillary Chromatography (MEKC):** Solutes are partitioning between micelles and the solvent in MEKC. When a surfactant is added to a solution, aggregates of surfactant molecules are formed above the critical micelle concentration. These aggregates are called micelles. The aggregates have polar negatively charged surfaces outside (Hydrophilic) and non-polar surfaces inside the micelle(hydrophobic).

   Hydrophobic molecules spend more time with micelles, while the hydrophilic molecule migrates faster with the solvent.

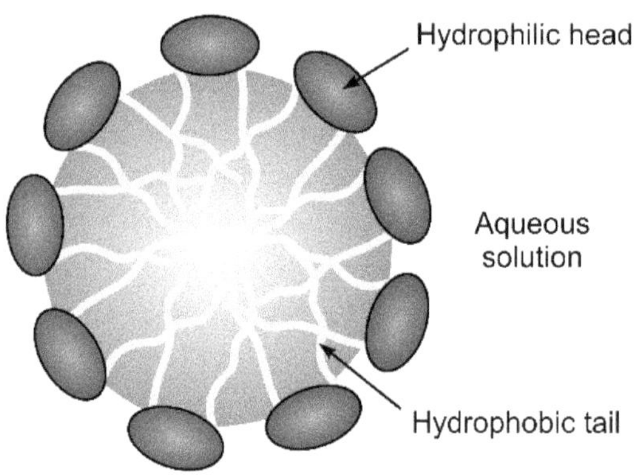

Fig. 16.15 Micelle formation.

   Factors that affect the electroosmotic flow in MEKC are pH, surfactant concentration, additives, and polymer coatings of the capillary wall.

4. **Capillary Electrochromatography (CEC):** The capillary is packed with silica particles. The separation principle is the same as column chromatography. Electroosmotic flow is present due to the charges on the silica. The flow obtained is a plug-type flow.
5. **Capillary Isoelectric Focusing (CIEF):** CIEF is commonly used to separate peptides and proteins. These molecules are zwitterionic in nature because they contain both positive and negative charges. Functional groups attached to the main chain and the pH of the environment determines the charge on the molecule. Each molecule

has a specific isoelectric point (pI). When the surrounding pH equals this pI, the molecule carries no net charge (zwitterion form).

At pH lower than pI – molecule exists as a positive ion

pH higher than pI – molecule exists as a negative ion.

Since the charge on the molecule changes with pH, a pH gradient can be used to separate molecules in a mixture. A pH gradient is maintained across the capillary and a voltage is applied. The anode (+ve voltage) of the capillary is situated in an acidic solution (low pH), while the cathode (-ve voltage) is situated in a basic solution (high pH). The components of the mixture migrate at different rates to the pH value that equals the pI value of each component. At pI, the molecule exists as a zwitterion, and its migration is stopped.

Pressure is applied to move the complete pH gradient through the capillary, and the components pass through the detection window.

6. **Capillary Isotachophoresis (CITP):** It is a discontinuous system based on the principle of moving boundary electrophoresis. The technique of isotachophoresis depends on the development of potential gradients.

   A leading electrolyte (e.g. chloride) with a higher mobility than the analytes and a trailing electrolyte (e.g. glycinate) with lower mobility is used. The solution in which the separation takes place is normally an aqueous medium containing sucrose to provide a higher density to the solution.

   The technique of isotachophoresis depends on the development of a potential gradient.

   The analytes are positioned between the electrolytes and when the voltage is applied, they migrate in order of decreasing mobility. This establishes the potential gradient and from that point on, all the analytes move at the same speed.

   Individual zones border one another but represent completely separated components without overlap.

   In isotachophoresis, no buffer is mixed with the sample, so current flow is carried only by charged sample ions.

7. **Electro Chromatography (EKC):** It is used to separate chiral compounds by differential interaction of enantiomers with cyclodextrins.

   Advantages of CE

   1. High separation efficiency
   2. Rapid technique and high resolution of separation
   3. Detection is simple.
   4. Easy operation and low waste generation,

Disadvantages

1. The small diameter of the capillary causes dissipation of heat, leading to increased diffusion.
2. Sample sticking to capillary walls.
3. Inconsistent retention times.

APPLICATIONS

1. **DNA fingerprinting:** Using CE, individual nucleotides can be identified.
2. **Drug analysis:** Drugs and related compounds can be identified with CE.
3. **To study the characteristics of protein:** Proteins are amphoteric in nature, and they can be separated and purified by CE using the isoelectric point pI.
4. **DNA sequencing:** DNA sequencing is the process of determining the order of nucleotides in DNA. This sequencing can be carried out with CE
5. Capillary electrophoresis is also used for the simultaneous estimation of NH^{4+}, Na^+, K^+, Mg^{2+} and Ca^{2+} in biological fluids.

CHAPTER 17

Gel Chromatography

Gel chromatography is a type of chromatography in which the separation of the molecules is based on **molecular size**. Gel chromatography is called Gel filtration chromatography, when the proteins and soluble polymers are separated using an **aqueous mobile phase.** When an **organic mobile phase** is used to separate **polar and organic soluble polymers,** the technique is called **Gel permeation chromatography. The gel chromatography is also called Size exclusion chromatography, Molecular exclusion chromatography, Molecular sieve chromatography.**

This technique uses porous particles as stationary phase and buffers as mobile phase. The stationary phase is a gel or a porous matrix with cross-linking in the form of beads.

PRINCIPLE AND MECHANISM

A mixture of compounds to be separated with different molecular sizes is passed through a porous matrix of stationary phase with buffer as mobile phase. The separation of the molecules is achieved on the basis of their molecular size and shape. The porous resins make use of their molecular sieving property to separate the components. The column packed with porous beads is equilibrated with the mobile phase (buffer), which fills the pores of the matrix and the interstitial spaces. Sometimes, the liquid inside the pores is referred to as the stationary phase, and this liquid is in equilibrium with the liquid outside the particles, referred to as the mobile phase.

Large molecular weight molecules are excluded from the pores, pass through the void space, interstitial spaces between the gel particles and they get eluted first. Smaller molecular weight particles pass through the porous matrix, enter into the pores of the gel and hence pass through the column at a slower rate, getting eluted later. Molecules with partial access to pores elute in the order of decreasing molecular size. Thus, larger molecules elute first, and smaller molecules elute later. Samples are eluted isocratically. (i.e.) There is no need of a different buffer for elution.

The distribution of molecules in gel filtration chromatography varies between 0 to 1. For larger molecules, K=0, which has no access to the mobile phase in the pores. For small molecules, K=1 can enter into the mobile phase in the pores. This variation of K between 0 and 1 helps in the separation of molecules based on their sizes, even with narrow molecular size variation.

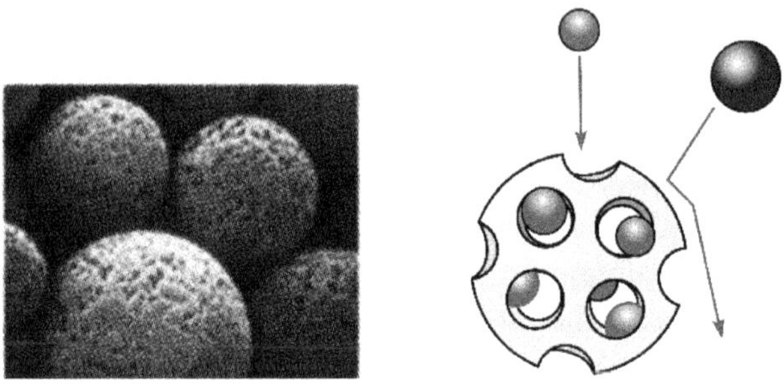

Fig. 17.1 Resin bead.

The resin bead is schematically represented as the ball. Large molecules cannot enter into the pore and travel with the mobile phase to get eluted quickly. But the molecules, which are smaller in size, enter in the pores and get eluted later.

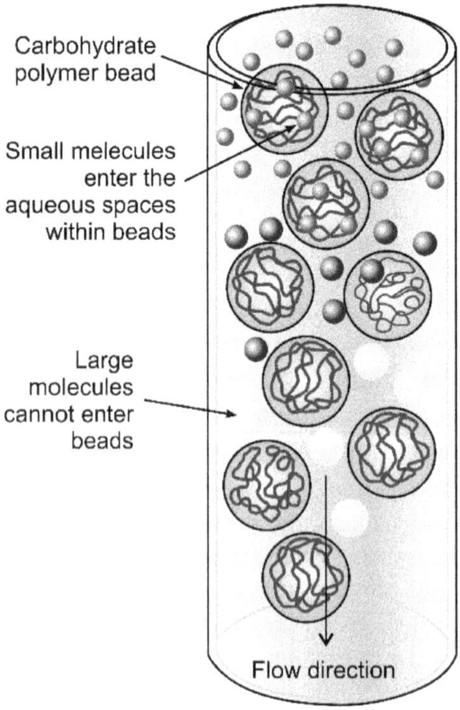

Fig. 17.2 Separation mechanism in Gel chromatography.

The eluted components can be detected by a suitable detector.

V_t = total column volume = $V_g + V_i + V_0$

V_g – Volume occupied by gel

V_i – Volume of the solvent in pores,

V_0 – Free solvent in column (space outside packing material)

V_e – elution volume of the compound

$V_e = V_0 + k_d V_i$

where k_d is distribution coefficient

V_c = Total (geometric) volume of the column

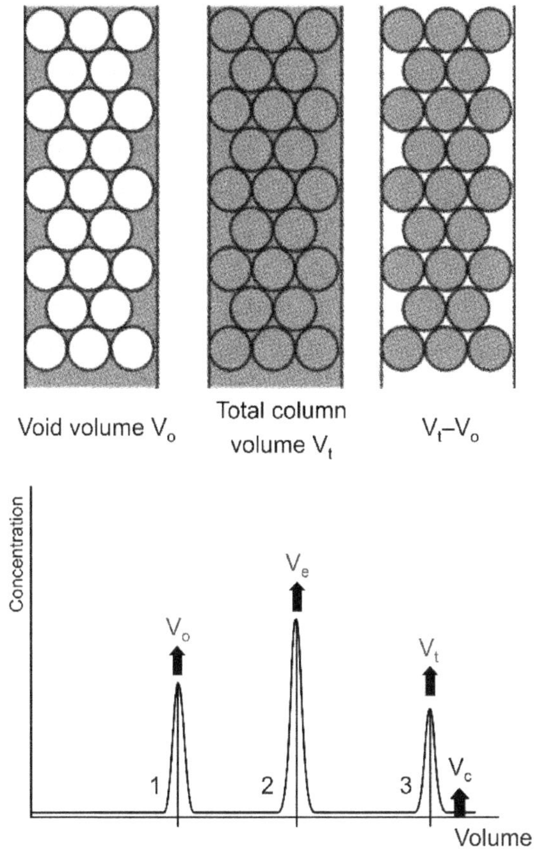

Fig. 17.3 Different volume terms used in Gel chromatography.

INSTRUMENTATION

The components of Gel chromatography are

1. Stationary phase
2. Mobile phase

3. Column
4. Pumps
5. Detectors

1. **Stationary phases:** These are semi-permeable, porous beads with a well-defined range of pore sizes. Cross-linked polymers are used as beads. The degree of cross-linking determines the pore size. Common stationary phases used are dextran, agarose or polyacrylamide. Some of the commercially available gel polymers are given below in table 14.1

Table 17.1 Some of the commercially available gel polymers.

Polymer gel	The molecular weight of molecules separated
Sephadex G (dextran based)	3000-70,000 >70,000 m.wt excluded from the column
Bio gel P150 (Polyacrylamide based)	15,000-1,50,000 m.wt
Sepharose 6B (agarose based)	10,000-4,00,000 m.wt

Smaller pore sizes are used for rapid desalting of proteins or protein purification

Intermediate pore sizes are used for small protein separation

Very large pore sizes are used for the separation of biological complexes.

Dextran: Dextran is a homo polysaccharide of glucose residues. It is available as dry beads, and the beads swell when water is added. The trade name is Sephadex. It is used to separate small peptides and globular proteins with small to average molecular mass.

Polyacrylamide: Cross-linking of acrylamide with N, N-methylene bis acrylamide gives these gels. They are used for the separation of small peptides and globular proteins. They are sold as bio-gel P. They are available in a wide range of pore sizes.

Agarose: Agarose is a Linear polymer of D-galactose and 3, 6 anhydro-1-galactose. The gel is held together with hydrogen bonds. The concentration in the gel determines the pore size. The pores of agarose gel are larger when compared with Sephadex or bio-gel P. Hence used for the separation of large globular proteins or long linear molecules such as DNA

Choice of the stationary phase depends on the molecular size, the shape of the molecules, operating pressure and temperature, flow rate, the viscosity of the sample, pH and tolerance for detergents and salts.

2. **Mobile phases:** Buffers are used as a mobile phase in gel filtration chromatography. E.g., phosphate buffer pH 7, Sodium chloride solutions, ammonium acetate, ammonium bicarbonate etc. Tris – HCl can also be used as a buffer.

   The sample is dissolved in the mobile phase and introduced into the column. Choice of the mobile phase depends on the type of separation and nature of the component to be separated.

3. **Columns:** Resolution increases with column length. Generally, long columns with small diameters are used. Length of the column can be 25,30,50,60 cm to 7.5-8 mm in diameter. Sometimes diameters of 2-3 mm are also used. If the column diameter increases, loading capacity increases as the bed volume of the column increases.

   V_t – total column volume, also called bed volume

   V_0 – void volume is the space between gel particles. It is usually 1/3rd of bed volume.

   The larger particles elute through void volume.

   Smaller molecules enter into the mobile phase present in the pores of the stationary phase and elute later.

   $V_t - V_0$ = volume occupied by the gel (V gel), including gel matrix

   V_s (stationary phase) = V_t-V_0-V_{gel}

   Column packing: There are three steps in column packing

   (a) Swelling of gel
   (b) Pouring of the gel into the column
   (c) Equilibration of the column.

   (a) Swelling of gel: It is done by two methods.

   Weighed quantity of the dried gel powder is mixed with the eluent (solvent) and allowed to swell. It is kept till equilibrium is obtained.

   The gel slurry is heated in a water bath at about 100° C. After swelling, the slurry is cooled and packed in the column.

   The gel and the entire buffer used in the chromatographic column have to be degassed to avoid air bubbles. This helps in uniform packing of column giving good resolution.

   (b) Pouring of gel in the column: The glass column is mounted vertically in a stand, and the buffer is poured through the column outlet to remove any air bubbles in the column. Now the gel slurry is poured with the help of a glass rod to avoid the trapping of air bubbles. The gel is allowed to settle down, and the excess buffer is decanted.

   (c) Equilibration of the column: The column equilibration is done with the mobile phase buffer with a slow flow rate. The column is equilibrated with 2-3 bed volumes of the buffer.

4. **Pumps:** The pumps used in the HPLC systems are used here. They are
    1. reciprocating piston pump,
    2. syringe pump
    3. constant pressure pump
5. **Detectors:** The detectors used in Gel filtration chromatography can be classified as

    I. Concentration sensitive detectors: These detectors are further classified as

    1. **Bulk Property Detectors-** e.g.-Refractive Index (RI) Detector
    2. **Solute Property Detectors-** e.g.-Ultraviolet (UV) Absorption Detector
    3. **Evaporative Detectors- e.g.,** Evaporative Light Scattering Detector (ELSD)

    II. Molar mass sensitive detectors: These detectors are classified as

    1. **Light Scattering Detectors:** Low Angle Light Scattering (LALS) Detectors
       Multi-angle Light Scattering (MALS) detectors
    2. **Viscosity Detectors- Differential Viscometers:** Other detectors used in Gel chromatography are Flame Ionization Detector (FID), Mass Spectrometer or Fourier Transform Infrared (FTIR) Spectrometer.

    1. **UV–visible detectors:** It is a photometric detector. Substances that absorb UV light can be detected by this solute property detector. These are versatile detectors with the best sensitivity and linearity. They are cost-effective, popular and widely used. There are three types of UV detector
        (a) Fixed wavelength detectors
        (b) Variable wavelength detectors
        (c) Photodiode array detectors

        (a) Fixed Wavelength detector: Detector operates at 254 nm only because most of the compounds absorb at this wavelength
        Simplest and cheapest of the UV/VIS detectors
        Limited in flexibility
        Limited in types of compounds that can be monitored

        (b) Variable Wavelength detector: In this detector, a single wavelength is monitored at any given time, but operates in the wavelength range 190-900 nm.
        More expensive requires more advanced optics
        More versatile, used for a broader range of compounds
        More sensitive due to photomultiplier tube

(c) **Photodiode Array Detector:** In this detector, the absorbance of solutes is measured simultaneously at several different wavelengths. Light from the emission source, such as a deuterium lamp, is collimated by an achromatic lens system. The total light passes through the sample cell and then to a holographic grating. In this way, all wavelengths of light emitted by the source are passing through the sample. The dispersed light from the grating is allowed to fall onto a diode array. The array contains many hundreds of diodes, and the output from each diode is processed by a computer and stored.

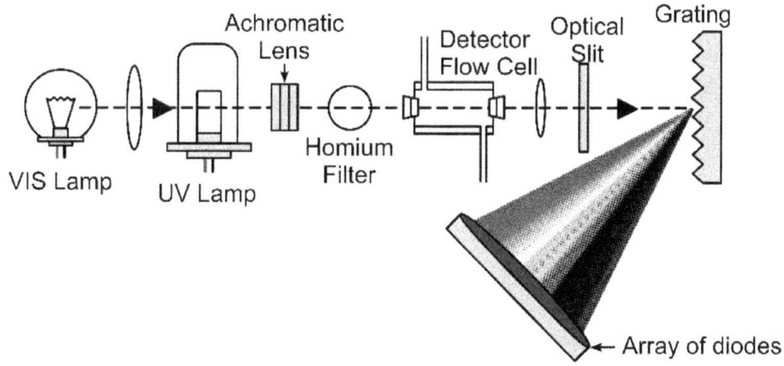

Fig. 17.4 Diode Array detector.

2. **Refractive index detector:** A Refractive index detector measures the molecule's ability to deflect light in a flowing mobile phase in a flow cell relative to a static mobile phase contained in a reference cell. The amount of deflection is proportional to the concentration of the solute in the mobile phase. The refractive index (RI) detector is one of the least sensitive LC detectors. This detector is extremely useful for detecting the compounds that are non-ionic, not showing ultraviolet light absorption and substances that do not exhibit fluorescence. E.g. sugar, alcohol, fatty acid and polymers.
3. **Fluorescence Detector:** These detectors are used for the substances that give fluorescence when subjected to radiation from a source. The excitation light is usually a low-pressure mercury lamp providing relatively high-intensity UV light at 253.7 nm. Many substances that fluoresce will be excited at this wavelength. The excitation light is focused by a quartz lens through the cell. A second lens, set normal to the incident light, focuses the fluorescent light onto a photocell. As it is very sensitive, its response is only linear over a relatively limited concentration range.

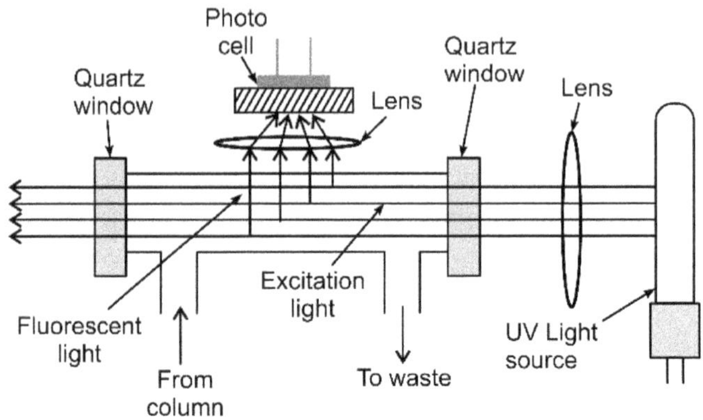

Fig. 17.5 Fluorescence detector.

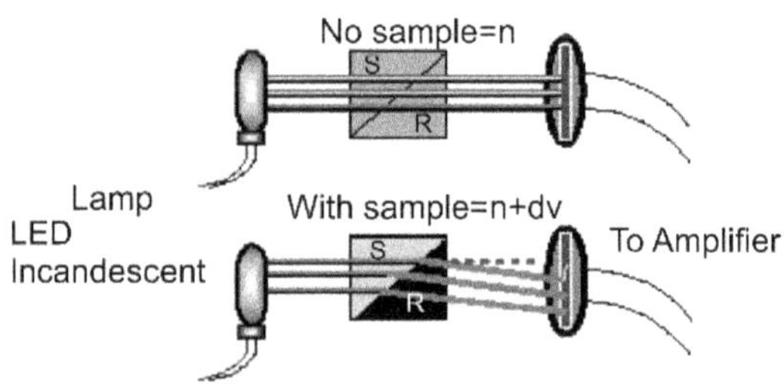

Fig. 17.6 Refractive index detector.

4. **Electrochemical detectors:** The current resulting from an oxidation/reduction reaction of the analyte at a suitable electrode is measured in this detector. The current produced is directly proportional to the analyte concentration.

   The eluent should be electrically conductive.

   E.g. of drugs detected using this detector are phenol, catecholamines, nitrosamines, and organic acids in the ng range.
5. **Conductivity detectors:** This detector is used in ion-exchange chromatography for the detection of ionic compounds. The ability of the mobile phase to conduct current when placed in a flow cell between two electrodes is measured. Conductivity detectors measure the resistance, which is directly proportional to the concentration of ions present in the solution. Two electrodes placed in mobile phase form each corresponding to one arm of a Wheatstone Bridge.
6. **Evaporative light scattering detector (ELSD):** Detection is based on the scattering of a beam of light by particles of the compound.

   The three steps involved in detection are

   Nebulisation

   Desolvation

   Detection

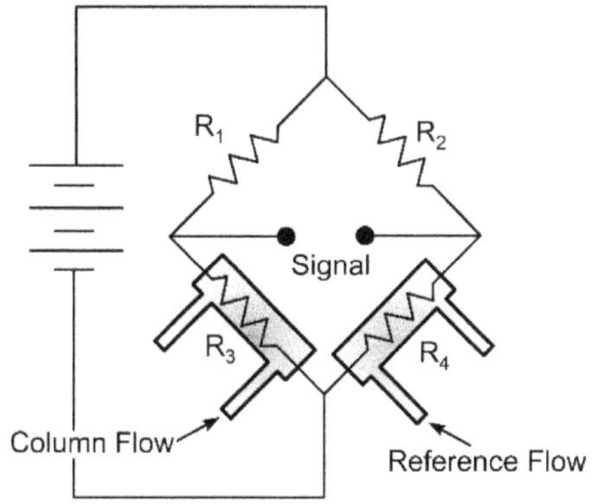

Fig. 17.7 Wheatstone Bridge.

A stream of inert gas nebulises the flow from the column. (Nebulizing is to convert a liquid into a fine spray or mist). The volatile mobile phase is evaporated, leaving tiny particles of the analytes. The particles, when passed through a laser beam, scatter the laser light. The scattered light is measured at right angles to the laser beam by a photodiode detector. It is a universal detector. The compound does not require a chromophore for detection by this detector.

7. **Mass spectrometer:** The HPLC system in which the Mass spectrophotometer is used as the detector is called LC-MS. In this method, the separation power of HPLC is combined with the detection power of Mass spectrometry. Mass spectrometry (MS) is a powerful analytical tool that can supply both structural information about compounds and quantitative data relating to mass.

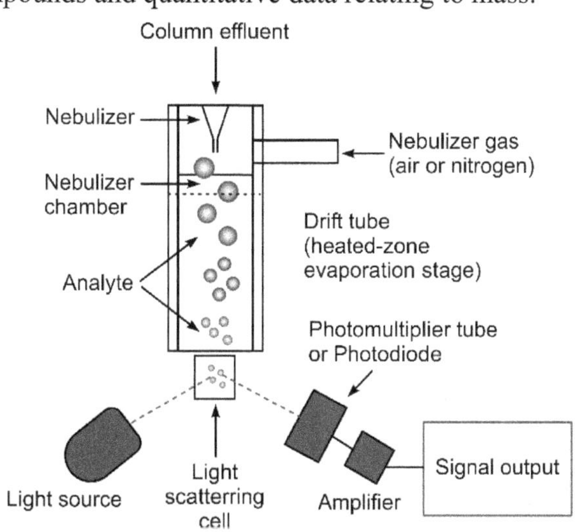

Fig. 17.8 Evaporative light scattering detector (ELSD).

8. **Chiral detectors:** Optically active compounds such as amino acids, sugars, terpenes and other compounds containing asymmetric carbon are detected by chiral detectors. There are two types of chiral detection techniques,
   1. Polarimetry or optical rotary dispersion (ORD)
   2. Circular dichroism (CD).

   ORD detectors are based on differences in refractive index

   CD detectors identify the enantiomers by measuring the differential absorption of right and left-handed circularly polarised light.

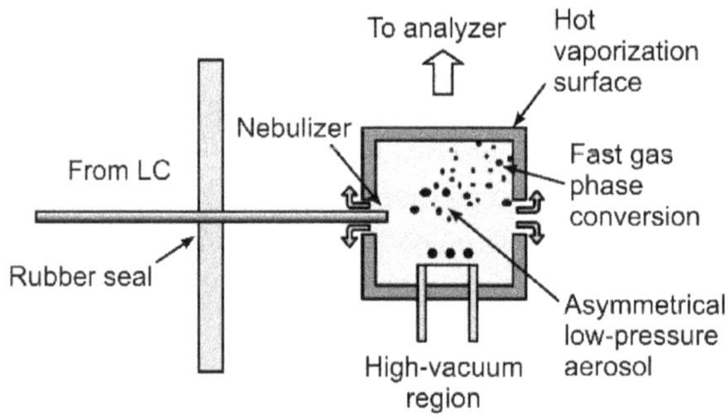

Fig. 17.9 Mass detector.

9. **Light Scattering Detectors:** An array of collimated detector elements is used to detect scattered light at discrete scattering angles.

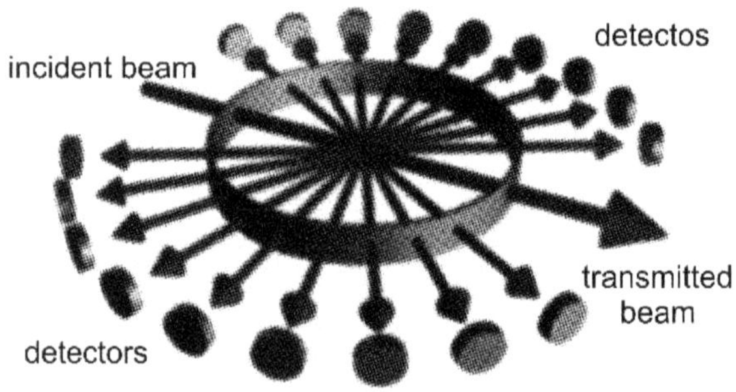

Fig. 17.10 Light Scattering devices.

Each sample is treated sequentially by a collimated light source, like a monochromatic laser, and the scattered light from each sample is measured as a function of scattering angle. This is shown schematically in figure 17.10, where an array of collimated diode detector elements detect scattered light at discrete scattering angles. This forms the basis of detection in these detectors.

A MALS detector employs three to twenty detectors arranged at various angles around the sample flow cell. A 90° detector is always included, and the remaining detectors are arranged as low as 12° and as high as 168°. A MALS detector measures the scattered light at a variety of angles, uses a model to extrapolate back to 0° to determine the molecular weight of the sample.

The RALS/LALS detector comprises of 90° and 7° detectors. For smaller samples of 10-15 nm in radius, the 90° detector is ideal because it is situated at a right angle to the incident beam, maximising the signal to noise ratio. The smaller samples scatter light with the same intensity in all directions. The RALS detector offers direct measurement of a sample's molecular weight. For samples with a radius larger than that 10-15 nm range displaying angular dependence, the LALS detector provides a measurement at 7°, which is the lowest detector position available.

Schematic diagram of Gel filtration chromatography instrumentation

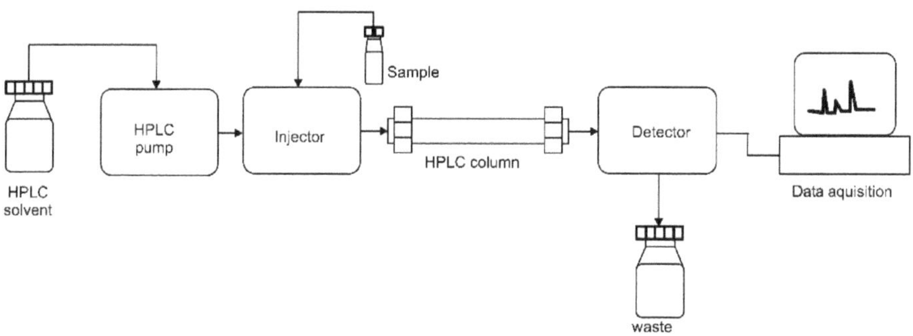

Fig. 17.11 Schematic diagram of Instrument in Gel filtration chromatography.

Working of gel filtration chromatography

1. **Preparation of column:** After packing the column as given above, it is equilibrated with the buffer.
2. **Loading of the sample:** The sample should be concentrated, and the sample size is normally 1% of bed volume. The sample should be filtered before loading. The sample is charged into the column, followed by the mobile phase.
3. **Elution:** Elution is carried out with the buffer, and the flow rate is maintained at 0.25 – 5ml/min. Fractions of individual components are collected separately. The same buffer is used for development as well as elution.

   V_e – elution volume is defined as the volume of the buffer that elutes from the column before a particular peak appears in the elution profile.

   K_d – distribution coefficient of the analyte

   $K_d = V_e\text{-}V_0/V_t\text{-}V_0$

After elution, the column is washed thoroughly with 1-2 bed volumes of the buffer.

4. **Detection:** UV detector is the commonly used detector. To determine the molecular weight of the unknown compound, a calibration graph is drawn in semi-log paper. For calibration of the gel in the column, logarithms of the molecular weights of standard proteins are plotted against their respective ratios of elution volume to column void volume, the column void volume being the elution volume of a very large molecule such as Blue Dextran. The standard markers used are Yeast alcohol dehydrogenase (1,50,000 daltons). Bovine serum albumin (66,000 daltons), carbonic anhydrase (29,000 daltons), cytochrome C (12,400 daltons).

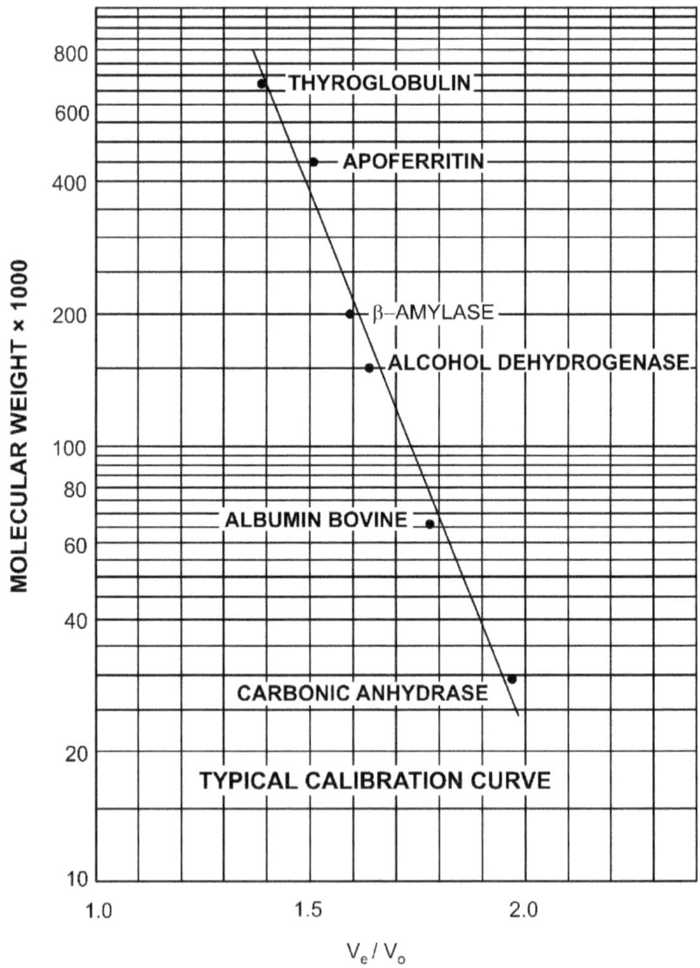

Fig. 17.12 Calibration graph used for molecular weight determination of unknown compound.

FACTORS AFFECTING RESOLUTION IN GEL FILTRATION

1. Column dimensions
2. Stationary phase packing density
3. Buffer composition
4. Sample volume and concentration
5. Particle size distribution
6. Flow rate of mobile phase
7. Pore size of packing
8. Viscosity of sample and buffer

Advantages

1. Biomolecules that are sensitive to changes in pH, the concentration of metal ions or cofactors and harsh environmental conditions can be analysed.
2. A significant advantage of gel filtration is that conditions can be varied to suit the type of sample without altering the separation.
3. Separations can be performed in the presence of essential ions or cofactors, detergents, urea, guanidine hydrochloride at a high or low ionic strength
4. Analysis can be performed at 37 °C or in the cold room according to the requirements of the experiment.
5. Molecules do not bind to the chromatography medium, so buffer composition does not directly affect resolution (the degree of separation between peaks).
6. Short analysis time and a small amount of mobile phase is sufficient.
7. Well defined separation with Narrow bands and good sensitivity.
8. There is no sample loss.

APPLICATIONS

1. **Molecular weight determination:** If the elution volume is known, the calibration graph can be used to determine molecular weight.
2. Separation of macromolecules like proteins and polypeptides, detection and separation of oligomers.
3. Purification of macromolecules, proteins, enzymes, amino acids, and polysaccharides. The impurities are separated based on their molecular weight.
4. Desalting- is the process of removal of salts from protein samples when salt is used in the separation of protein fraction. Salts travel slowly, whereas the large molecules get eluted faster in gel chromatography.

CHAPTER 18

Affinity Chromatography

Affinity chromatography is a sample purification technique, used mainly for biological molecules like proteins, enzymes etc. It is a type of chromatography that makes use of a specific affinity between the component to be isolated and a molecule that can bind to it (ligand).

PRINCIPLE

In this method, a mixture of proteins or nucleic acid molecules are separated by specific interactions with a compound known as ligand. Biological interactions between ligand and target molecule can be a result of electrostatic or hydrophobic interactions, Vander Waals' forces and hydrogen bonding.

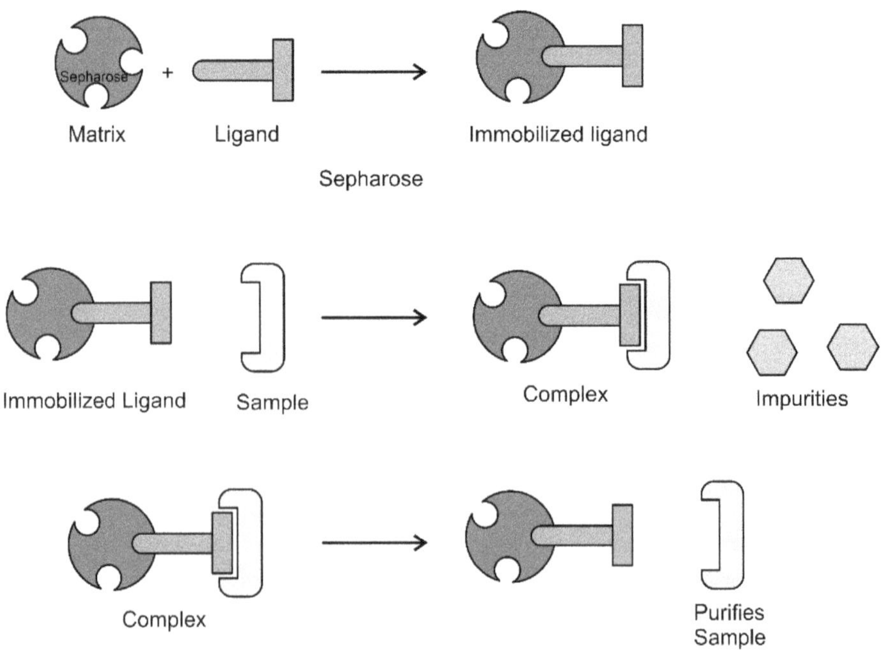

Fig. 18.1 Principle of Affinity chromatography.

The ligand is immobilized on a support. The interactions are specific biological interactions like enzyme-substrate, receptor-ligand or antigen-antibody reactions. These reactions are reversible reactions used for purification. The ligand which is attached to the solid matrix acts as the stationary phase. Ligand coupled matrices are commonly available.

The molecule to be separated is dissolved in the suitable solvent and injected into an equilibrated column. The molecules with more affinity for the ligand are retained in the column and the substances with no affinity for the ligand are washed through the column.

The reversible binding of the ligand to the specific molecule or group of molecules form the basis of affinity chromatography

The elution of the retained molecules can be carried out by

1. Altering pH
2. Changing temperature
3. Changing ionic strength
4. Changing the organic solvent concentration

COMPONENTS OF AFFINITY CHROMATOGRAPHY

1. Matrix (support)
2. Spacer arm
3. Ligand

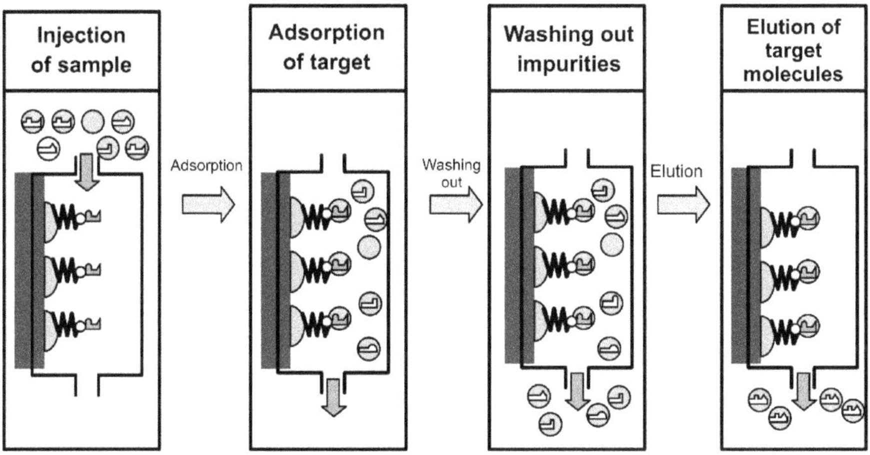

Fig. 18.2 Steps involved in Affinity chromatography.

1. **Matrix (support):** Matrix is the solid support to which the specific ligand is bonded covalently.

The characteristics of the matrix are

1. It should not be soluble in solvents and buffers used in the chromatographic development
2. It should not adsorb molecules to itself
3. It should be chemically and mechanically stable
4. The ligand or the spacer arm should be able to couple without undergoing any changes in its binding properties.
5. It should have a large surface area for the attachment of the ligand.

Agarose and polysaccharide are the most commonly used matrix materials. The other support materials used are Agarose (Sepharose), cross-linked dextran (Sephadex), Polyacrylamide, cross-linked cellulose, silica, methacrylate and polystyrene. They are usually used in the form of beads.

2. **Spacer arms:** Attachment of the ligand directly to the support matrix may alter the binding property of the ligand with macromolecules. To prevent this alteration, spacers or spacer arms are used.

The optimum length of the spacer arms can be 6-10 carbon atoms or equivalent to it. Spacers are used for small immobilized ligands. Eg of spacers :1, 6 diamino hexane and 6-amino hexanoic acid.

For agarose matrix, spacers like cyanogen bromide, 2-thiopyridyl, 1, 6 diamino hexane and 6-amino hexanoic acid can be used.

For polyacrylamide matrix, aminoethyl and hydrazide spacers can be used.

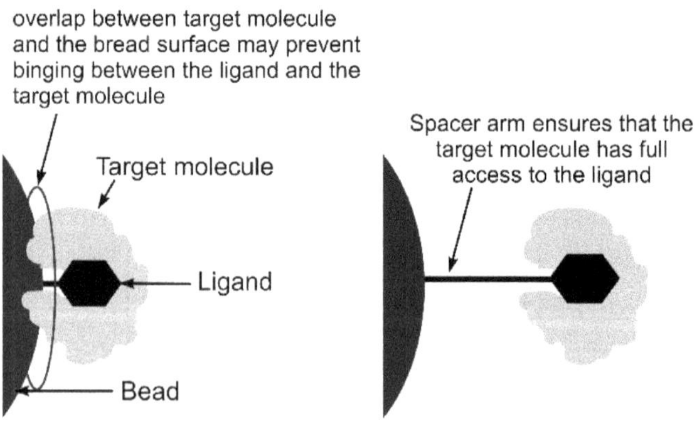

Fig. 18.3 Spacer arm.

3. **Ligand:** The ligand binds reversibly to the specific molecule or group of molecules and this forms the basis of affinity chromatography.

The choice of the ligand depends on

1. The binding affinity of the ligand and the target molecule.

2. The ligand should have a chemically modifiable group so that it can get attached to the support matrix without losing binding activity.
   E.g., of ligands: coagulation factors
   Heparin for lipoproteins, Proteins A and G for immunoglobulins
   Antigen for antibody
   Hormone for the purification of hormone receptor protein
   Substrate for enzyme

SAMPLE PREPARATION

Samples should be clear and free from particulate matter. Sample preparation techniques including clarification are used to remove the components that interfere with binding (the interaction between the target molecule and the ligand).

The column must be pre-equilibrated in the binding buffer before sample application. Samples are applied at a high flow rate if there is a strong affinity between the ligand and the target molecule that quickly reach equilibrium. However, for interactions with weak affinity or slow equilibrium, a lower flow rate should be used.

PROCEDURE FOR AFFINITY CHROMATOGRAPHY

1. The affinity stationary phase is equilibrated with binding buffer
2. The sample is applied under the conditions required for the specific binding of the target molecule to the ligand. Reversible binding of the target molecules occurs, and the unbound material is washed through the column.
3. Elution of the bound protein is carried out by changing the working conditions.
   Elution can be performed by three methods
   (a) Specific method – competitive binding
   This method is carried out by using a substance that has more binding affinity for the ligand than the target compounds
   (b) Non –specific methods
      1. Changing pH
      2. Changing ionic strength or polarity
      3. Adding free ligands
   (a) Specific method – competitive binding: In this type of competitive binding, A ligand with more binding affinity either for the ligand or for the target compound is used. These free ligands, when added to the column with ligand-target compound

bindings, compete for binding with ligand or target compounds depending on their affinity. The figure shows the addition of a competitive free ligand with binding affinity for the target compound.

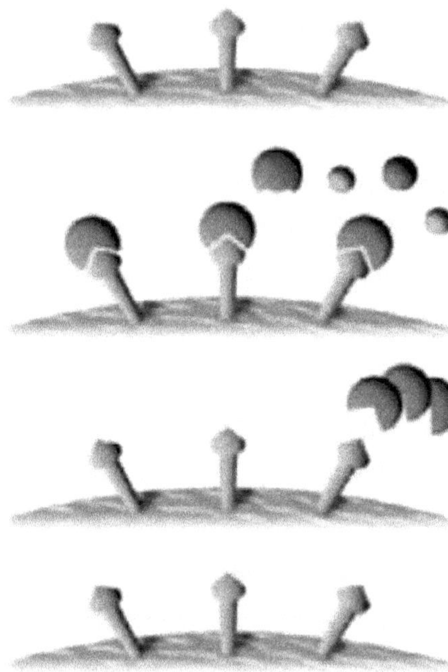

Fig. 18.4 Diagrammatic representation of procedure in affinity chromatography.

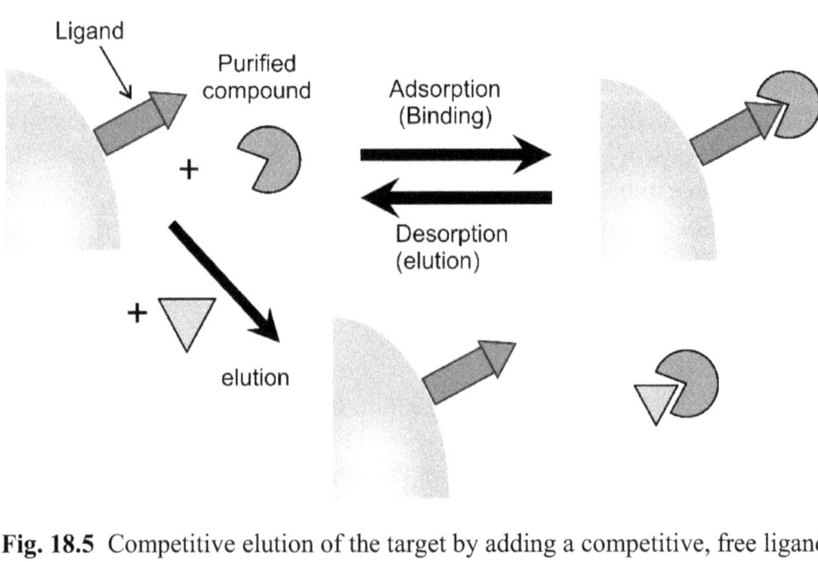

Fig. 18.5 Competitive elution of the target by adding a competitive, free ligand (triangle).

(b) Non –specific methods

pH elution: A change in pH alters the degree of ionization of charged groups on the ligand or the bound protein. This change may affect the binding sites directly, reducing their affinity, or cause indirect changes in affinity by alterations in conformation. A stepwise decrease in pH is the most common way to elute bound substances. The chemical stability of the matrix, ligand and target protein determines the limit of pH that may be used.

If low pH is used, the fractions are collected in neutralization buffer such as 1 M Tris-HCl, pH 9 (60–200 µl per ml eluted fraction) to return the fraction to a neutral pH. The column should also be re-equilibrated to neutral pH immediately.

Ionic strength elution: The exact mechanism of elution by changes in ionic strength depends on the specific interaction between the ligand and target protein. This is a mild elution using a buffer with more ionic strength, usually, NaCl is applied as a linear gradient. Enzymes usually elute at a concentration of 1 M NaCl or less.

Competitive elution: Selective eluents are used to separate substances when the binding affinity of the ligand/target protein interaction is relatively high. The eluting agent competes either for binding to the target protein or for binding to the ligand. Substances maybe eluted either by a concentration gradient of a single eluent or by pulse elution. In competitive elution, the concentration of the competing compound should be similar to the concentration of the coupled ligand. If the free competing compound shows weak binding than the ligand to the target molecule, a concentration of ten-fold higher than that of the ligand is used.

The reduced polarity of eluent: The polarity of the eluent is reduced to promote elution without inactivating the eluted substances. Dioxane 10% or ethylene glycol (up to 50%) are, e.g. of this type of eluent.

Chaotropic eluents: If other elution methods fail, deforming buffers, which alter the structure of proteins, can be used, e.g. chaotropic agents such as guanidine hydrochloride or urea. Chaotropes are likely to denature the eluted protein, and hence their usage is very limited.

4. Re-equilibration of the column by the binding buffer

The flow chart of the steps involved in affinity chromatography is given below.

equilibration → adsorption of sample and elution of unbound material → wash away unbound material → elute bound protein(s) → re-equilibration

Advantages of affinity chromatography

1. Specificity is high and yields products of high purity.
2. Single-step purification and reproducible.
3. Matrix is reusable
4. The binding sites of the biological molecules can be studied.

Disadvantages of affinity chromatography

1. Ligands are expensive
2. Leakage of ligands in the mobile phase.
3. Solid support degradation causing limited lifespan
4. Possibility of non-specific adsorption

APPLICATIONS

1. Isolation and purification of biological macromolecules
2. Purification and concentration of enzymes
3. To study the binding of the compounds
4. To remove impurities in a mixture
5. Nucleic acid purification in genetic engineering
6. Antibody purification from blood serum in vaccine production.

SECTION – III: Electrometric Methods

19. Potentiometry
20. Conductometry
21. Polarography
22. Amperometry

CHAPTER 19

Potentiometry

Potentiometry is one of the electroanalytical techniques. It is used to find out the concentration of the solute in solution. In this technique, the potential of the electrochemical cell is measured under static conditions. A high impedance voltmeter is used to maintain the static conditions. The high impedance voltmeter ensures negligible current flows through the system. The current flow is negligible and no electrochemical reactions are involved. Thus the composition of the electrochemical cell remains unchanged.

A potentiometer consists of two electrodes in two different solutions connected by a salt bridge. The voltmeter attached to the electrodes, measure the potential difference between the electrodes. One of the electrodes is the working electrode called as indicator electrode and it responds to the concentration of analyte. The second electrode is the standard electrode or reference electrode and it has known fixed potential.

The electrochemical cell is made up of two half-cells. Each half cell contains an electrode immersed in a solution of ions whose activities will determine the potential of the electrode. A salt bridge connects the two half cells. The salt bridge contains an inert electrolyte like KCl and the function of the salt bridge is to connect the two half cells and it aids in the exchange of ions. The salt bridge ends are fitted with porous frits, through which the movement of the electrolyte ions is facilitated between the half cells through salt bridge. This movement of ions in the salt bridge completes the electrical circuit

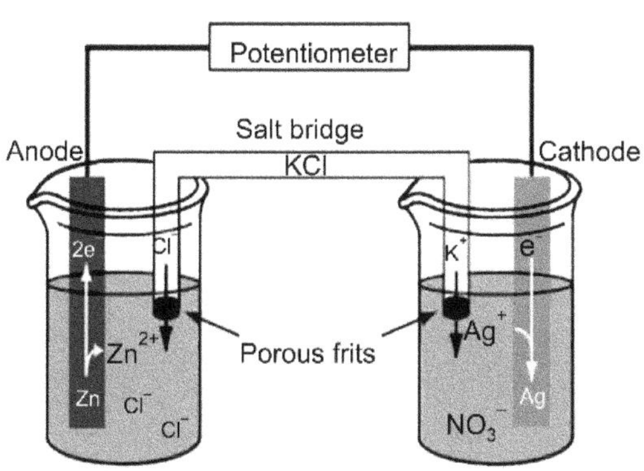

$ZnCl_2$ & $AgNO_3$ Electrochemical cell.

PRINCIPLE

The Nernst equation forms the basis of quantitative potentiometric applications. This Nernst equation gives the relationship between electrochemical cell potential and the concentration of the electroactive species in the cells.

By convention, the electrode on the left side is anode where the oxidation takes place and it is the reference electrode. The electrode on the right side is cathode where the reduction occurs and it is the indicator electrode.

The electrochemical cell in the figure is represented as

$$Zn(s)\left|ZnCl_2\left(aq.a_{zn}{}^{2+}=0.0667\right)\right|\left|AgNO_3\left(aq,{}^{+}=0.100\right)\right|Ag(s)$$

The double vertical line (| |) represents the salt bridge and it also denotes that there is a potential difference between the salt bridge and each halfcell.

NERNST EQUATION

The potential of potentiometric electrochemical cell is

$$E_{cell} = E_{\text{ cathode}} - E_{\text{ anode}} \qquad .....(19.1)$$

Where the E_{cathode} and E_{anode} are the reduction potentials of the redox reactions at the cathode and anode respectively.

Each reduction potential is given as

E= E° - (RT/nF) In Q where

E° - Standard reduction potential of reference standard electrode (anode)

It is a constant value for each electrode and different for different electrodes used in different cells.

R-Gas constant

T-Temp in Kelvin

n-no of electrons involved in redox reactions.

F-Faraday constant.

Q-reaction quotient

At a temp of 298K (25° C) the Nernst equation becomes as

$$E= E° - (0.05916//n) \log_{10} Q \qquad .....(19.2)$$

where E is in volts.

The potential of E_{anode} in this cellis

$$E_{\text{anode}} = E^0{}_{Zn^{2+}/Zn} - (0.05916/2) \log (1/a_{Zn^{2+}})$$

$$E_{\text{cathode}} = E^0{}_{Ag+/Ag} - (0.05916/1) \log (1/a_{Ag+})$$

Substituting these E_{anode} and E_{cathode} in equation (19.1)

$E_{cell} = [E^0_{Ag+/Ag} - (0.05916/1) \log (1/a_{Ag+})] - [E^0_{Zn^{2+}/Zn} - (0.05916/2) \log (1/a_{Zn^{2+}})]$

By substituting standard electrode potentials, the equation becomes

$E_{cell} = [0.7996 - (0.05916/1) \log (1/a_{Ag+})] - [0.7618 - (0.05916/2) \log (1/0.0167)]$

with the known cell potential, it is easy to calculate the concentration of Ag^+ i.e. the concentration of Ag^+ ions.

JUNCTION POTENTIAL

A small junction potential is always present in the salt bridge. The potential difference across the membrane is called as junction potential and is represented as E_j.

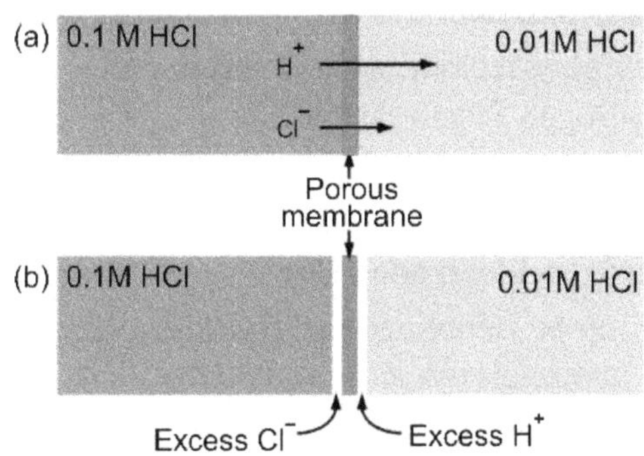

Due to the difference in the concentration and mobility of the ions, a potential develops at the interface between two ionic solutions. This potential is called as junction potential. The example shown here in the figure depicts the movement of H^+ & Cl^- ions across a porous membrane separating two ionic solutions. H^+ ions mobility is more compared to Cl^- ions leading to excess H^+ ions on right side causing positive charge and move Cl^- ions on the left side leading to negative charge. This difference in potential across the membrane is called junction potential. The junction potential may be around 30-40 mV.

This junction potential also contributes to the potential of the cell. So to minimize the effect of junction potential in salt bridge, a salt like KCl is used where the mobility of K^+ & Cl^- are almost equal. Even the salt bridge containing KCl, always presents a small junction potential.

Thus the cell potential is

$E_{cell}=E_{cathode} - E_{anode} + E_j$

But mostly junction potential is ignored because it remains almost constant. Potentiometric methods are the most accurate method for determining pH of the solution. An electrode reversible to H^+ ions is used. The common electrodes used for this purpose are **Hydrogen electrode,**

Quinhydrone electrode, glass electrode, antimony-antimony oxide electrode and ion selective electrodes like glass membrane electrodes

THE REFERENCE ELECTRODES

In potentiometric electrochemical cell, two half cells are present. One half cell maintains a fixed reference potential. The electrode of this half cell is the reference electrode and it acts as the anode. The other half cell contains the indicator electrode, whose potential varies with the analyte concentration and this electrode is the cathode of the cell.

Characteristics of ideal reference electrode are

1. It should be stable
2. It should have known potential.
3. Should be easy to make

The most commonly used reference electrodes are

1. Standard Hydrogen Electrode (SHE)
2. Calomel electrode.
3. Silver/Silver chloride electrode.

1. Standard Hydrogen Electrode (SHE)

SHE can be set up by bubbling pure Hydrogen gas through a solution of an acid whose hydrogen ion activity is unity. The standard H_2 electrode potential is defined as the potential that is developed between the adsorbed H_2 gas on the platinum metal and H^+ of the solution when the H_2 gas is maintained at a pressure of 760 mm of Hg and is in equilibrium with H^+ of unit concentration.

The electrode potential of this electrode is determined by a platinised platinum plate dipped partly in acid and hydrogen gas is allowed to bubble on it at a slow rate.

$$Pt(s), H_2H^+_{(a=1)} \| H_2, H^+_{(a=x)} \ |Pt$$

The standard electrode potential E^0=0.00V for Hydrogen electrode.

Thus applying Nernst equation

$$E = E^o - \frac{0.0591}{1} \log (1/a^+)$$

$$E = 0 - \frac{0.0591}{1} \log (1/a^+) \qquad [E^o = 0]$$

$$E = -0.0591 \log (1/a^+)$$

The activity of a^+ions can be calculated by the known electrode potential. If the detected ions are H^+ ions, then the equation becomes as

$$E = -0.0591pH$$

$$pH = - E/0.0591$$

Thus the emf of the cell is used to measure the pH of the solution. Thus SHE can be used for both pH and potentiometric measurements.

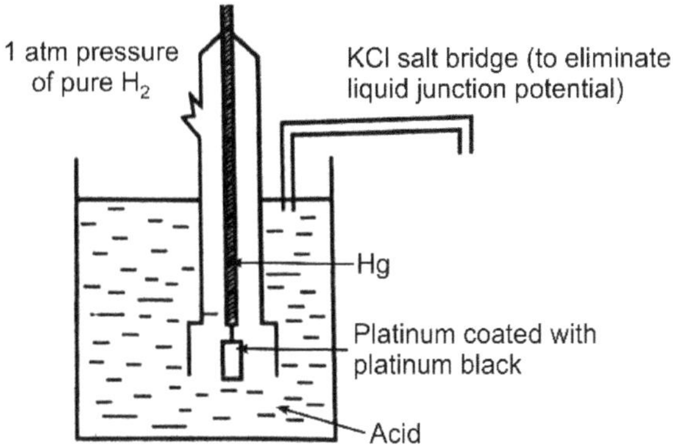

Hydrogen electrode

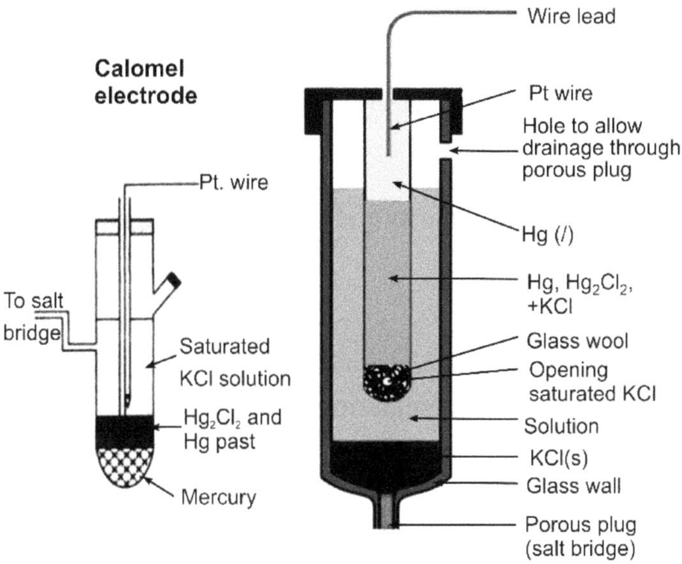

Advantages of Hydrogen electrode

1. It is the fundamental electrode against which all other potentials are measured.
2. It can be used for the pH measurements over entire pH range.
3. No salt error.

Disadvantages

SHE cannot be used in presence of air, dissolved oxygen, oxidising or reducing agents.

The platinum black coating is poisoned due to compounds like alkaloids, sulphides, cyanides, arsenic and antimony salts. The deteriorated coating should be removed from time to time.

It is difficult to maintain the pressure of hydrogen gas at a fixed value.

It is difficult to get pure hydrogen.

2. Calomel Electrode – Saturated (SCE) [HG_2CL_2]

The electrode consists of a inner jacket and outer sleeve. Inner jacket has a wire contact with Hg and plugged with a mixture of Hg_2Cl_2 and KCl. Outer sleeve is filled with either saturated KCl or 1N KCl or 0.1N KCl. A small hole connects the two tubes and a porous wick serves as a salt bridge to the solution in which the SCE is immersed. Mercuric chloride [Hg_2Cl_2] is called as calomel.

The calomel electrode is represented as

Hg (l) | Hg_2Cl_2 (sat'd), KCl (aq, sat'd) || Hg_2Cl_2(s) +2e– ↔2Hg(l) + 2Cl^-(aq)]

Redox reaction happening at calomel electrode

The half cell reaction is

Hg (l) | Hg_2Cl_2 (sat'd), KCl (aq, sat'd)

Applications

1. Used in pH measurement
2. Used in Cyclic voltammetry and general aqueous electrochemistry

Advantages

1. Ease of construction
2. Stability of potential.

3. Silver-Silver Chloride Electrode

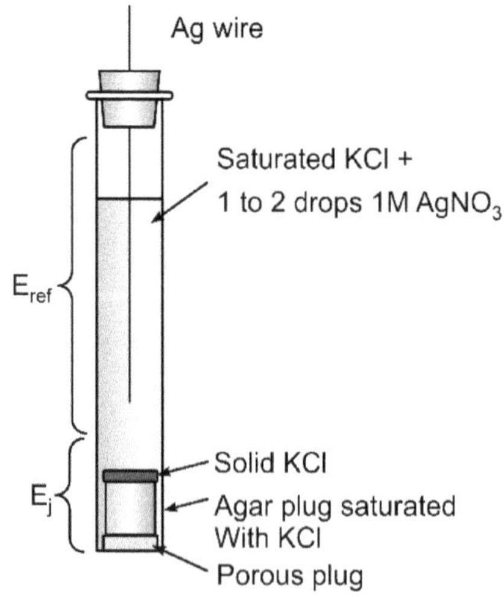

This electrode is based on the reduction of AgCl to Ag

$$AgCl(s) + e^- \leftrightarrow Ag(s) + Cl^- (aq)$$

The activity of Cl^- determines the potential of Ag/AgCl electrode. The electrode consists of a silver wire coated electrolytically with silverchloride and dipped in to saturated KCl solution. It consists of a porous plug (salt bridge) for contact with the ions of the solution in which it is dipped. The half cell is represented as

Ag(s) | AgCl (sat'd), KCl (x M)

Advantages

1. Easy to use.
2. Simple and inexpensive
3. Very stable and nontoxic

Disadvantages

It is difficult to prepare.

INDICATOR ELECTRODES

The potential of the indicator electrode is proportional to the analyte concentration. The indicator electrodes are broadly classified as Metallic electrodes, ion-selective electrodes and molecular sensing electrodes.

Metallic indicator electrodes

The metallic indicator electrodes are further classified as

A. Electrodes of the First Kind
B. Electrodes of the Second Kind
C. Electrodes of the Third Kind
D. Inert Metallic Electrodes (for Redox Systems)

A. Electrodes of the First Kind

These kinds of electrodes are the indicator electrodes, in which the metal is in contact with solution containing the same metal ion. E.g. use of copper electrode to detect Cu^{2+} ions in solution

It involves a single reaction

$$Cu^{2+} + 2e^- \leftrightarrow Cu\ (s)$$

This electrodes potential gives the direct measurement of Cu^{2+} ions.

$$E_{ind} = E^o_{Cu} - (0.0592/2) \log a_{Cu(s)}/a_{Cu2+}$$

Since $a_{Cu(s)} = 1$, the equation becomes as

$$E_{ind} = E^o_{Cu} - (0.0592/2) \log 1/a_{Cu2+}$$

$$= 0.3419-(0.0592/2) \log 1/a_{Cu2+}$$

The reference electrode used in the cell is SCE.

$$E_{cell} = E_{ind} - E_{SCE} + E_j$$

$$E_{cell} = \underbrace{0.3419 - (0.0592/2)\log 1/a_{Cu2+}}_{E_{ind}} \underbrace{-0.224 + E_j}_{E_{SCE}}$$

Disadvantages

1. Not very selective. These electrodes respond to other cations also. E.g. Copper electrodes cannot be used for Cu^{2+} in presence of Ag^{+}
2. As metals are soluble in acids, they can be used only in neutral pH.
3. Formation of metal oxides on metal electrode surface.
4. Certain metals do not provide reproducible potentials. E.g. Fe, Cr, Co, Ni.

These disadvantages lead to the limited usage of these electrodes for the detection of metals like Ag, Bi, Cu, Hg, Pb, Sn, Ti and Zn in deaerated solutions.

$$E_{ind} = E^{o} - (0.0592/n) \log 1/[M^{n+}]$$

B. Electrodes of the Second Kind

These electrodes are the metal electrodes which can act as indicator electrode for their own cations and also for the anions which can form precipitates or stable complexes with its own cations. These electrodes respond to the activity of an anion in equilibrium with the cation.

These electrodes are made up of a metal wire coated with one of its salts. E.g. Silver electrode coated with AgCl.

E.g. Detection of Cl^{-} with silver electrode.

The electrode is used to measure the activity of chloride ions in a solution

$$AgCl(s) + e- \rightarrow Ag(s) + Cl^{-}(aq) \qquad E^{0}_{AgCl/Ag} = 0.222 \text{ V}$$

The nernst equation for this process is given as

$$E_{ind} = E^{0}_{AgCl/Ag} - 0.0592 \log a_{Cl-}$$

In a solution saturated with AgCl, this electrode can serve as an indicator electrode. This is an electrode of second kind for Cl^{-} ions.

C. Electrodes of third kind

These are the metal electrodes which respond to a different cation other than the cation of the electrode metal in solution. The potential of the electrode depends on the concentration of the cation and the concentration of this cation is controlled by the anion concentration. If another common cation is used in this solution the anion concentration is controlled by the second cation. These are very slow and unstable electrodes.

1. Metal electrodes that respond to different cation
2. Linked to cation by an intermediate reaction

E.g. Detection of EDTA ion (y^{4-}) with Hg electrode

Half reaction $Hg\ y^{2-} + 2e^{-} \leftrightarrow Hg(l) + y^{4-}$

$$E_{ind} = E^0 - (0.0592/2) \log a_{Hg\,(l)} . a_{y}^{4-} / a_{Hg\,y}^{2-}$$ the equation becomes

$$E_{ind} = E^0 - (0.0592/2) \log a_{y}^{4-} / a_{Hg\,y}^{2-} \text{ as } a_{Hg\,(l)} = 1$$

A small concentration of $Hg\ y^{2-}$ is introduced in to the analyte solution to use this electrode system. The complex is highly stable and its activity remains constant.

Now the equation is given as

$E_{ind} = K - (0.0592/2) \log a_{y}^{4-}$ where $K = 0.21 - (0.0592/2) \log 1/ a_{Hg\,y2}^{-}$ as ($\log a_{y}^{4-} = 1$)

To the equilibrium of EDTA complex, calcium solution is added leading to the formation of new equilibrium

$$Cay^{2-} \leftrightarrow Ca^{2+} + Y^{4-}$$

$$E_{ind} = K - (0.0592/2) \log K\, a_{Ca\,y}^{2-} / a_{Ca}^{2+}$$

Thus the mercury electrode becomes an electrode of the third kind for Ca.

These electrodes can detect a linked cation in an intermediate reaction.

E.g. Detection of EDTA by Hg electrode. It can be made to detect other cations that bind to EDTA, which affect the concentration of first cation.

D. Inert metallic electrodes (for Redox electrodes)

Inert conductors are made up of materials like platinum, gold, palladium, and carbon and they can respond to redox systems. These electrodes are used as redox electrodes and they act as electron sink or source.

The inert metal electrode is in contact with a solution containing soluble oxidized and reduced forms of redox half reaction. The reaction may not be reversible. The potential of the electrode is determined by the ratio of oxidized species to the reduced species in half reaction.

E.g. of redox electrodes Hydrogen electrode, platinum, gold, palladium, and carbon

E.g. of the reaction

Detection of Ce^{3+} with Pt electrode

Half reaction is given as $Ce^{4+} + e^{-} \leftrightarrow Ce^{3+}$

$$E_{ind} = E^{o} - (0.0592/1) \log a_{Ce}^{3+} / a_{Ce}^{4+}$$

Disadvantages

1. Irreversible reaction
2. Half reactions are not predictable.

Membrane indicator electrodes/ Ion selective electrodes

Membrane indicator electrodes are classified as

A. Glass pH indicator electrodes
B. Glass indicator electrodes for other cations
C. Liquid Membrane indicator electrodes
D. Crystalline-Membrane indicator electrodes
E. Molecular selective electrode

In membrane indicator electrodes, the cations or anions are detected by selective adsorption of these ions to a membrane surface. These ion selective electrodes are also called as P ion electrodes and the data obtained from these electrodes are presented as p-functions. For E.g. (pH, pCa, pNO_2). In membrane electrodes, the observed potential is a type of junction potential which develops across a membrane separating the analyte solution from reference solution. A metallic electrode potential arises due to the oxidation reduction reaction occurring on the electrodes surface where as the potential developing in the membrane depends on the nature of the membrane.

A. Glass pH indicator electrodes

These are similar to the glass electrodes used in pH meter.

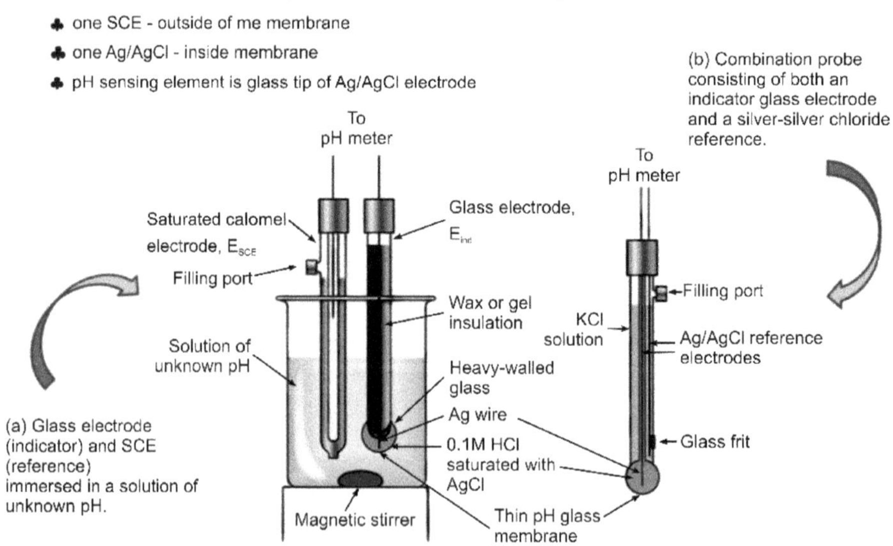

(a) Glass electrode (indicator) and SCE (reference) immersed in a solution of unknown pH.

(b) Combination probe consisting of both an indicator glass electrode and a silver-silver chloride reference.

Construction and working

A glass membrane that binds to H^+ ions is used preferentially. The typical pH electrode system consists of

Two reference electrodes

1. SCE – outside the membrane
2. Ag/AgCl – inside the membrane.
3. The pH sensing element is the glass membrane present at the tip of Ag/AgCl electrode.

Combination probes consist of indicator glass electrode and silver/silver chloride reference electrode both inside and outside the bulb.

Glass electrode is the most commonly used indicator electrode which involves ion exchange reaction. The glass membrane is made up of chemically bonded Na_2O, CaO, SiO_2 and $Al_2 O_3$. The glass bulb is filled with HCl and KCl solution. The silver wire coated with AgCl acts as the internal reference electrode. The internal reference electrode is not the pH sensing element. The glass membrane bulb at the tip is the electrode that responds to pH.

THE COMPOSITION AND STRUCTURE OF GLASS MEMBRANE

The sensitivity of the membrane to protons and other cations depends on the composition of the glass. For membranes, Corning 015 glass is widely used and it exhibits specificity of H^+ ions up to pH 9.

The cross sectional view of silicate glass structure shows three Si-O bonds in the same plane and an additional oxygen atom attached to Si either below or above the plane of paper. Each silicon atom is bonded to four oxygen atoms and each oxygen is shared by two silicon atoms. There are sufficient cations in the interstices of the structure to balance the negative charge of the silicate groups. Mono valent cations, such as sodium and lithium are mobile in the lattice and are responsible for electrical conduction within the membrane.

The hygroscopicity of glass membranes

The surface of the glass membrane must be hydrated well to function as pH electrode. The exchange reaction between singly charged cations in the interstices of the glass lattice and H^+ ions in solution is called as Hydration of the pH sensitive glass membrane.

$$H^+ + Na^+Gl^- \rightarrow Na^+ + H^+Gl^-$$

This process involves only mono valent cations because divalent and trivalent cations are strongly held within the silicate structure. The entire surface of hydrated glass membrane consists of silicic acid (H^+Gl^-). In highly alkaline solutions significant H^+ ions are replaced by Na^+ ions.

Determination of pH

The charge imbalance across the membrane leads to an electrical potential across the material. Both the inside and outside interfaces of glass membrane in glass electrode bulb have Si OH groups. The inner surface of the membrane is in contact with a fixed concentration of HCl and thus the number of SiO^-

groups in the inner surface of the membrane remains constant. Against this, the number of SiO^- groups on the outside of the glass membrane change with the solution of the pH in which it is immersed. This creates a difference in charge between the inside and outside of the glass membrane leading to membrane potential. The developed potential is the boundary potential to give the concentration of H^+ ions (pH) of the solution in which the glass electrode is immersed. The surface of the glass in contact with the solution forms the hydrated layer by absorbing water where the ions are exchanged. Therefore, pH electrodes made of glass must be always dipped in water, so that it will not get dried up.

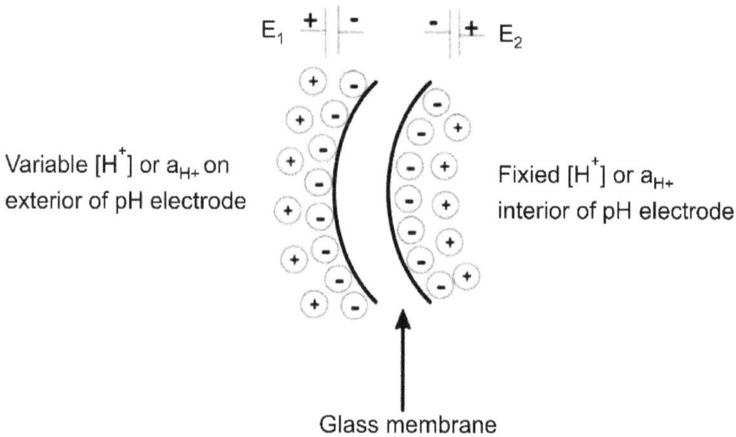

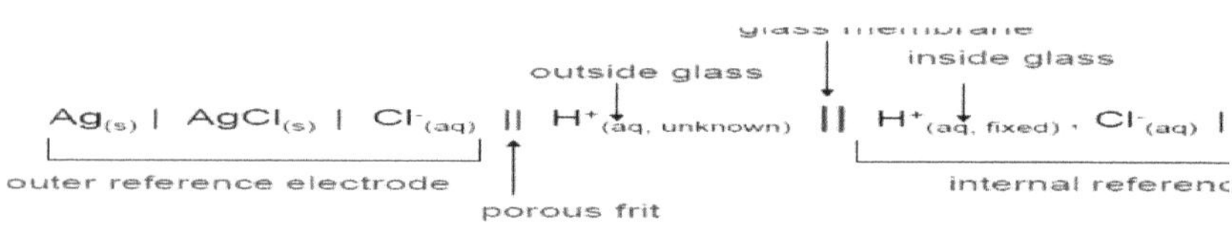

$$E_b = E_1 - E_2$$

$$E_b = C - 0.0592pH$$

where

C is a constant, pH is $-\log a_+$ (analyte solution/exterior solution)

Advantages

1. It can be used in the presence of oxidising and reducing agents.
2. It is used for pH values 2-10. Can be extended up to 14 with special glass.
3. No electrode poisoning
4. Simple operation and equilibrium reached faster

Disadvantages

1. Fragile
2. Can be used only in electronic potentiometers, due to high resistance

3. Requires frequent standardisation
4. Cannot be used with ethyl alcohol ,acetic acid and gelatine

There are four potentials in Glass electrode

1. $E_{Ag/Agcl}$ (internal reference electrode) and E_{SCE} (External reference electrode) potential and both are constants.
2. Third potential is the Ej (junction potential) across the salt bridge.
3. The fourth potential is the boundary potential E_b and this is the important potential that varies with the pH of the analyte solution.

Formation of boundary potential across the glass membrane is used to determine pH.

Applying Nernst equation

$E_b = E_1 - E_2 = 0.0592 \log a_1/a_2$ where a_1-activity of analyte solution and a_2 – activity of internal solution.

For glass pH electrode

$$E_b = L' + 0.0592 \log a_1$$

$$= L' - 0.0592pH, \text{ where } L' = -0.0592\log a_2$$

Thus the boundary potential E_b is the measure of activity of external solution. (a_1).

The glass electrode potential

$$E_{ind} = E_b + E_{Ag/AgCl} + E_{asy}$$

E_{asy} is the asymmetric potential. It is the change in potential due to the imperfections in membrane developed during usage over time.

Substituting the value of E_b, the equation becomes

$$E_{ind} = L^1 + 0.0592 \log a_1 + E_{Ag/AgCl} + E_{asy}$$

$$E_{ind} = L + 0.0592 \log a_1 = L - 0.0592pH, \text{ where } L = L^1 + E_{Ag/AgCl} + E_{asy}.$$

B. Glass indicator electrodes for other cations

Cation sensitive type

In basic solutions, glass electrodes respond to the concentration of other alkali metal ions along with H^+ions. At higher pH, electrodes indicate less pH than the actual value and this is called as alkaline error.

To eliminate alkaline error in glass electrodes, different electrodes are developed with different compositions like Al_2O_3 or B_2O_3.This results in enhancement of binding towards other ions

Thus cation sensitive glass electrodes are used for the determination of singly charged cations like Na^+, K^+, NH_4^+, CS^+ and Ag^+.

C. Liquid membrane indicator electrodes

These electrodes are formed from immiscible liquids that selectively bond to certain ions. The membrane consists of organic liquid (insoluble in sample) held in porous disc between aqueous reference solution and sample solution. The membrane has ability to bind to the ions of interest selectively.

Liquid membrane electrode

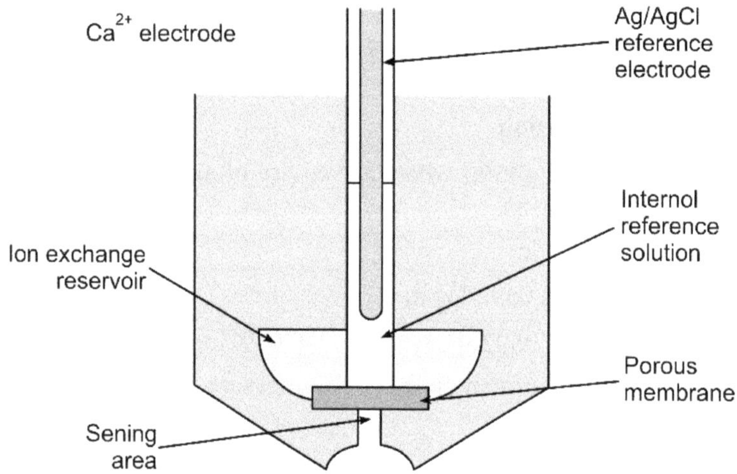

A Potential develops across the interface between the analyte solution and the liquid ion exchanger that bond with analyte. The membrane is an organic polymer saturated with a liquid ion exchanger. It is used for polyvalent ions as well as some anions.

E.g.: Calcium dialkyl phosphate Liquid membrane electrodesbind to Ca^{2+} strongly.

Calcium dialkyl phosphate is insoluble in water, but binds withCa^{2+}strongly. The liquid membrane consists of cation exchangers for cation detection, anion exchangers for anion detection and macro cyclic compounds for complexing certain cations.

D. Crystalline Membrane indicator electrodes

These are solid state electrodes, usually made of ionic compounds. The crushed powder of the compound is melted and formed into a membrane. Working of these electrodes is similar to glass membrane electrodes. In some instances single crystal is used as the membrane. The diameter of the crystal is about 10 mm and thickness is about 1 to 2 mm.

The membrane is sealed to the end of a tube made of chemically inert plastic such as Teflon or poly vinyl chloride.

E.g. AgX membrane used for the determination of X^-

Ag S membrane used for the determination of S^{-2}

LaF_3 membrane used for the determination of F^-

E. Molecular selective electrodes

These electrodes detect the molecule instead of ions.

Gas sensing electrodes (probes)

These electrodes are hydrophobic polymers which are microporous in nature. The pore size is less than 1 μm, and is about 0.1 mm thick.

The analyte gas passes through the membrane and dissolves in the internal solution.

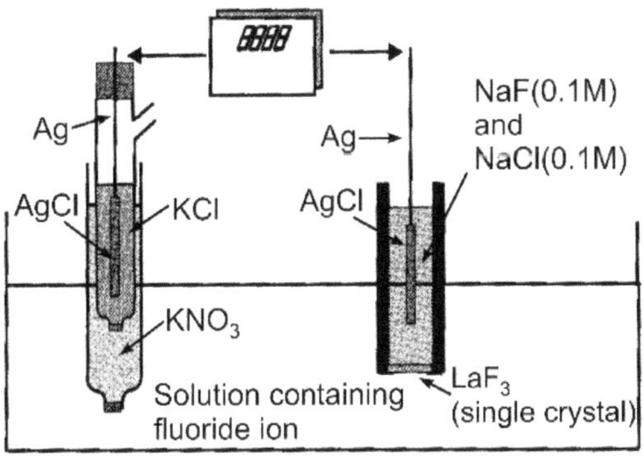

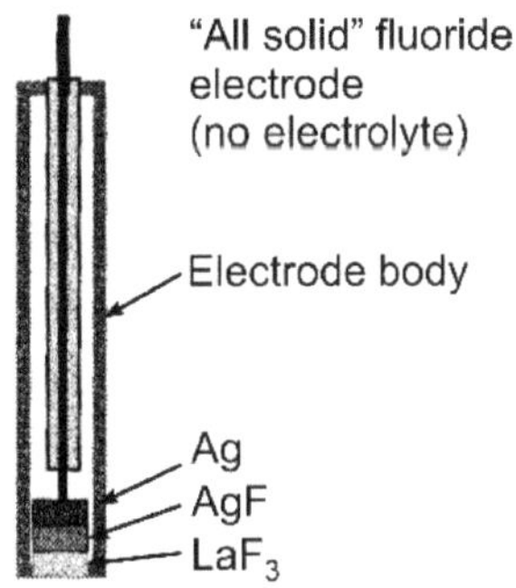

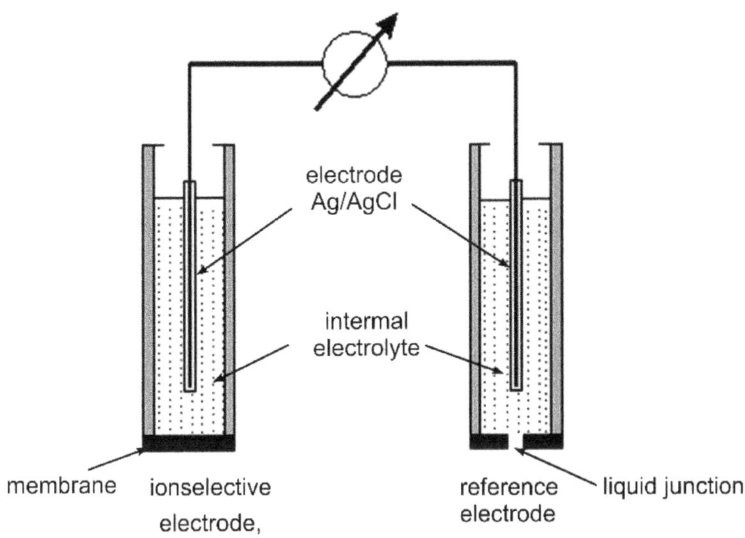

Crystalline membrane electrodes

Fluoride electrode

Gas diffuses through the membrane

$$\underset{\text{External solution}}{CO_2(aq)} \leftrightarrow \underset{\text{membrane pores}}{CO_2(g)} \leftrightarrow \underset{\text{internal solution}}{CO_2(aq)}$$

In internal solution, pH changes because of the dissolved gas and this is detected by the ISE probe.

$$CO_2(aq) + H_2O \leftrightarrow HCO_3^{+} + H^{+}$$

Overall reaction

$$\underset{\substack{\text{External}\\\text{solution}}}{CO_2(aq) + H_2O} \leftrightarrow \underset{\substack{\text{Internal}\\\text{solution}}}{HCO_3^{+} + H^{+}}$$

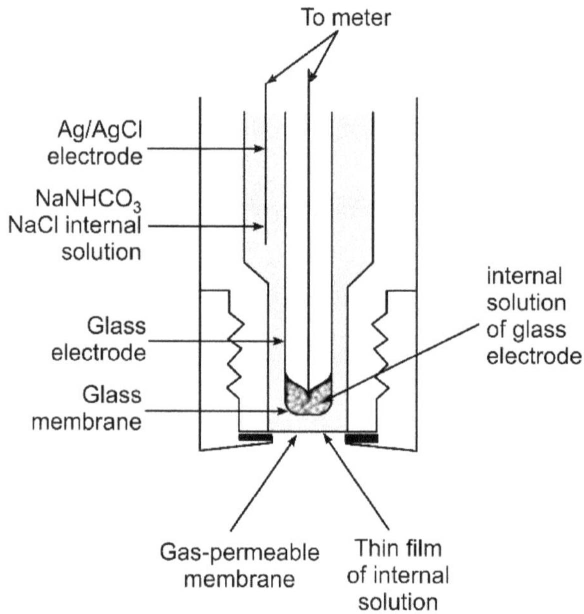

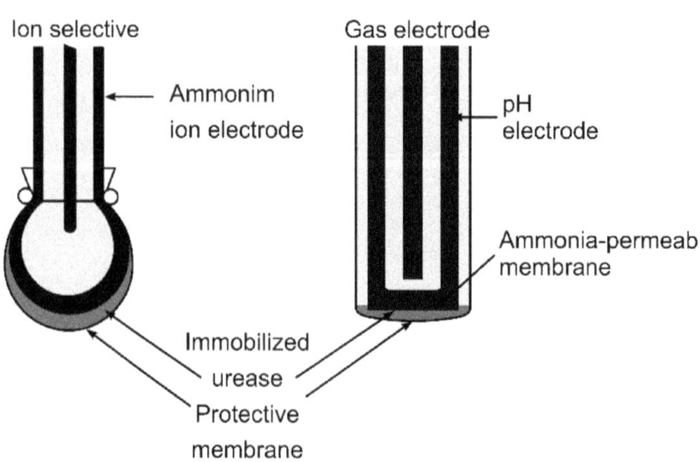

ENZYME ELECTRODES (BIOCATALYTIC MEMBRANE ELECTRODES)

An immobilized enzyme is used in these electrodes. The enzyme converts the molecular analyte to a form that can be followed electrochemically. They are very selective.

E.g. Urea enzyme electrode

In this electrode, urea is hydrolyzed to give Ammonia and H^+ by the enzyme urease.

$$(NH_4)CO + 2H_2O + H^+ \leftrightarrow 2NH_4^+ + HCO_{3-} \leftrightarrow 2NH_3 + 2H^+$$

Amount of Ammonia gas produced is monitored using Ammonia gas sensing probe.

Measurement of emf and pH

The emf or pH of a solution is given in mv and it is measured using a potentiometer. As the modern instruments are capable of measuring both emf and pH, they are called as potentiometer or pH meter.

pH indicator electrodes

1. **Hydrogen electrode**
   It has got very limited usage because of the reactivity of hydrogen.
2. **Glass electrode**
   Explained under glass membrane electrodes

Quinhydrone electrode

Quinhydrone consists of 1:1 molar compound of quinine and hydroquinonein a solution. A reversible redox system is formed by Quinone, hydroquinone and hydrogen ions.

$$C_6H_4O_2 + 2H^+ + 2e^- \rightarrow C_6H_4(OH)_2$$

Quinone Hydroquinone

The Nernst equation is given as

$$E = E^0 \text{ -0.0591pHat25°C}$$

The equation clearly states that the electrode potential changes with change in the concentration of hydrogen ions.

Advantages:

1. It has got low resistance and it quickly reaches equilibrium.
2. It is not affected by dissolved oxygen.
3. Micro determinations can be done.

Disadvantages:

1. pH values of less than 8 alone can be determined by this electrode

2. The analyte solution gets contaminates
3. Salt error
4. It cannot be used if oxidising and reducing substances are present in the solution.

Antimony antimony oxide electrode

An antimony rod is placed in a solution having hydrogen ions.

The reaction is

$$Sb + H_2O \rightarrow SbO+ +2H^+ +3e^-$$

The potential of the electrode is

$$E = E^0 + (0.0592/3) \log [SbO^+][H^+]^2$$

$$E = 0.255 - 0.0592 \text{ pH}$$

Thus the electrode can be used for the determination of pH.

Advantages

1. Robust
2. pH in the range of 4-12 can be determined.
3. It has low resistance and does not contaminate the solution

POTENTIOMETRIC TITRATIONS

In potentiometric titrations, the concentration of one or more of the species is followed potentiometrically. The titration beaker forms one half cell.

Potentiometric titrations are the titrations where the change in electrode potential on the addition of titrant is observed against the volume of the titrant added. Potentiometer is the instrument used for the measurement of potentials in potentiometric titrations. The endpoint is obtained by plotting a graph of potential versus the volume of the titrant.

Potentiometric titrations can be applied to all types of reactions. The titrations are carried out well beyond the endpoint.

Apparatus and working

The apparatus consists of a beaker with a stirrer. The indicator and reference electrodes (SCE) are dipped in to the analyte solution. The potential is noted after the addition of each increment of the titrant. A graph is plotted as potential against volume of the titrant. The indicator electrode is varied depending on the analyte.

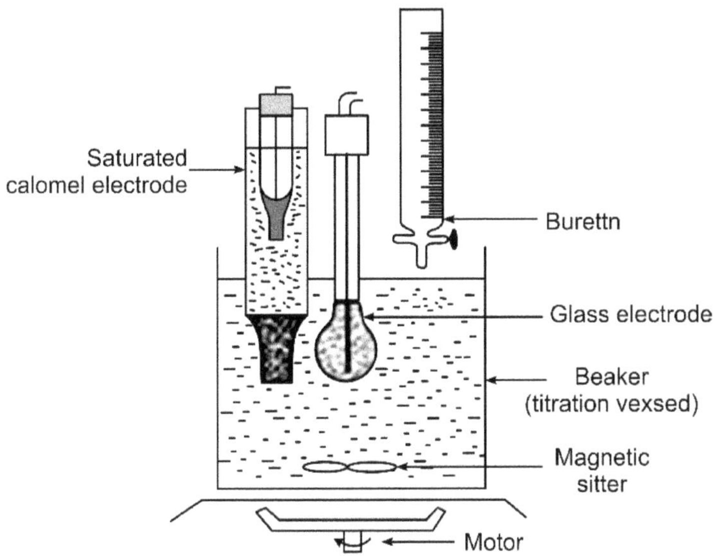

Apparatus for Potentiometric titration

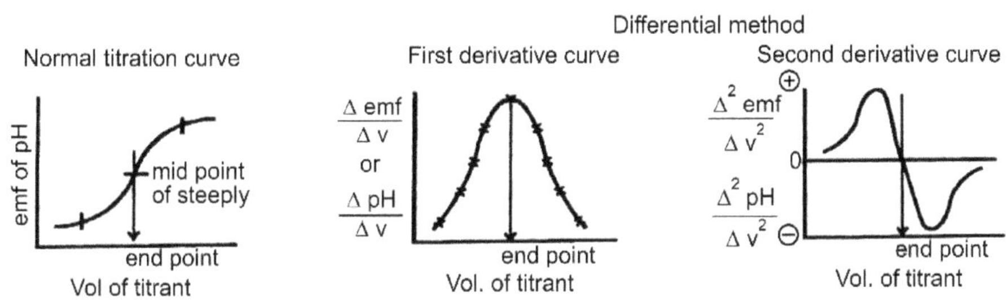

The endpoint detection in the potentiometric titrations are

1. **Normal titration curve**

   In this method the emf (potential) is plotted against the volume of the titrant. The endpoint is determined by extrapolating the midpoint of steeply rising portion of the curve to meet the x axis. This gives the endpoint of the titration. At endpoint the rate of change of potential is maximum.

   The first derivative curve is the curve in which $\frac{\Delta E}{\Delta V}$ is plotted against volume of titrant. The peak of the curve gives the endpoint.

   The second derivative curve in which the $\Delta^2E/\Delta V^2$ is plotted against volume gives the endpoint at the zero crossing of the curve

   Types of potentiometric titrations

   The different types of Potentiometry are

   1. Acid base titrations
   2. Redox titrations

3. Diazotization titrations
4. Precipitation titrations
5. Complexometric titrations
6. Dead stop end point technique.

1. Acid Base Titrations

Acid base titrations involve neutralization of the acids and bases. These titrations are accompanied by changes in the concentration of H^+ and OH^- ions. Reference Electrode is saturated Calomel electrode. Glass electrode is used as the indicator electrode. A known volume of the acid to be titrated is taken in a beaker and the indictor and reference electrodes are immersed in the acid. Both the electrodes are connected by salt bridge. The electrodes are connected to the potentiometer and after addition of each increment of the base, the emf is measured. A graph of emf versus volume of the titrant is recorded.

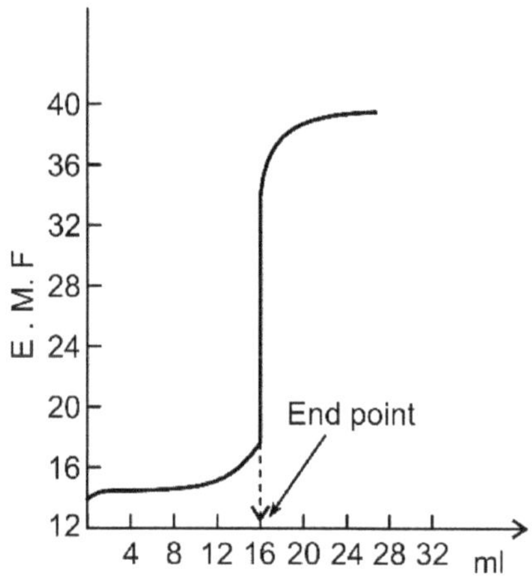

$$E = E_0 - 0.0591 \log a_{H^+}$$

$$E = E_0 - 0.0591 pH$$

Thus the changes in emf of the cell are proportional to the pH changes during titrations. The midpoint of the rising portion of the curve gives end point.

E.g. there are two types of Acid base titrations that can be carried out by potentiometry. They are

1. Titrations in aqueous medium

(i) Weak acid vs. weak base (Acetic acid vs. Ammonium hydroxide)
Weak acid vs.Strong base (Acetic acid vs. Sodium hydroxide)
Strong acid vs.strong base (Hydrochloric acid vs. Ammonium hydroxide)
Strong acid vs. Strong base (Hydrochloric acid vs. Sodium hydroxide)

(ii) Mixture of acids vs.bases (mixture of acetic acid and Hydrochloric acid against sodium hydroxide
Mixture of bases vs. acid (mixture of Ammonium hydroxide and sodium hydroxide against Hydrochloric acid

(iii) Poly basic acids vs. bases (citric acid vs. sodium hydroxide)
(Tartaric acid vs. Sodium hydroxide)

2. **Titrations in non- aqueous medium (Non-aqueous titrations)**

   The same electrode system is used.

   (i) Weak acids vs. potassium or lithium methoxide (barbituric acid against lithium methoxide)

   (ii) Weak bases vs. perchloric acid (Ephedrine hydrochloride, Quinine sulphate, metronidazole or chloroquine phosphate vs.0.1N $HClO_4$.)

2. **Redox Titrations**

   These titrations involve the transfer of electrons from the substance being oxidised to the substance being reduced. Redox titration can be generally represented as

   $$\text{Reductant} + ne \rightarrow \text{oxidant}$$

   $$Ce^{4+} + Fe^{2+} \rightarrow Ce^{3+} + Fe^{3+}$$

   The oxidising agent (Ce^{4+}) oxidises ferrous ions (Fe^{2+}) to ferric ions (Fe^{3+}) while it gets reduced to cerrous (Ce^{3+}) in the process. The reference electrode used is SCE or silver-silver chloride electrode. A platinum wire or foil is used as indicator electrode.

   The potential E of the redox reaction is represented by

   $$E = E^0 + (0.0592/n) \log ([OX]/[RED])$$

   Where E^0- standard potential

   n- no of electrons involved in the reaction.

   [OX] – Concentration of oxidant

   [RED] – Concentration of reductant

   Detection of emf is done on each addition of titrant and a graph is plotted with emf against volume of the titrant. The endpoint is determined from the graph.

   E.g. of other redox titrations are

   Ferrous ammonium sulphate in dil.sulphuric acid vs. Potassium permanganate.

   Ferrous ammonium sulphate in dil.sulphuric acid vs. Potassium dichromate

3. **Diazotization Titrations**

   Diazonium salts are formed by the titration of aromatic primary amine against sodium nitrite in acidic medium. Endpoint can be determined either by external indicator method (using starch iodide paper) or using potentiometric endpoint. Reference electrode used is SCE and the indicator electrode is glass electrode.

   E.g. of substances titrated by diazotisation method are alkaloids, amines, sulpha drugs etc.

4. **Precipitation Titrations**

   SCE, Hydrogen electrode and silver silver chloride electrodes can be used as the reference electrode. The metal involved in the reaction is used as indicator electrode.

E.g. of ions that can be titrated by precipitation titrations are Mercury, Silver, lead, copper. They are titrated against precipitants to form insoluble salts. The end point is determined by potentiometric endpoint

The solubility of the substance precipitated and its concentration decides the potential change at the endpoint

Ex: Titration of chloride ions with silver nitrate using silver metal indicator electrode.

The other electrode is reference electrode.

The potential of silver electrode is governed by the Nernst equation

$$E_{Ag^+/Ag} = E^o_{Ag^+/Ag} + \frac{0.0591}{1}\log_{10}\left[Ag^+\right]$$

5. **Complexometric Titrations**

   Metallic ions including divalent cations are titrated against EDTA and the endpoints are determined potentiometrically. Any reference electrode can be used including the SCE. Silver, mercury electrodes are used as indicator electrode.

   E.g. Titration of cyanide ion with EDTA

Advantages of Potentiometric titrations

1. Coloured solutions, turbid and dilute solutions can be titrated.
2. Potential of the reference electrode need not be known as it is a constant throughout the process.
3. Automation is possible
4. Titrations of mixtures is possible
5. Accurate and inexpensive.

Applications

1. To determine endpoints in titrations
2. To determine the concentration of ions using ISE.
3. Determination of pH.
4. Determination of equilibrium constants.
5. Determination of electrolytes in clinical chemistry.
6. Monitoring of waste water systems.
7. Analysis of CN^-, F^-, NH_3 and NO_3 in water and waste water.
8. Used for the analysis of salt, calcium, potassium and NO_3, NO_2 in food industry

CHAPTER 20

Conductometry

It is a method of electrochemical analysis in which the conductance of the solution is measured. The conductivity of the solution is due to the movement of the ions in the solution. The mobility of the ion dictates the ability of the ion to transport charges. The mobility of ion is defined as the rate of movement of the ion, under the influence of applied field.

PRINCIPLE

Conductometry is based on the principle of determination of changes in conductivity. These changes in conductance are due to the mobility of ions under the influence of applied field. The factors affecting mobility of ions are charge, size, mass and salvation. Ionic conductance is different for different ions.

Conductance is defined as the flow of current through an electrolyte solution due to migration of ions, when a potential difference is applied between two electrodes. The positively charged cations will move towards the cathode (-ve electrode) and the negatively charged anions will move towards anode (+ve electrode). Conductance is denoted as C.

Important terms and laws

1. **Ohm's Law:** The law states that the strength of current (I) flowing through a conductor is directly proportional to the potential difference E applied across the conductor, and is inversely proportional to the resistance (R) of the conductor. The mathematical expression is given as

   $$I = \frac{E}{R}$$

2. **Conductance**: It is the ease with which the current can flow through a conductor. It is the reciprocal of resistance. Mathematically

   $$C = \frac{1}{R}$$

   Unit of conductance is reciprocal ohms or mhos

3. **Specific Resistance:**

   The resistance R of the conductor is directly proportional to the length (l) and inversely proportional to its area of cross section. (a)

   So $R \propto l$ and $R \propto \frac{1}{a}$

   $\therefore R \propto \frac{l}{a}$

   $R = \rho \frac{l}{a}$

   Where ρ is specific resistance or resistivity.

   Where l=1cm and a=1 sq.cm, R=ρ

   Hence the **specific resistance ρ is defined as the resistance of the conductor having 1cm length and 1sq.cm as area of cross section**

   Therefore $\rho = R\,\frac{a}{l}$ .The Unit of ρ is ohm-cm

4. **Specific conductance:** The specific conductance of any conductor is the reciprocal of specific resistance and it is denoted by the letter K. (Kappa)

   $$R = \frac{\rho l}{a}$$

   $$R = \frac{1}{k} \times \frac{l}{a}$$

   $$k = \frac{1}{R} \times \frac{l}{a}$$

   The unit for specific conductance is $ohm^{-1}\ cm^{-1}$

   When l=1 cm and a=1sq.cm then

   $$\boldsymbol{k = \frac{1}{R} = C}$$

   Thus specific conductance is defined as the conductivity of a solution of length 1cm and area of cross section 1 sq.cm. Its unit is mhos/cm.

5. **Equivalent conductance:** It is the conductance of the solution containing 1 gm equivalent of an electrolyte placed between two electrodes which are 1 cm apart. It is denoted by λ_v, where v is the volume in ml containing 1gm equivalent of the electrolyte. The unit is mhos.

6. **Molecular conductance/Molar conductance:** It is the conductance of a solution containing 1 gm mole of the electrolyte held between two electrodes which are 1cm apart from each other. It is denoted by μ_v and the unit is mhos.

Specific conductance vs Equivalent conductance

If 1 ml of 1 gm equivalent solution is placed between electrodes which are 1 cm apart, then the conductance of the solution is equal to specific conductance

$$\lambda = k$$

Diluting the solution 10 times, the equivalent conductance $\lambda = k \times 10$

If the dilution is made 100 times, then $\lambda = k \times 100$.

Thus $\lambda = k \times v$, where v is the volume of the solution containing 1gm equivalent of the electrolyte.

Equivalent conductance = specific conductance × volume of solution containing 1gm equivalent of the electrolyte.

Molecular conductance and specific conductance

$$\mu_v = k \times v$$

Molecular conductance = specific conductance × volume of solution containing1gm mole of the electrolyte.

Thus both equivalent and molar conductance are directly proportional to volume of the solution and so both equivalent and molar conductance increase with increase in dilution.

EFFECT OF DILUTION

On Conductance

The degree of dissociation of electrolyte increases with dilution. This produces more ions in solution. As the conductance of the solution is dependent on concentration of ions, the conductance increases with dilution.

On specific conductance

Specific conductance depends on the number of ions per ml of the solution. Though there is an increase in degree of dissociation with dilution, the number of ions per ml decreases. Thus the specific conductance decreases with increase in dilution.

On Equivalent conductance and molar conductance

Equivalent conductance and molar conductance both are dependent on specific conductance and volume of the solution. The increase in volume v is more than the decrease in specific conductance on dilution. Thus both equivalent conductance and molar conductance increase on dilution.

Conductance Measurements

The conductance of the solution is measured using wheat stone bridge arrangement. The different conductance bridges are

1. Kohlrausch conductance bridge
2. Direct reading conductance bridge

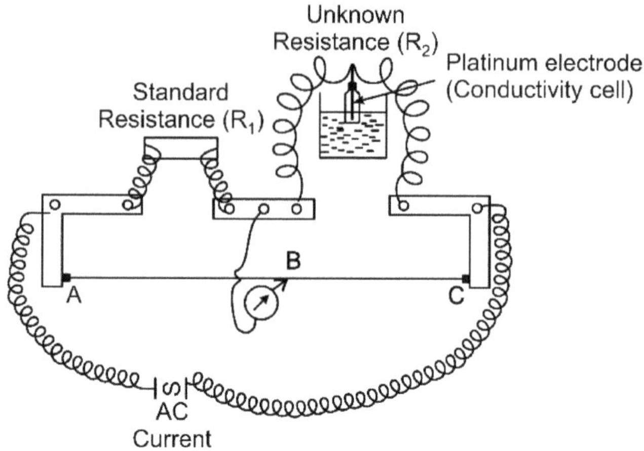

Circuit diagram of conductance bridge

INSTRUMENTATION

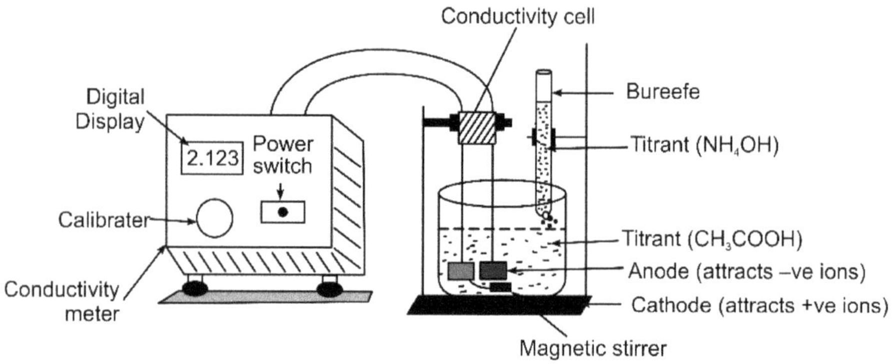

The components of conductometer are

(i) Current source
(ii) Conductivity meter
(iii) Conductivity cell
(iv) Electrodes

(i) Current source

A high frequency alternating current generator is employed to supply alternating current. When electrical potential is applied, ions move towards the respective electrodes and conductance takes place.

(ii) Conductivity meter

This consists of

1. Digital Display
2. Calibrator
3. Power switch

Power switch is used to apply potential to the conductivity cell. The calibrator is used for the calibration of the instrument. The conductance of the solution is displayed in the digital display.

(iii) Conductivity cell

The sample solution whose conductivity is to be measured is taken in conductivity cell. The cells are made of pyrex glass or quartz. They contain the platinum electrodes.

(iv) Electrodes

The electrodes are two parallel sheets of platinum foil. The distance between the electrodes is 1 cm and it is always a constant. To remove the polarization of the electrodes, the electrodes are coated with finely divided platinum black.

The platinization of electrodes are carried out by the electrolysis of chloro platinic acid (2-3%) containing 0.02 to 0.03 gms of lead acetate, using the electrodes. The electrodes are coated with finely divided platinum and they get blackened. They are washed repeatedly with water and finally with conductivity water.

CONDUCTIVITY WATER

Conductivity of the solution is sensitive to the presence of impurities. Thus the water used in conductometric measurements should be free from impurities. To avoid the conductance due to dissolved impurities, the conductivity water should be of high degree of purity. The conductivity water is prepared by the distillation of water containing small quantities of sodium hydroxide and potassium permanganate.

CELL CONSTANT

The electrodes in the conductivity cell are not always 1 cm apart and their surface area may not be one sq.cm. Hence, the observed conductivity is not equal to specific conductivity, but it is proportional to it. The cell constant is a factor for conductivity cell. This factor when multiplied by the observed conductivity, gives the value for specific conductivity.

It is known that

$$R = \rho \frac{1}{a}$$

$$R = \rho x \left[x = \frac{1}{a} = \text{cell constant} \right]$$

$$x = \text{cell constant} = \frac{R}{\rho}$$

$$\text{Cell constant} = \frac{1/\text{observed conductivity}}{1/\text{specific conductivity}}$$

$$= \frac{\text{Specific conductivity}}{\text{Observed conductivity}}$$

∴ Specific conductivity = cell constant × observed conductivity

$$\text{Cell constant} = \frac{0.002765}{\text{Observed conductivity}}$$

Where 0.002765 is the specific conductivity of N/50 KCl solution at 25° C.

EFFECT OF TEMPERATURE

Temperature should be monitored during conductivity measurements as the temperature coefficient for conductivity measurements is about 2% per degree Celsius.

Applications

1. Determination of basicity of organic acids
2. To determine the solubility of sparingly soluble salts.
3. To determine the ionic product of water.
4. Determination of degree of dissociation of weak electrolytes
5. Degree of hydrolysis
6. Determination of vanillin in vanilla essence
7. Conductometric titrations.
8. Determination of atmospheric sulphur dioxide

CONDUCTOMETRIC TITRATIONS

The substances which show a sharp change in conductivity at the endpoint can be determined by conductometric titrations. The titrations in which the endpoint is determined using conductivity measurements are called as conductometric titrations.

In conductometric titrations, the titrant is added from the burette and the conductivity of the titrand (titrated substance) is followed during the course of the titration even after the endpoint is reached.

The conductivities are plotted against the volume of the titrant in ml. The measured conductivity varies linearly with the concentration of ions present. The endpoint is determined by the extrapolation of point of intersection of lines in the graph to meet the x axis.

To get straight line graphs, the total volume of the solution should be maintained constant. To achieve this, the concentration of the titrant should be 10 times stronger than the solution (titrand). This makes the change in volume negligible.

Types of conductometric titrations

The different types of conductometric titrations are

1. Acid –base or neutral titrations
2. Replacement or displacement titrations
3. Precipitation titrations
4. Redox titrations
5. Complexometric titrations
6. Non-aqueous titrations

1. Acid base titrations

These titrations are well adapted to conductometric endpoints. The conductance of hydroxide and hydronium ions are compared with the conductance of reaction products. The different types of acid base titrations carried out by conductometry are discussed below

These titrations are further subdivided into

(i) STRONG ACID-STRONG BASE E.g.: HCL vs. NaOH
(ii) STRONG ACID-WEAK BASE E.g. HCL vs. NH_4OH
(iii) WEAK ACID-STRONG BASE E.g. CH_3COOH vs. NaOH
(iv) WEAK ACID -WEAK BASE E.g. CH_3COOH vs. NH_4OH

(i) Strong acid against strong base

Consider the titration of Hydrochloric acid (HCl) with Sodium hydroxide (NaOH)

$$\mathbf{HCl + NaOH \rightarrow NaCl + H_2O}$$

Before starting the titration, the high conductivity of the solution is due to the high mobility of H^+ ions (hydrogen). The Chloride ions (Cl^-) do not contribute much to the conductivity due to their less mobility. When the titrant NaOH is added to HCl, the highly mobile hydrogen ions are replaced by sodium ions (Na^+) which are less mobile. This leads to rapid decrease in conductance. At neutralization point (endpoint) only sodium and chloride ions are present and because of this, the conductivity is at its minimum. On the addition of more NaOH, the conductivity again increases due to the Hydroxyl ions (OH^-)

The titration is carried out at constant temperature. The conductivity is plotted against volume of sodium hydroxide. The point of intersection of the two lines gives the endpoint.

If the lines are curved at the endpoint, they are extrapolated to get the intersection (end point).

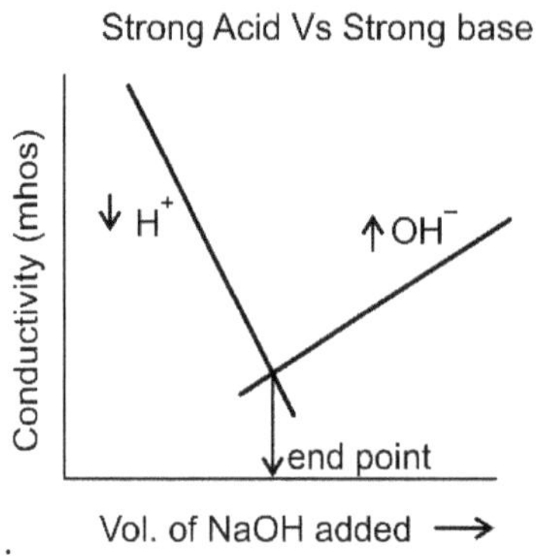

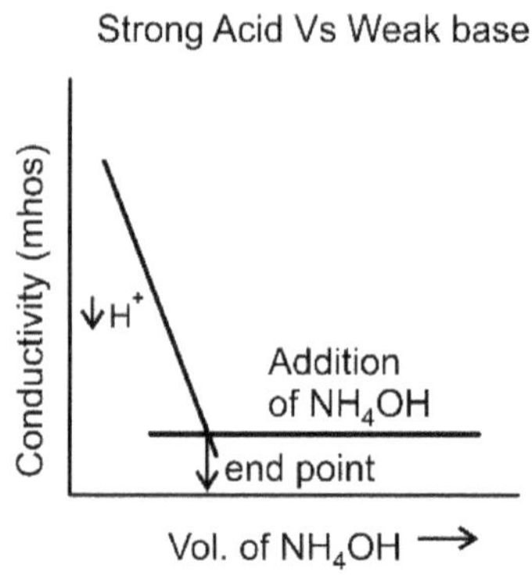

(ii) Strong acid against weak base

Consider the reaction of Hydrochloric acid with Ammonium hydroxide

$$\mathbf{HCl + NH_4OH \rightarrow NH_4Cl + H_2O}$$

Ammonium hydroxide (weak base) is added to strong acid (HCl) during titration. As the titration proceeds, fast moving Hydrogen (H^+) ions are replaced with slow moving ammonium ions (NH_4^+).So there is a decrease in conductance in the first part of the curve. After the endpoint, further addition of ammonium hydroxide does not change the conductance, because it is a weakly ionized electrolyte.

(iii) Weak acid against a strong base

Consider the reaction of Acetic acid (weak acid) with sodium hydroxide (strong base)

$$\mathbf{CH_3COOH + NaOH \rightarrow CH_3COONa + H_2O}$$

The titration starts with low conductivity as acetic acid is a weak acid which is poorly ionized. As NaOH (strong base) is added, initially due to neutralization, the conductivity decreases. After the end point when the neutralization is complete, further addition of sodium hydroxide increases the conductivity. This increase in conductivity is due to the excess of OH^- ions.

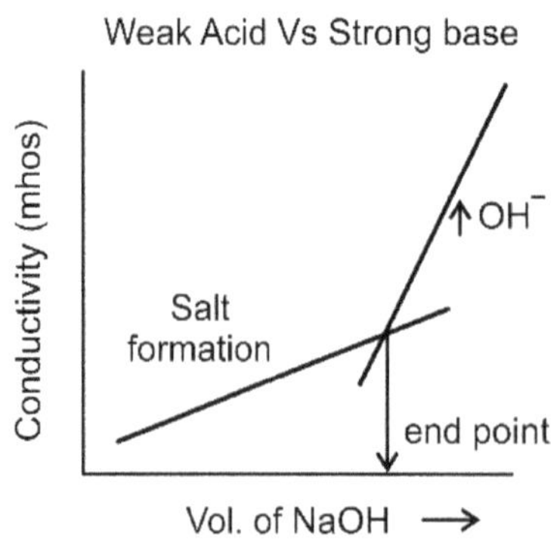

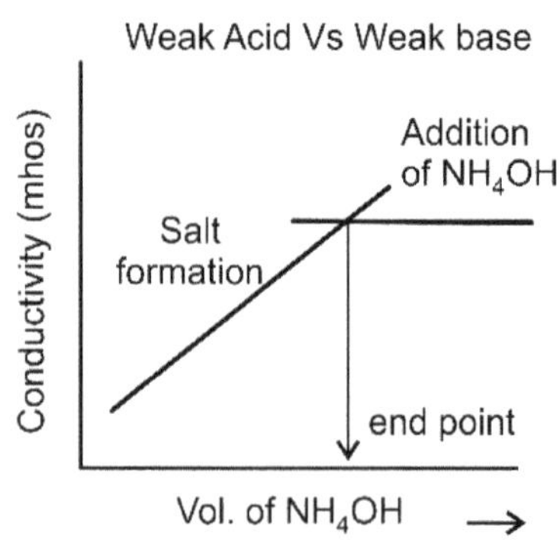

(iv) Weak acid against a weak base

Consider the reaction of acetic acid against Ammonium hydroxide

$$CH_3COOH + NH_4OH \rightarrow CH_3COONH_4 + H_2O$$

The initial conductivity is low, due to the weak dissociation of weak acid (acetic acid). When ammonium hydroxide (weak base) is added as the titrant, ammonium acetate salt is formed. This salt has better conductivity than both the reactants and there is an increase in conductivity after each addition of titrant. When all acetic acid is consumed after the endpoint, further addition of ammonium hydroxide causes no increase in conductivity and hence a plateau is obtained.

The first part of the graph shows increase in conductivity because of the salt formation and after the endpoint the graph shows a plateau because of the poor dissociation of weak base ammonium hydroxide.

2. Replacement or displacement titrations

In these titrations one ion is replaced by the other ion.

E.g. Salt of strong base and weak acid against strong acid

Consider the titration of sodium acetate with HCl

$$CH_3COONa + HCl \rightarrow CH_3COOH + NaCl$$

The titration starts with gradual increase in conductivity when the titrant HCl is added. This is due to the replacement of the acetate ions by chloride ions. After the endpoint, further addition of HCl causes a steep rise in conductivity due the H^+ ions. The graph is shown below

Salt of Strong acid and weak base against strong base

$$NH_4Cl + NaOH \rightarrow NH_4OH + NaCl$$

Initially the graph shows a plateau, because the ammonium ions are replaced with sodium ions till the endpoint. After the endpoint addition of further sodium hydroxide causes an increase in conductance. The graph is given in the figure

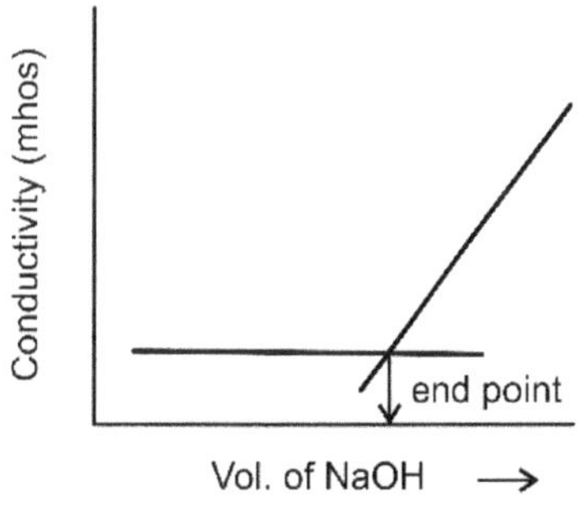

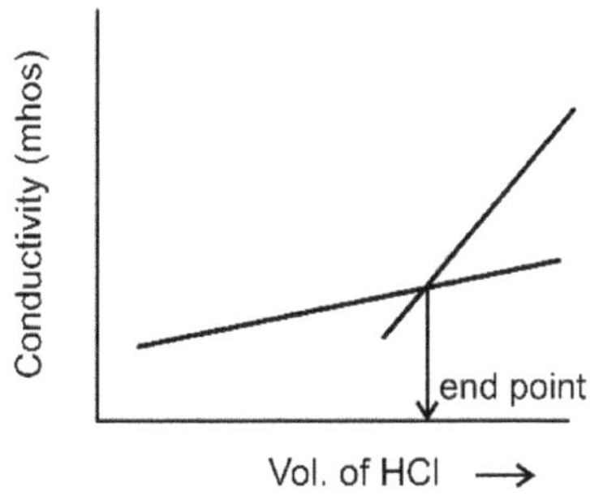

Salt of Strong acid and weak base against strong base

Salt of strong base and weak acid against strong acid

3. Precipitation titrations

In this type of the titrations, both products formed can be precipitates or one product is precipitate and the other one is a soluble product. Precipitation titrations are not very sensitive because of the adsorption of solutes on to the precipitate and slow precipitation.

Consider the titration of potassium chloride with silver nitrate - only one product is a precipitate

$$KCl + AgNO_3 \rightarrow AgCl\downarrow + KNO_3$$

Initially when silver nitrate is added, there is not much change in conductance. This is due to the fact that the Cl^- ions are replaced with NO^3 ions and both ions are having equal conductance. After the endpoint, addition of excess silver nitrate causes a sharp rise in conductance

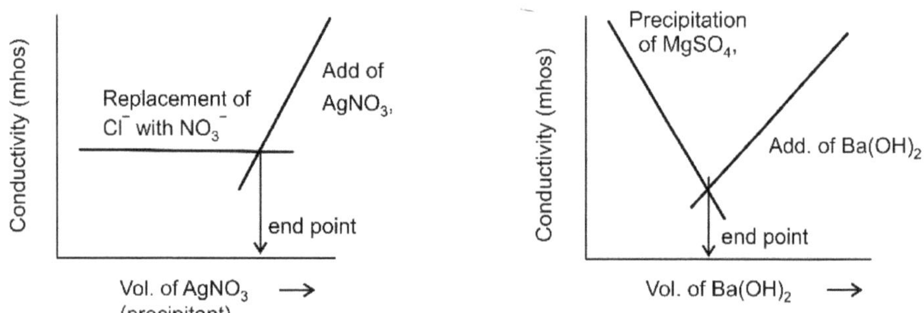

Precipitation titrations

Titration of magnesium sulphate with barium hydroxide – Both the precipitates are sparingly soluble

$$MgSO^4 + Ba(OH)_2 \rightarrow BaSO_4 + Mg(OH)_2$$

Magnesium sulphate is the titrand titrated with the titrant –barium hydroxide. The products barium hydroxide and magnesium hydroxide both are sparingly soluble precipitates. As the titration proceeds initially there is a decrease in conductivity due to the decrease of conducting Magnesium sulphate. After the endpoint the conductivity increases due to the excess of Barium hydroxide.

4. Redox titrations

$$6\,Fe^{2+} + Cr_2O_7^{2-} + 14H^+ \rightarrow 6Fe^{3+} + 2Cr^{3+} + 7H_2O$$

Redox titrations are carried out in the presence of acid. A decrease in conductance is observed as there is a decrease in concentration of hydrogen ions. After the end point there is not much change in conductivity.

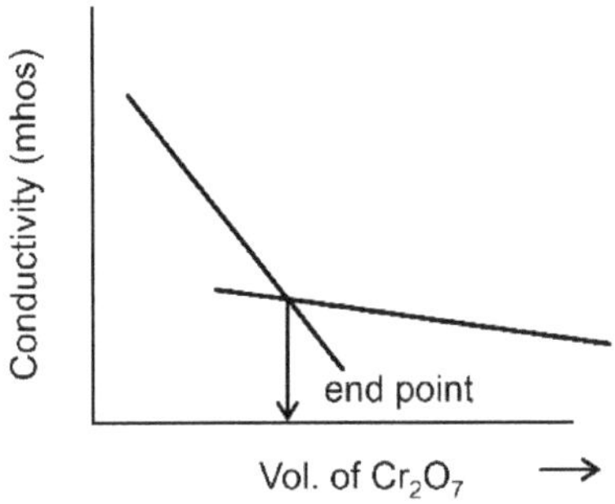

Redox titration curve

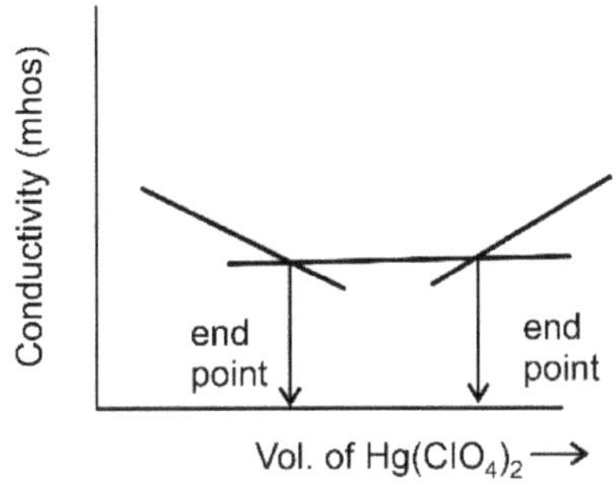

Complexometric titration curve

5. Complexometric titrations

Titration of Potassium chloride with Mercuric chlorate

$$Hg(ClO_4) + 4\,KCl \rightarrow (HgCl_4)^{2-} + 2K^+ + 2KClO_4$$

$$(HgCl_4)^{2} + 2K^+ \rightarrow K_2HgCl_4$$

There are two breaks in the curve. The first break indicates the formation of $(HgCl_4)^2$ and the second break indicates the completion of the reaction by forming K_2HgCl_4

6. Non-aqueous titrations

Titration of weak acids and weak bases are carried out by this method.

E.g. Weak organic acids are titrated in methanol, pyridine or dimethyl formamide against tetra methyl ammonium hydroxide in benzene containing methanol or pyridine.

Weak bases are titrated against perchloric acid in dioxin formic acid.

Advantages of conductometric titrations

1. Coloured solutions where indicators cannot be used can be titrated by conductometry.
2. Dilute solutions and weak acids can be titrated.

Disadvantages

1. It cannot give accurate results with concentrated electrolyte solutions.

Not much suitable for redox titrations

CHAPTER 21

Polarography

Polarography is defined as the method of instrumental analysis where the potential difference is measured as the current flows in solution. A plot of current against voltage gives the nature and amount of the substance present. The instrument used is polarograph and the curves obtained are called polarograms. Polarography is an electrochemical method of analysis in which the solution is electrolyzed and the electro reducible or oxidisable substances are determined qualitatively or quantitatively.

PRINCIPLE

A gradually increasing negative potential (voltage) is applied between two electrodes, of which one electrode is polarisable and the other electrode is nonpolarisable. The current flowing through the system is recorded as the voltage is varied. Both electrodes are mercury electrodes. A pool of mercury acts as the anode (large) and a mercury drop from a fine capillary tube acts as the cathode (negatively charged). The anode is the non polarisable electrode and the cathode is the polarisable electrode. The analyte is the dilute solution of the electro active material i.e. the electrolyte.

The solution contains an excess of a different electrolyte which is the supporting electrolyte. The bulk of the current is carried by the supporting electrolyte and it increases the conductivity of the solution.

If a steady increasing negative voltage is applied to this cell, the positive ions of the analyte diffuse in the solution towards the dropping mercury electrode. Current is flowing through the solution due to the diffusion of ions. This current is called as diffusion current (i_d). From the current voltage curves, the nature and concentration of the substance present can be obtained.

CONSTRUCTION OF THE APPARATUS

The apparatus used in polarography consists of a dropping mercury electrode (DME) which is polarisable and saturated calomel electrode as the reference electrode which is non-polarisable. The pool of mercury at the bottom of the beaker can also be used as the reference electrode. Its surface area is large and hence it is nonpolarisable. The beaker or the sample cell contains the sample to be analyzed. The capillary is dipped into the analyte solution. A drop time of 2-12 sec is obtained by adjusting the height of mercury reservoir.

Both the cathode and anode are connected to a battery and an increasing negative potential is applied across the electrodes. The current is measured with a galvanometer G. Nitrogen gas is passed through the sample, to remove dissolved oxygen from the sample.

DROPPING MERCURY ELECTRODE (DME)

DME is made up of a fine capillary with an inner diameter of 20-50μ and it is connected to a mercury reservoir on top. The time taken for a new mercury drop to form, grow and fall from the capillary is called drop time. The drop time can be altered by adjusting the height of the mercury reservoir. Usual drop time set is 2-12 sec. The size of the capillary determines the size of mercury drop. Wire contacts are provided through the tube through which the mercury flows. DME acts as the cathode and it is a polarisable electrode. The potential range that can be applied is given +0.4 to -1.8 V. The tip of the capillary should be kept clean to avoid clogging.

ADVANTAGES OF DME

1. Reproducible surface area with any capillary.
2. Mercury lowers the reduction potential of metals by forming amalgams so that they can be analyzed by polarography
3. Diffusion current is reproducible and steady value is reached instantaneously.
4. Poisoning effects can be eliminated by constant renewal of electrodes.
5. Surface area of the drops can be calculated from weight of the drops.

DISADVANTAGES OF DME

1. The electrode can be used only in the range of +0.4 to -1.8V. Above 0.4 V mercury dissolves and anodic wave is recorded. Below -1.8 V, hydrogen is liberated.
2. Easy oxidation of mercury limits the usage of the electrode.
3. Plugging of the capillary due to foreign material is a drawback
4. As the size of the drop changes, the surface area also changes.

WORKING OF THE APPARATUS (POLAROGRAPH)

A potential is applied to the cell containing the solution of the analyte. The electrical force attracts the positively charged ions towards DME. A diffusive force is also acting from the concentration gradient formed at the surface of the electrode. Voltage is increased gradually and the current is recorded. The graph obtained is called as **polarogram.**

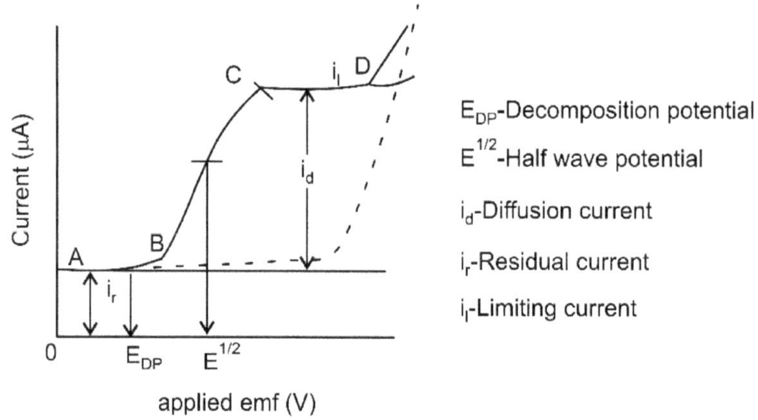

Current voltage curve (Polarogram)

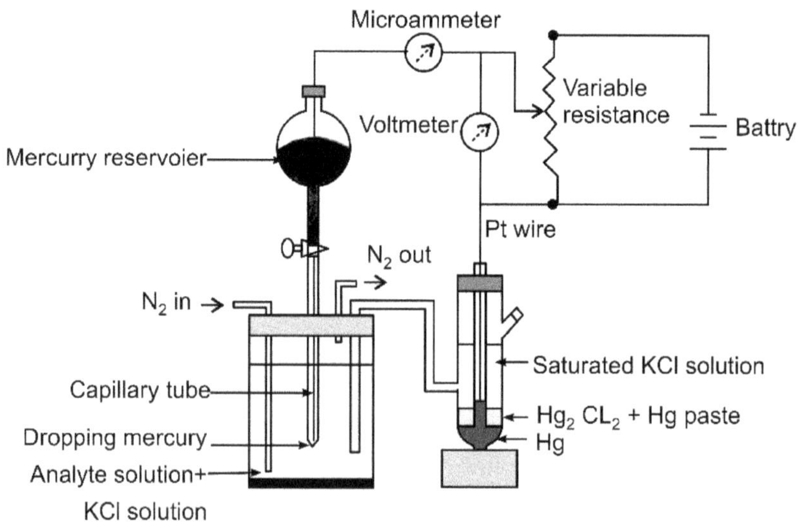

Schematic representation of polarographic circuit

In the figure the current flowing from A to B is called as residual current. This current is due to the supporting electrolyte and impurities in the sample. The supporting electrolyte concentration is 100 times greater than the analyte. The potential of the electrode becomes equal to the decomposition potential of the analyte at point B. There is an increase in current from B to C.

After the point C there is no linear increase in current with increase in voltage and the current reaches a steady limiting value at D. After D there is no increase in current even at higher cathode potentials. The curve CD is called as limiting current.

The diffusion current is the difference between residual current and limiting current and it is designated as i_d.

The factors (different currents) affecting current voltage curves are

(i) Residual current

(ii) Migration current

(iii) Diffusion current

(iv) Kinetic current

(i) Residual current

The current is a combination of current produced by reduction of impurities and the condenser current produced by the helmhaltz double layer.

The current produced by the impurities is called as Faradiac current. The condenser current is produced by the migration of positively charged K^+ ions towards the negatively charged growing mercury drop. These K^+ ions are not reduced to K atoms and they form a layer around the mercury drop surface, creating a electrical double layer. This effect resembles charging of a condenser. When the drop falls of, the whole process starts again and a new condenser is charged up. There is a continuous flow of current due to this process, and there is an increase in current as the potential of the drop is increased.

Residual current = Faradiac current + Condenser current.

(ii) Migration current

The migration current is produced by the migration of charged particles of electro active material in presence of electric field produced by the potential difference between the electrode surface and solution. The diffusion process of particles also carries a part of migration.

Migration current can be eliminated by increasing the concentration of supporting electrolyte.

(iii) Diffusion current

The current is due to the diffusion of the analyte and it is directly proportional to the concentration of the analyte getting reduced or oxidized at the dropping mercury electrode. Diffusion current is given by the ilkovic equation

$$I_d = 607_n CD^{1/2} m^{2/3} t^{1/6}$$

where

I_d - diffusion current in microamperes

n - no of electrons transferred per ion.

C - Concentration in milli moles /litre.

D - Diffusion coefficient of reducible ion in $cm^2\ sec^{-1}$

M - mass of mercury flowing per second in mg

t - drop time in seconds.

The ilkovic equation states that the diffusion current is directly proportional to the concentration of electro active material. This forms the basis of quantitative analysis by polarography.

Factors affecting diffusion current

1. **Concentration**

   The quantitative analysis is based on the principle that the **diffusion current increases with an increase in the concentration** of the electro-reducible ion.

2. **Temperature**

   Diffusion current varies with temperature as the diffusion of ions is dependent on temperature.

3. **Viscosity of the medium**

   Diffusion current varies with the viscosity of the medium as the diffusion coefficient depends on the viscosity of the medium.

4. **Capillary characteristics**

   The flow characteristics of the capillary vary with the bore size of the capillary and drop time in seconds and the pressure of mercury. These factors in turn will affect the diffusion current.

5. **Presence of agents like maxima suppressors**

   The presence of maxima suppressors like gelatin, dye, and surfactants also affect the diffusion current.

(iv) Kinetic current

This current is due to the equilibrium of the oxidized or reduced form of the analyte with other substances. Because these are rate processes, the resulting current is called Kinetic current. It is dependent on the size of the mercury drop but is independent of the rate of flow of mercury from the capillary.

HALF WAVE POTENTIAL

It is the characteristic property of the electroactive material. The potential at one-half of the distance between the residual and limiting current is called half-wave potential. It is found on the steeply rising portion of the current-voltage curve. It is denoted as $E_{1/2}$. At half-wave potential 50% of oxidized and 50% of reduced form are present. It is used for the identification of the substances by comparison with a standard value (qualitative analysis).

The reduction at the DME is represented as

Oxidant + ne ↔ reductant

Ox + ne ↔ red

$$E = E^0 + (0.0591/n)\,(\log[\,(ox)_0/(red)_0]$$

By definition, half wave potential is $i = \frac{1}{2}\, i_d$.

$$E_{1/2} = E^0 + (0.0591/n)\log[\,D_{red}/D_{ox}]$$

$E_{1/2}$ is the half-wave potential. The equation shows that polarographic wave potential is related to the standard reduction potential of the oxidation-reduction system.

The half-wave potential of a reducible substance is independent of concentration and is characteristic of the nature of the reacting material. This forms the basis of quantitative and qualitative polarographic analysis

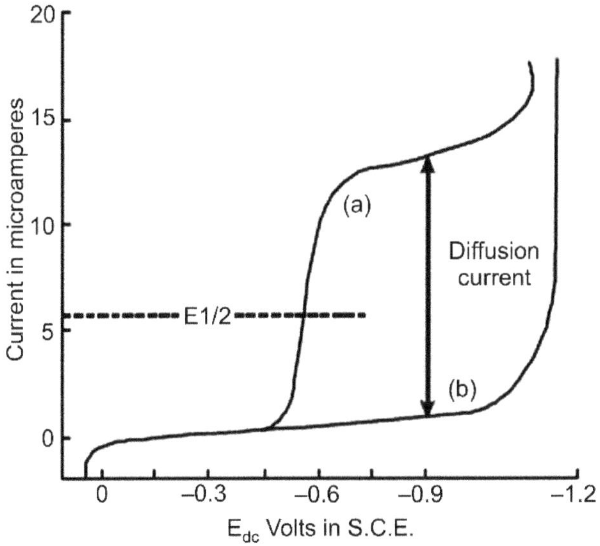

Half wave potential

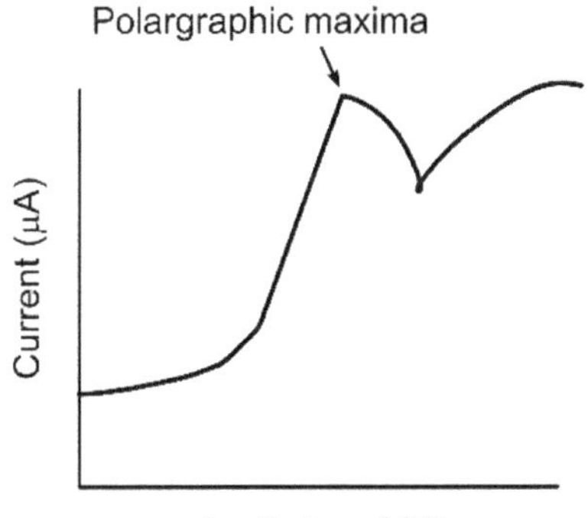

Polarographic maxima

FACTORS THAT AFFECT THE HALF-WAVE POTENTIALS

1. The temperature coefficient of the half-wave potential is mostly between –2 and +2 mv/degree
2. The half-wave potential is almost always independent of the concentration of the electroactive species
3. The half-wave potential of a reversible wave is nearly independent of the capillary characteristics
4. The half-wave potential of a totally irreversible wave, however, varies significantly with *t*
5. Changes in the nature and concentration of supporting electrolytes may affect the half-wave potential in many ways.
6. Complex formation may cause the half-wave potential
7. Temperature

POLAROGRAPHIC MAXIMA

Current-voltage curves obtained using DME are sometimes distorted by small or more pronounced maxima. They can be sharp peaks or rounded humps. The current rises abnormally until a critical value is reached and then rapidly decreases to normal limiting current corresponding to the normal diffusion current plateau.

These are the abnormal peaks that appear on the polarogram above the limiting current. It occurs in concentrated solutions.

Two types namely (1) Maxima of the first kind and (2) Maxima of the second kind

MAXIMA OF THE FIRST KIND

In dilute solutions of supporting electrolytes this kind of maxima is usually observed on the rising portion of the polarographic wave. It increases rapidly with voltage to larger values than the limiting current and falls discontinuously to the normal limiting current. Thus, the first kind of maxima is characterized by a sharp current peak.

The maximum is called positive or negative depending on whether the half-wave potential of the depolarizer lies on the positive side of the electro-capillary curve or on the negative side. Streaming of the solution past the electrode surface causes these maxima.

MAXIMA OF THE SECOND KIND

These maxima are observed in concentrated solutions of the supporting electrolyte (>0.1 N). This appears on the limiting current region and it depends on the purity of the solution. This maximum appears as an increase in the original wave or forms a new wave and the current does not fall abruptly in contrast to the first kind of maxima.

The occurrence of the maximum of the second kind depends on the mercury flow rate. By reducing the mercury flow rate the maximum can be suppressed.

MAXIMA SUPPRESSORS

Maxima of both kinds are causing obstacles to quantitative polarographic analyses. They can be eliminated by the addition of a small number of maximum suppressors to the solution. The maxima suppressor is the substance that gets adsorbed onto the surface of the dropping electrode and then retards or prevents the motion of the solution past the drop surface. The most common maximum suppressors are some of the surface-active reagents like gelatin, agar, organic dyes, and Triton-X-100. The suppressors must be present in smaller concentrations.

At higher concentration, the suppressors make the interpretation of polarograms difficult by diminishing the limiting current of the substance itself. The effectiveness of a suppressor can be expressed as the maximum dilution or the minimum necessary for complete suppression of a given maximum. Maxima suppressors belong to the following categories

1. Gelatin
2. Dyes
3. Surfactants.

Gelatin is used in the concentration of 0.002 to 0.01% Agar, methyl cellulose, methyl red, acid and basic fuschine dyes are used as suppressors.

APPLICATIONS OF POLAROGRAPHY

1. **Application to Inorganic Compounds**
   Used in the estimation of cations and anions in the presence of interfering ions. E.g. Estimation of Li in presence of other alkali metals.
2. **Application to Organic compounds**
   Organic polarography is useful for the structure determination, Qualitative and quantitative analysis.

3. **Determination of Dissolved oxygen**

   The dissolved oxygen is measured by measuring the oxygen waves. Oxygen is not swept out with nitrogen. Combined oxygen does not interfere in this method,

4. **Studies of complexes**

   Useful in studying the composition of complexes.

5. **Determination of plant content**

6. **Application to pharmaceuticals**

   For the determination of Dissolved oxygen and peroxides, trace metals and metal containing drugs, Antiseptics and insecticides, Vitamins, Hormones, Antibiotics, Alkaloids, Blood serum and cancer diagnosis.

CHAPTER 22

Amperometry

Polarography forms the basis of amperometric methods. This method is comparable with Potentiometric, conductometric and photometric methods.

PRINCIPLE

In amperometric methods, the voltage applied across the electrodes is kept constant and the diffusion current is measured. The measured diffusion current is plotted against the volume of the reagent added.

In Polarography only electro reducible ions can be detected whereas in amperometry both electro reducible and non-reducible substances can be detected. From polarography it is known that the diffusion current is proportional to the concentration of electro active material in the solution. If some of the electro active material is removed by any means, there will be a decrease in diffusion current. This forms the basis of amperometric titrations. The current is measured in the ampere units. Diffusion current is because of polarization at the micro electrode. These titrations are more accurate than polarography because they are not much dependent on the characteristics of capillary and supporting electrolyte

APPARATUS

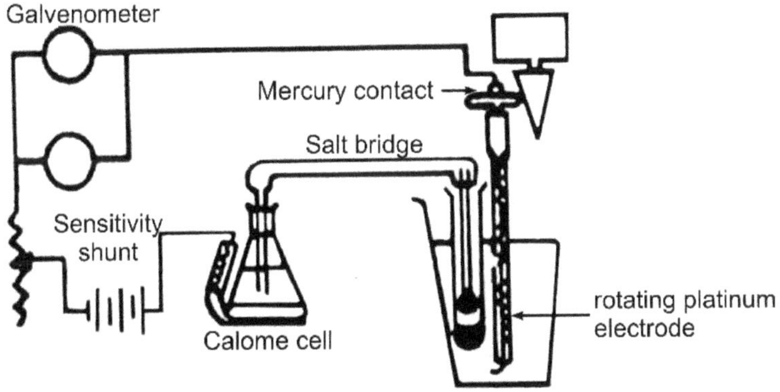

The apparatus used is same as the Polarography apparatus. It consists of a dropping mercury electrode or a rotating platinum electrode which act as the

cathode. Calomel electrode is used as the reference electrode. The galvanometer measures the current. During amperometric titrations, the voltage applied between the electrodes is kept constant and the diffusion current is measured after each addition of the titrant. A burette for delivering the titrant is included and a stirrer is also present to mix the contents.

ROTATING PLATINUM MICRO ELECTRODE

Construction and working

It consists of a glass tube of about 15-20 cm in length and mm in diameter. A platinum wire of length 5-10 +mm extends out from the tip of the glass tube. The electrode is mounted on a shaft the motor and it is rotated at a constant speed of about 600 rotations per minute.

Advantages of rotating platinum electrode

1. Construction is simple
2. Workable range on the +ve voltage side up to 0.9V. This electrode can work in positive potentials where as mercury electrode cannot be used in +ve potentials (-2 volts to 0.4V)
3. Rotation of the platinum electrode increases the volume of diffusion current 20 times more than that obtained in polarography, making amperometric titrations more sensitive than Polarography.

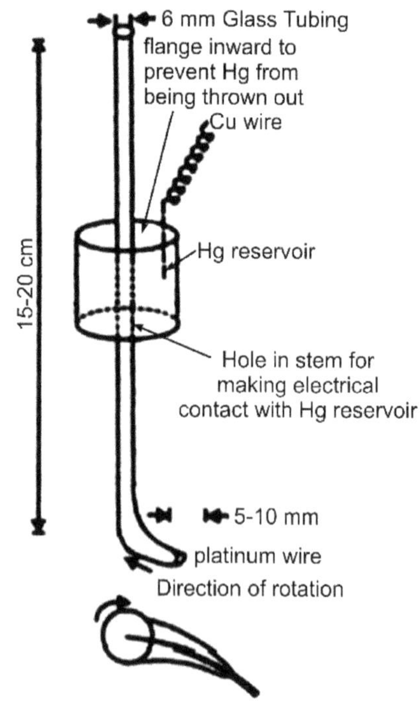

The diffusion current flowing through the system is proportional to the concentration the electro active species. The titrant is added in predetermined increments and the diffusion current decreases due to the removal of the electro active species by reaction with the titrant. The diffusion current is measured after each addition of the titrant. The titration is continued even after the end point is reached. The diffusion current is plotted against volume of the titrant added and the intersection of the curves gives the endpoint. Removal of oxygen is done by bubbling purified nitrogen through the solution before the start of the titration and for1 minute after each addition of the titrant.

The addition of the titrant instalments, dilute the experimental solution. Because of this dilution, the observed current is smaller than the actual value. Hence a correction factor is applied.

AMPEROMETRIC TITRATIONS

The amperometric titrations can be performed only if either the titrated ion or titrant or both are electro reducible. The potential applied during the titration should correspond to the limiting current.

The different types of amperometric titrations are dependent on the nature of the electro active species and the titrant.

1. **Reducible titrate and non reducible titrant**

   Titration of electro reducible ion against Non-reducible titrant.

   Example: Pb $^{2+}$ with SO_4 $^{2-}$

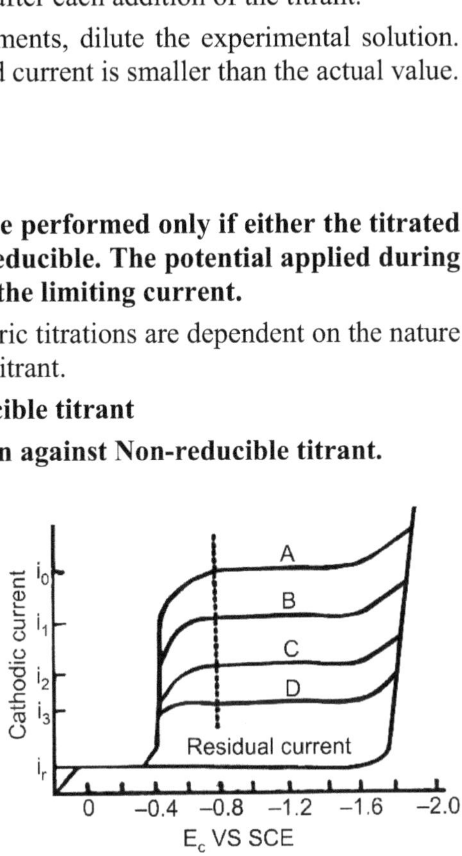

   The Pb^{2+} ions undergo reduction at the cathode giving diffusion current. The sulphate ions are non-reducible and no diffusion current is produced by them.

   As the titrant is added, the sulphate ions $(SO_4)^{2-}$ remove some of the electro reducible lead ions (Pb^{2+}) leading to decrease in concentration of Pb^{2+} ions. Voltage is kept constant.

   To find out the working voltage range, initially cathode current is plotted against voltage.

   Curve A- is the current due to reducible Pb^{2+} ions before the addition of sulphate ions. (current i_O)

   Curve B- is the current due to reducible Pb^{2+} ions after the addition of some sulphate ions. There is a small decrease in the initial current. (current i)

   Curve C and D –are current i_2 and i_3 which are the currents after the further additions of sulphate ions.

During this stage, the current flowing is the residual current due to the supporting electrolyte because all Pb^{2+} ions are consumed

From the graph it is known that, there is a decrease in current with decrease in concentration of electro reducible ion. The working voltage region is determined from the plateau of voltage curve. From the range of -0.6 to 1.2 volt, the volt -0.8 is selected for this titration.

After finding the working voltage, the diffusion current is plotted against the volume of the titrant. The curve is shown in the figure.

The intersection of the extrapolated curves gives the end point.

2. **Non-reducible titrate and electro reducible titrant**

Example: Titration of Cl^- with Ag^+

The titration curve is initially horizontal line, not showing any change in diffusion current with the addition of titrant. The titrand is non-reducible and the diffusion current is equal to the migration current. After the end point the diffusion current increases with the addition of the titrant. The concentration of the electro reducible Ag^+ ions increases after the addition of titrant leading to increased diffusion current after the endpoint.

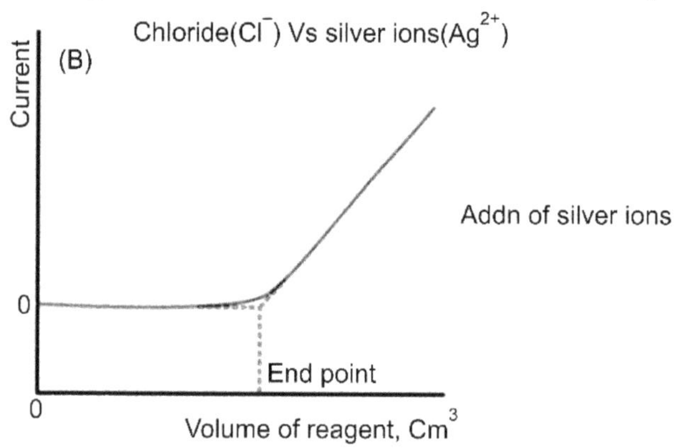

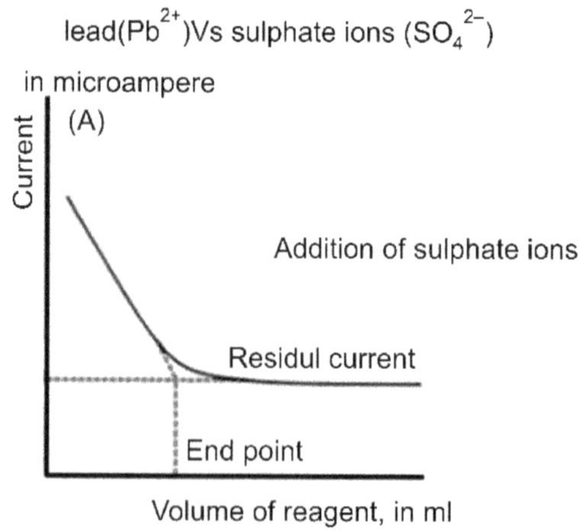

3. Titration of reducible titrate with reducible titrant (both are reducible)

Example: Titration of Pb^{2+} vs. $Cr_2O_7^{2-}$

Both the titrated ion and the titrant ion are reducible at the cathode. The initial high diffusion current decreases as the titrant is added from the burette. Dichromate ions remove the Pb^{2+} ions and the diffusion current decreases till the endpoint is reached. After the endpoint, the diffusion current increases due to increase in electro reducible dichromate ions. The titration curve looks like V shape curve. The intersection of the lines gives the endpoint.

Ex: lead(Pb^{2+})Vs dichromate ions($Cr_2O_7^{2-}$)

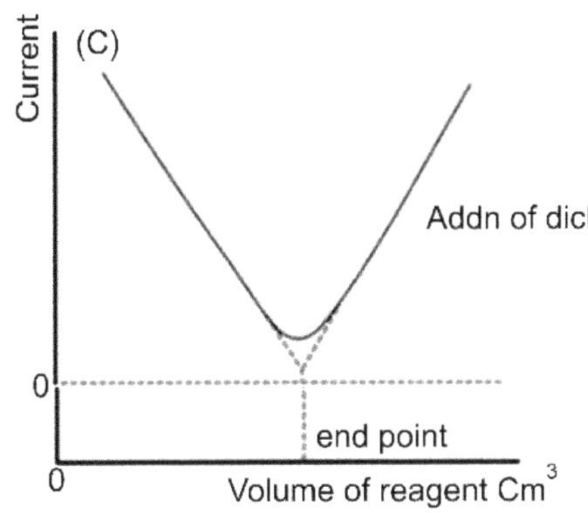

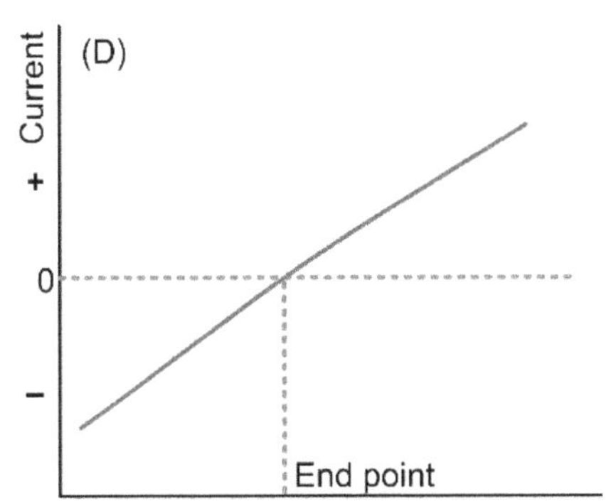

4. Redox titrations

In these titrations both the oxidant and the reductant are giving diffusion current

Ferric ions titrated against titanous ions

Initially the diffusion current decreases linearly with the addition of titrant (T_i^{3+} ions). The ferric ions are reduced by titanous ions until all the ferric ions are consumed. The diffusion current reaches a zero value at the endpoint. The diffusion current due to T_i^{3+}ions is shown as a change in slope of the curve after the endpoint. The point of intersection of two curves gives the endpoint.

Dead stop endpoint technique (Bi amperometry)

When an oxidation-reduction system is involved before and after the endpoint, dead stop endpoint technique is used.

The cell consists of two similar platinum electrodes. The two electrodes are dipped in two different solutions in two different vessels and are linked by a salt bridge. A constant voltage is applied between these two electrodes.

When the reactant involves a reversible system, the amount of oxidised form reduced at the cathode is equal to the reduced form oxidised at the anode. Both electrodes are depolarised at this stage. When the oxidised / reduced form is consumed by the titrant (at the end point) only one electrode is depolarised as if the titrant does not involve a reversible system. The current is equal to zero or nearly zero at the endpoint and after the endpoint both the electrodes are depolarized and the current shoots up as shown in the figure.

At the start of titration, one electrode is depolarized, and as titration proceeds, both electrodes are depolarised. Near the endpoint, as one of the reactant is depleted, only one electrode is depolarised and no current is flowing through the system. As the system involves a redox system before and after the endpoint, immediately both electrodes become depolarised and there is a sudden increase in current.

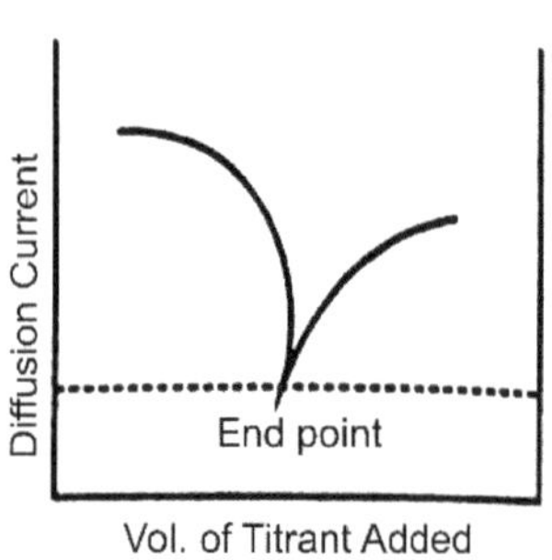

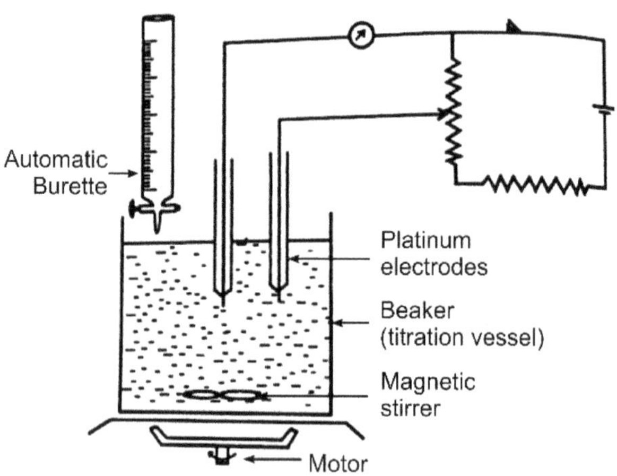

Apparatus for
dead stop end point technique

Example of dead stop endpoint technique is determination of water with Karl Fischer reagent. The apparatus consists of two platinum electrodes, and an emf is applied between the electrodes. As long as water is present both electrodes are depolarised and current is flowing. Current flows only when both electrodes are depolarised. There is a decrease in current as the water molecules are consumed by the KF reagent which is the titrant. KF reagent consists of iodine and sulphur dioxide in pyridine and methanol. Titrant is added from the burette. At the end point only one electrode remains depolarized and the current reaches zero value and there is a sudden increase in current. Thus, at the endpoint, the decreased current suddenly increases.

Karl fischer titration is a titration in which either volumetric or coulometric titration is used to determine the quantity of water present in the given sample.

PRINCIPLE

The principle is based on the oxidation reaction between sulphur dioxide and iodine. Water reacts with sulphur dioxide and iodine to form hydrogen iodide and sulphur trioxide. During the titration iodine is added to the sample and the amount of iodine required to consume all the water in the analyte is noted. The titration is a biamperometric titration and the end point is determined electrometrically

A constant volt of 500mV is applied between the two platinum electrodes and the current flowing through the system is measured. The iodine added, consumes the water. When all the water is consumed, there is no free iodine in solution and when the endpoint is reached, the current increases suddenly from almost nil.

$$3C_5H_5N + SO_2 + I_2 + H_2O \longrightarrow 2\ C_5H_5NHI + C_5H_5NOSO_2$$

$$C_5H_5NOSO_2 + CH_3OH \longrightarrow C_5H_5NHSO_4CH_3$$

Preparation of KF reagent

KF reagent is a solution containing a mixture of 170 ml of pyridine and 70ml of methanol. To this solution125g of iodine is added and cooled. This solution is taken in a 250 ml graduated cylinder and 100ml of pyridine is added. Cooled in ice bath and sulphur dioxide gas (dry) is passed through the solution till the volume reaches 200ml.

The KF reagent is standardised using sodium tartrate dehydrate. It has got 15.66 % stoichiometric water content. The equivalence factor is 0.1566 X W/V in mgs of water per ml of reagent, where w-wt of sodium tartrate in mgs, V is the reagent volume in ml.

Applications

It is used for water determination in plastics, oils, gases. It is also used for determination of water in pharmaceutical products, cosmetic products and other industries.

Advantages of amperometric titrations

1. Apparatus is simple
2. Few disturbing factors
3. More accurate than polarography

4. Temperature is constant
5. Sensitivity is more than conductometric or Potentiometric titration
6. Capillary characteristic does not affect the titrations
7. Constant current need not be maintained
8. Both reversible and irreversible titrations can be done
9. The depolarising substances can be titrated by amperometry
10. Endpoint is more accurate because it is determined graphically
11. No interference from foreign salts
12. Dilute solutions can be titrated accurately
13. Applicable to precipitation titrations

Disadvantages

1. Co-precipitation gives inaccurate results
2. Foreign substances should not be present in large concentration as the relative current becomes smaller

Applications of amperometric titrations

1. Titrations involving slightly soluble precipitates. E.g. Titration of Pb^{2+} against $K_2Cr_2O_7$.
2. Used as detectors in liquid chromatography
3. Titrations involving electro reducible and non-reducible ions

SECTION – IV: Spectroscopy

23. UV Visible Spectroscopy
24. IR Spectroscopy
25. Fluorimetry
26. Flame Photometry
27. Atomic Absorption Spectroscopy
28. Atomic Emission Spectroscopy
29. NMR and ESR Spectroscopy
30. Mass Spectroscopy
31. Polarimetry
32. X-Ray Diffraction
33. Thermal Methods

CHAPTER 23

UV Visible Spectroscopy

INTRODUCTION

Spectroscopy is the branch of science that deals with studying the **interaction of matter with electromagnetic radiation**. Due to this interaction, energy is either absorbed or emitted by the matter in discrete amounts called quanta. The measurement of this absorbed or emitted radiation by the matter forms the basis of spectroscopic techniques. Spectroscopic techniques are helpful in the study of atomic and molecular structures. Spectroscopy is one of the most powerful tools available for the qualitative and quantitative analysis of different samples.

Spectroscopy can be studied under two major headings

1. **Atomic spectroscopy** – deals with the interaction of electromagnetic radiation with atoms in the ground energy level (lowest energy).
   E.g., Atomic absorption spectroscopy, Atomic emission spectroscopy, Flame emission spectroscopy
2. **Molecular spectroscopy** – deals with the interaction of electromagnetic radiation with molecules.
   E.g., IR spectroscopy, Raman spectroscopy.

Spectroscopy can also be classified based on the measured mode of interaction of matter with electromagnetic radiation, which is given in the Table 23.1.

Table 23.1 Instrumental Methods based on measurement of property.

Absorption of radiation	Emission of radiation	Scattering
Absorption spectroscopy: X-ray, UV, IR, Colorimetry, Atomic absorption, Nuclear magnetic resonance, and electron spin resonance spectroscopy	**Emission spectroscopy:** Flame emission photometry, Fluorescence spectroscopy	Turbidimetry, Nephelometry, Raman spectroscopy.

PROPERTIES OF ELECTROMAGNETIC RADIATION

Electromagnetic radiation is an energy form that travels with enormous velocity in space. Electromagnetic radiation (EMR) possesses both wave and particle nature. These properties are a distinct feature of EMR, and they are inseparable.

Wave properties of Electromagnetic radiation

Electromagnetic radiation has an electrical component and a magnetic component oscillating in perpendicular planes and also perpendicular to the direction of propagation. The wave nature of EMR shows properties like refraction, reflection, constructive and destructive interferences.

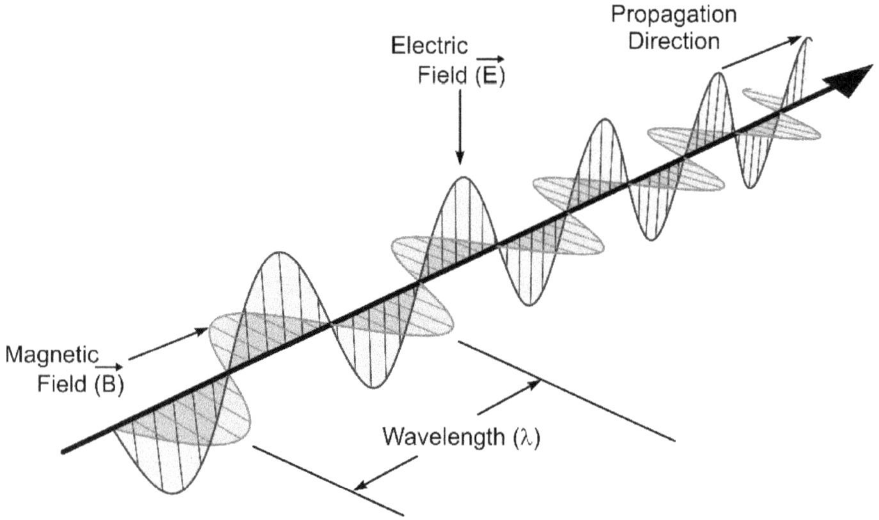

Fig. 23.1 Electromagnetic wave with its components.

The electromagnetic wave parameters are

(a) **Wave length, λ:** Is the **distance between two successive maxima or minima in an electromagnetic wave**. It is denoted by the Greek letter lambda. Units of wavelength are meters (m), centimeter (cm), millimeter (mm), micrometers (μm), nanometers (nm) and angstrom (Å).

$$1\text{Å} = 10^{-8}\text{ cm} = 0.1\text{nm} = 10^{-10}\text{m}$$

A beam of radiation with only one wavelength is called **monochromatic radiation,** and the beam consisting of several wavelengths is called **polychromatic or heterochromatic radiation.**

(b) **Frequency, υ:** Is the **number of wavelength units passing through a given point in unit time.** It is denoted by the Greek letter υ.Unit is cycles per second or Hertz.

(c) **Wave number $\bar{\upsilon}$:** Frequency is usually a large number making its use more difficult in regular practice. To overcome this problem, frequency is usually expressed as wave number. **The wave number is the number of waves in vacuum**. The symbol is $\bar{\upsilon}$. Unit for wave number is cm^{-1}

$$\bar{\upsilon} = 1/\lambda$$

Particle properties of electromagnetic radiation

When electromagnetic radiation hits a material, it emits electrons called photoelectrons. This **photoelectric effect** is due to the particle properties of EMR. To explain this property, it is assumed that EMR consists of a stream of discrete packets (particles) of energy called photons or quanta. The energy of the photon is proportional to the frequency of the radiation and is given by the relationship

$$E = h\upsilon, \text{ where,}$$

E is the energy of a photon in ergs, υ is the frequency of the EMR in cycles per second, and h is called Planck's constant (6.624×10^{-34} joules/second).

EMR of longer wavelength (low frequency) has lower energy than the shorter wavelength (high frequency).

Electromagnetic spectrum

The entire range of EMR is called as EMR spectrum.

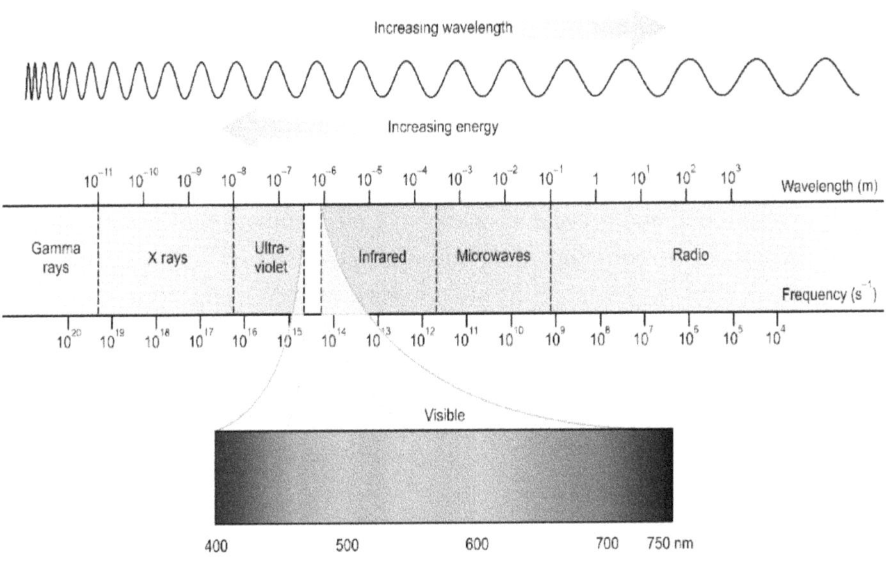

Fig. 23.2 Electromagnetic spectrum showing different regions of EMR.

The various spectral regions are

γ(Gamma) ray region – lies between 0.02 to 1 angstrom. These are the shortest waves.

X-ray region –This region lies between 1 to 10 angstrom. These rays cause core electron excitation.

Visible and Ultra violet region – These rays cause valence electron excitation. This region consists of three parts

Vacuum UV	:	**1 - 180 nm**
Ultraviolet	:	**180 - 400 nm**
Visible	:	**400 - 800 nm**

Infrared region – This region is subdivided into three regions

Near IR	:	**0.7 - 2.5 μm**
Mid IR	:	**2.5 - 15 μm**
Far IR	:	**15 - 200 μm**

Microwave region – 0.1 mm – 1 cm

Radiofrequency region – 100m – 1 cm

INTERACTION OF ELECTROMAGNETIC RADIATION WITH MATTER

When electromagnetic radiation passes through matter, a variety of events may occur. Some of them are

1. **Absorption of radiation:** If the radiation of appropriate energy is used, they may be absorbed by the matter resulting in electronic, vibrational, and rotational changes or a combination of these changes. After absorption, the molecules become excited and go to a high energy level (low stability). They lose energy in the form of heat or re-emit EMR to come back to the ground state (high stability).

   The total energy of the molecule at the ground state is given as

   $$E_0 = E_{electronic} + E_{vibrational} + E_{rotational}$$

   The schematic energy level diagram for a simple diatomic molecule is shown in the figure.

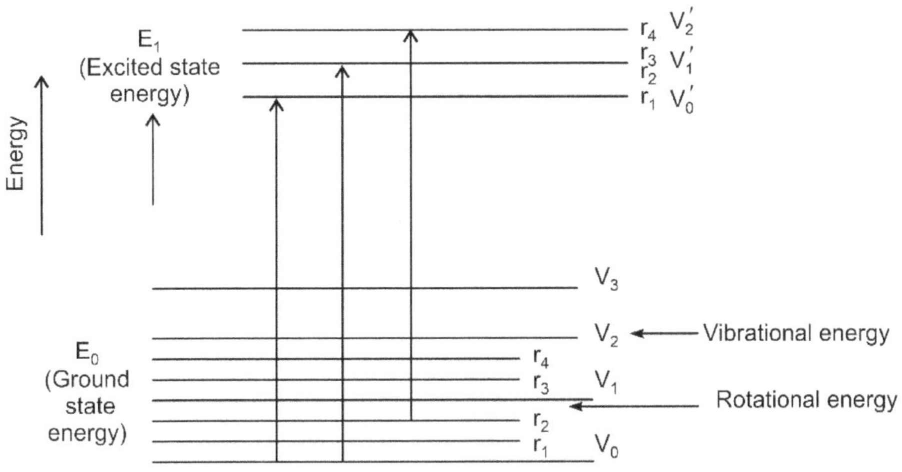

Fig. 23.3 Energy level diagram of a molecule showing vibrational and rotational energy level.

An electronic transition due to absorption of light may include vibrational or rotational changes.

2. **Scattering**: Sometimes, the radiation is not absorbed completely by the matter, and a portion of it may undergo scattering or reflection
3. **Emission:** In some cases, the molecules become excited after absorbing the radiation, and they lose energy by re-emitting radiation either instantaneously or with a time delay.

Franck–Condon principle

Franck–Condon principle gives the interaction between the electronic and vibrational motions. It states that the timescale of electronic transitions are so rapid when compared with the nuclear motion and the mass of the nuclei are heavy compared with electrons. An electronic transition is therefore considered to be a vertical transition. The light is absorbed in femtoseconds to nanoseconds, and within this timescale, electrons move, but the nuclei cannot. The heavier atomic nuclei cannot adjust during the absorption but readjust after the absorption process, creating vibrations. Simultaneous occurrence of electronic and vibrational transitions is called vibronic transitions, which give rise to the vibrational structure of the electronic bands.

The quantum mechanical formulation of this principle is that the **intensity of a vibronic transition is proportional to the square of the overlap integral between the vibrational wave functions of the two states that are involved in the transition.**

The Figure illustrates the Franck–Condon principle for vibronic transitions in a molecule. Potential energy functions in both the ground and excited electronic states are shown. In the low temperature, the molecule in the $v = 0$ vibrational level of the ground electronic state absorbs a photon of the necessary energy, makes a transition to the excited electronic state. The electron configuration of the excited state results in a shift of the equilibrium position of the nuclei of the molecule. In the figure, this shift in nuclear coordinates between the ground and the first excited state is labeled as q_{01}. In a simple case of a diatomic molecule, the nuclear coordinate axis refers to the internuclear separation. The vibronic transition is indicated by a vertical arrow, assuming constant nuclear coordinates during the transition. In the electronic excited state, molecules quickly relax to the lowest vibrational level of the lowest electronic excitation state (Kasha's rule). From there, they decay to the electronic ground state through photon emission. The Franck–Condon principle is applied equally to absorption as well as fluorescence.

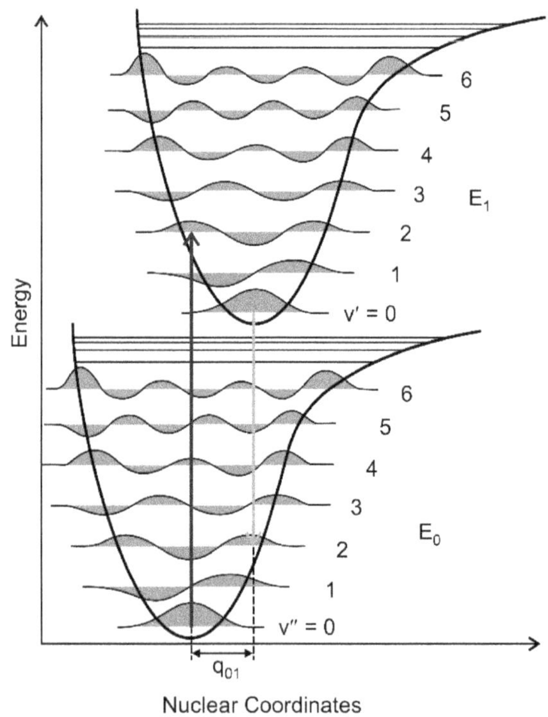

Fig. 23.4 Franck-condon principle for vibronic transitions in a molecule.

23.1 VISIBLE SPECTROPHOTOMETRY AND COLORIMETRY

UV-Visible Spectroscopy is one of the important absorption spectroscopic techniques, and it is most commonly employed for quantitative and qualitative analysis. It is also playing a role in the structural elucidation of organic compounds.

The wavelength range of visible light is 800-400 nm (8000-4000 Angstrom). This range of visible radiation is used for colorimetric analysis. Determination of concentration of coloured_compounds in solution is called colorimetry. A colorimeter is a device used to test the concentration of a solution by measuring its absorbance at a specific wave length of light.

Coloured substances absorb in the visible region, and the colorless substances absorb in the UV region. The amount of light absorbed differs with the wavelength, and a plot of absorbance vs. wavelength is called an absorption spectrum. **In the absorption spectrum, the wavelength at which maximum absorption occurs is called λ_{max}.** This λ_{max} is characteristic or unique for every substance and is used to identify the substances (qualitative analysis). **λ_{max}** is **independent of concentration, meaning that the λ_{max} will not change** even if the concentration is changed.

A calibration graph is a plot of concentration vs. absorbance. This graph helps to determine the concentration/amount of the drug present in the given sample solution (quantitative analysis).

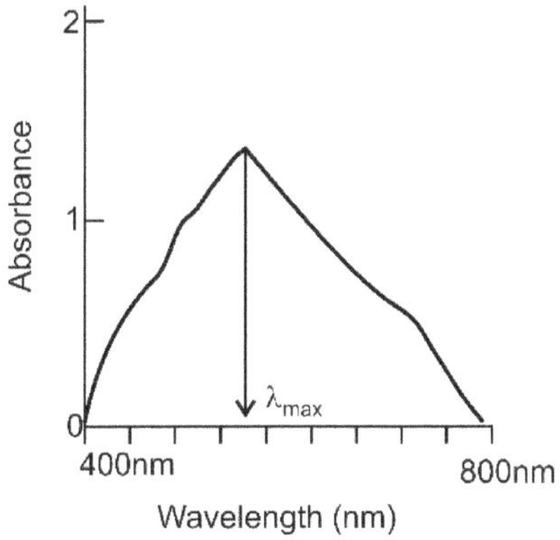

Fig. 23.5 Absorption spectrum.

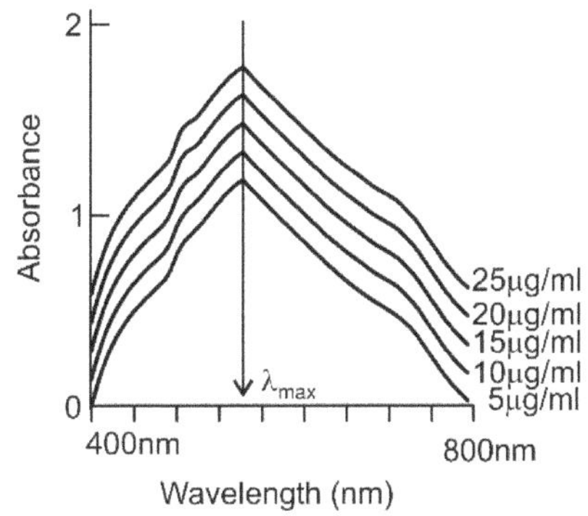

Fig. 23.6 Absorption spectrum of a substance in different concentrations.

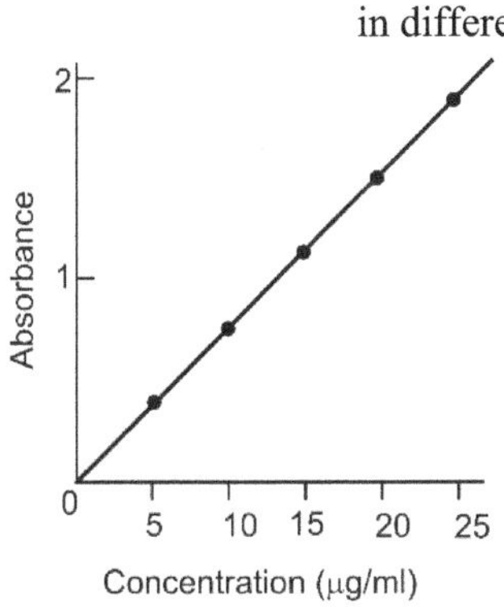

Fig. 23.7 Calibration curve.

THEORY OF SPECTROPHOTOMETRY & COLORIMETRY (ABSORPTION LAWS)

When light is incident upon a homogenous medium, a part of the incident light is reflected, a part is absorbed, and the remainder is transmitted so

$$\mathbf{I_0 = I_a + I_t + I_r} \qquad .....(23.1)$$

Where $\mathbf{I_0}$ – incident light; $\mathbf{I_a}$ – absorbed light; $\mathbf{I_t}$ – transmitted light and $\mathbf{I_r}$ – is reflected light. The value of I_r is minimal (about 4%), and it is eliminated for air-glass interfaces if a comparison cell is used. So, equation (1.1) becomes as

$$I_0 = I_a + I_t \qquad .....(23.2)$$

The two laws governing the absorption of light are:

1. **Beer's law** (concentration-dependent)
2. **Lambert's law** (Thickness/path length dependent absorbance)

Lambert's law states that when a beam of monochromatic light is allowed to pass through a transparent medium, **the rate of decrease of intensity with the thickness of the medium is directly proportional to the intensity of incident light.**

$$-\frac{dI}{dt} \alpha\, I$$

$$-\frac{dI}{dt} = k\,I \qquad .....(23.3)$$

$$-\frac{dI}{I} = kdt \qquad \text{(rearranging the equation)}$$

On integration

$$-\ln I_t = kt + b \quad (\ln - \text{natural logarithm}) \qquad .....(23.4)$$

where b is the integration constant

When thickness is zero, there is no absorbance. So $I_t = I_0$

Substituting this in equation 23.4

$$-\ln I_0 = k \times 0 + b$$

$$-\ln I_0 = b$$

Substituting this value of b in equation 23.4

$$-\ln I_t = kt - \ln I_0$$

On rearranging

$$\ln I_0 - \ln I_t = kt$$

$$\ln \frac{I_0}{I_t} = kt$$

Removing natural logarithm

$$I_0/I_t = e^{kt}$$

Taking inverse on both sides

$$I_t/I_0 = e^{-kt}$$

$$\mathbf{I_t = I_0.e^{-kt}} \qquad .....(23.5)$$

This equation is called as Lambert's law where I_0 is intensity of incident radiation, I_t is transmitted radiation and k is a constant.

Lambert's law shows the logarithmic relationship between transmittance and the optical path length

Beer's law: Beer observed a similar relationship between transmittance and the concentration of a solution. Beer's law states that the **intensity of a beam of monochromatic light decreases** exponentially with an **increase in the concentration of absorbing species arithmetically**.

$$-\frac{dI}{dc} \alpha I$$

$$-\frac{dI}{dc} = k'I \qquad .....(23.6)$$

Rearranging the equation

$$-\frac{dI}{I} = k'dc$$

On integration

$$-\ln I_t = k'c + b \text{ (ln – natural logarithm)} \qquad .....(23.7)$$

where b is the integration constant

When concentration is zero, there is no absorbance. So $I_t = I_0$

Substituting this in equation 1.7

$$-\ln I_0 = k' \times 0 + b$$

$$-\ln I_0 = b$$

Substituting this value of b in equation 23.7

$$-\ln I_t = k'c - \ln I_0$$

On rearranging

$$\ln I_0 - \ln I_t = k'c$$

$$\ln \frac{I_0}{I_t} = k'c$$

Removing natural logarithm

$$I_0/I_t = e^{k'c}$$

Taking inverse on both sides

$$I_t/I_0 = e^{-k'c}$$

$$\mathbf{I_t = I_0 . e^{-k'c}} \qquad .....(23.8)$$

This equation is called as Beer's law equation where I_0 is intensity of incident radiation, I_t is intensity of transmitted radiation and k is a constant.

On combining equations 23.5 and 23.8, we get

$$\mathbf{I_t = I_0 . e^{-Kct}}$$

on changing from natural logarithms to base 10,

$$\mathbf{I_t = I_0 . 10^{-Kct}} \text{ where } K = k \times 0.4343$$

Rearranging terms

$$I_t/I_0 = 10^{-Kct}$$

Taking inverse on both sides

$$I_0/I_t = 10^{Kct}$$

Taking log on both sides

$$\log I_0/I_t = Kct \qquad .....(23.9)$$

Transmittance $T = I_t/I_0$, Absorbance $A = \log 1/T$

Substituting for T in absorbance A, the equation becomes

$$A = \log I_0/I_t \qquad .....(23.10)$$

From equations 23.9 and 23.10

$$A = Kct.$$

If a is used instead of K, then

$$A = act$$

$$\mathbf{\log I_0/I_t = act}$$

is the mathematical expression of Beer Lambert's law,

Where A= absorbance, a = absorption coefficient or absorptivity, c= concentration of the substance and t = path length in cm.

Absorptivity reflects the sensitivity of the procedure. Sensitivity increases with an increase in absorptivity.

If the concentration is expressed in moles/liter, then a is replaced with ε.Then the equation becomes

$$\mathbf{A = \varepsilon ct} \qquad .....(23.11)$$

where

A = absorbance, ε = molar absorption coefficient or Molar absorptivity, c = concentration of the substance in mol/lit, t = path length in cm.

A = ε, when the concentration is one mole per liter and the path length is one centimeter.

Thus **Molar absorption coefficient** is defined as the absorption of a one molar solution when the path length is one cm. The molar absorption coefficient is otherwise called molar absorptivity.

The value of **molar absorptivity is constant** even if the concentration of the solution and the thickness of the container change. But it **differs with different wavelengths**.

Absorbance also varies with wavelength. For this reason, only monochromatic light is used in spectrophotometry and colorimetry.

Molar absorption coefficient **ε** is expressed as

$$\varepsilon = A^{1\%}_{1\,cm} \times \frac{\text{Molecular weight}}{10}$$

Where, $A^{1\%}_{1\,cm}$ is the **specific absorbance which is the absorbance of 1% w/v solution, using a path length of 1cm**. It is a constant for each drug at the given wavelength. This specific absorbance can be used for the quantitative estimation of formulations. ε_{max} is the value of ε at λ_{max}.

DEVIATIONS FROM BEER'S LAW

According to Beer's law, the plot of concentration Vs. absorbance should give a straight line passing through the origin. The straight line can also be obtained by using the line of best fit or method of least squares or by joining the maximum number of points so that the positive and negative errors are balanced or minimized. The regression line obtained can also be used for determining the concentration of a solution. When a nonlinear curve (not a straight line) is obtained in a plot of concentration vs. absorbance, the system is said to have deviations from Beer's law.

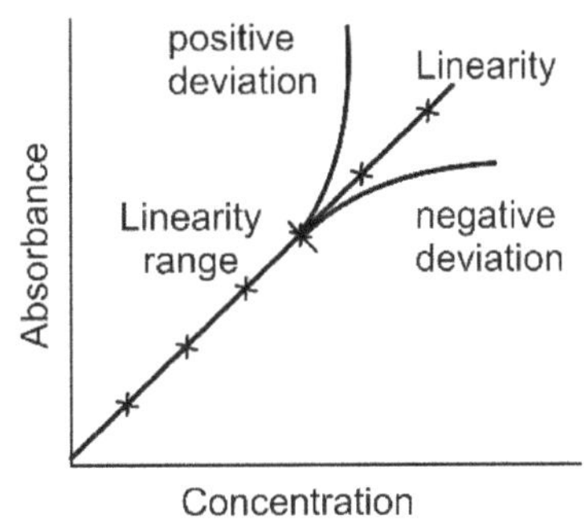

Fig. 23.8 Real deviations.

Beer's law is normally obeyed only in a certain concentration range, and above or below it may exhibit deviation.

The reasons for the deviations may be classified as

1. Real Deviations
2. Instrumental Deviations
3. Chemical Deviations
4. Incomplete reaction

1. **Real Deviations:** There are two types of real deviations from Beer's law
   - **(i) Positive deviation (concave upwards):** It occurs when a small change in concentration produces a great change in absorbance.
   - **(ii) Negative deviation (concave downwards):** It occurs when a large change in concentration produces a small change in absorbance.
2. **Instrumental deviations:** Factors like stray radiation, improper slit width, fluctuation in a single beam, and the type of light used can influence the deviation.
   - If monochromatic light is not used, deviation may occur.
   - If the width of the slit is not proper and if it allows undesirable radiations to fall on the detector, these undesirable radiations might be absorbed by the impurities present in the sample leading to changes in absorbance.
   - The possibility of error due to monochromatic radiation may be minimized by selecting a spectral region, where the change in absorptivity with a change in wavelength is very small.
   - This dictates that wavelength selection should be from a broad band (close to λ_{max}) rather than a sharply rising or sharply falling section of the absorption curve.
   - It is necessary to prepare a calibrated curve for the absorbance concentration relationship at the chosen wavelength to avoid errors.
3. **Chemical deviations:**

   Physicochemical changes in solution: Factors like association, dissociation, ionization (change in pH), faulty development of colour (incompletion of reaction), and refractive index at high concentration can influence such deviation.
   - **Association:** Methylene blue at a concentration of 10^{-5} M exists as monomer and has λ_{max} of 660nm. But methylene blue at a concentration above 10^{-4} M exist as a dimer or trimer and has a λ_{max} of 600. If the shift of this λ_{max} is not considered during absorbance measurements, then deviations occur.
   - **Dissociation**: Benzyl alcohol in chloroform exists in a polymeric equilibrium;

     $4C_6H_5CH_2OH \leftrightarrow (C_6H_5CH_2OH)_4$.

     Dissociation of the polymer increases with dilution. The monomer absorbs at 2.750 to 2.765 μ, where as the polymer absorbs at 3.0 μ. Hence absorption at 2.75 micron shows a negative deviation whereas at 3.0 μ gives a positive deviation.

Potassium dichromate at high concentration exists as an orange solution (λ_{max} of 450nm). But on dilution, dichromate ions are dissociated into chromate ions which is yellow in color (λ_{max} of 410nm)

$$Cr_2O_7^{2-} \text{ (orange)} + H_2O \rightarrow 2H^+ + 2CrO_4^{2-} \text{ (yellow)}.$$

If 450 nm is used for absorbance measurement for dilute solutions, then it leads to deviations from Beer's law.

- **Coloured solute ionization or dissociation** in solution leads to deviation in Beer's law. Colour change of dichromate ion on dilution can be given as an example.
- The deviation may also occur due to the **presence of impurities** that fluoresce or absorb at the absorption wavelength. This interference introduces an error in the measurement of absorption of the sample.
- If the solute undergoes **polymerization**, Ex Benzyl alcohol in carbon tetrachloride in high concentration exists in polymeric form. Dissociation of this polymer increases with dilution, which causes changes in absorbance, causing deviation.
- Beer's law can't be applied for suspensions, but colorimetry can be used with different known concentrations to prepare the reference curve.

4. **Incomplete reaction:**
   - Sufficient time should be allowed before taking absorbance for the reaction to complete so that the colour will be formed completely.
   - If the readings are taken after the colour fades away (instability), deviations can occur. Ex: Limit test for iron: reaction of iron with thioglycolic acid.

INSTRUMENTATION

Table 23.2 Summary of instrumentation.

Source of light	Filters and Monochromators	Sample cells	Detectors
Tungsten lamp Carbon arc lamp	Absorption filters. Interference filters Prisms Grating	Glass cuvettes Polystyrene cells for aqueous solutions	1. Barrier layer cell or Photo voltaic cell 2. Photo tubes or Photo emissive cells 3. Photomultiplier tubes.

The common instruments used for measuring emission or absorption of radiant energy are

(i) Photometer (ii) Spectrophotometer

Photometer: These are inexpensive and less accurate instruments. Filters are employed to isolate a wave length region, and a photocell or photo tube is used as a detector. A commercial photometer with filters is called **colorimeter**. It measures either absorbance or transmittance. The working range of wavelength for these instruments is 400-700nm.

Spectrophotometer: These are a little more expensive than colorimeters. They are used for wider wavelength regions, i.e., 360 nm- 900nm or 1000nm. Since these instruments employ **grating monochromators** for scanning and **photomultipliers** as detectors, they are highly accurate. The modern spectrophotometers are microprocessors or computer-based for easy handling of data.

The basic components of both types of instruments are

(a) Source of light
(b) Filters or monochromators
(c) Sample cells
(d) Detectors

Now we will discuss these components

(a) Source of light /radiation sources: The visible region extends from 400-800nm

The requirements of the radiation sources are

1. It must be stable and no fluctuations should be there.
2. It should provide continuous radiation from 400-800nm.
3. The intensity should be adequate.

The common radiation sources used in colorimetry (visible region) are

1. **Tungsten lamp:** Most widely used. The lamp consists of a tungsten filament in a vacuum bulb. It provides sufficient intensity.

Advantages

(i) Stable, robust and easy to use.
(ii) The Emission intensity varies with wavelength.

Disadvantages

(i) The intensity at the shorter wavelength is less
(ii) Difficult to maintain a constant intensity

2. **Carbon arc lamp:** This lamp is used for high intensity. It provides an entire range of the visible spectrum.

(b) Filters and Monochromators: The source emits continuous spectra from 400-800nm. This is called Polychromatic light consisting of several wavelengths. A colorimeter or spectrophotometer works only with a monochromatic light consisting of a single wavelength. A filter or a monochromator is used in these instruments to convert the polychromatic light into monochromatic light.

(a) Filters: There are two types of Filters

1. Absorption filters.
2. Interference filters

1. Absorption filters: These filters are made of a solid sheet of glass coloured by dissolved or dispersed pigments. Dyed gelatin is also used as an absorption filter.

The selection of filters is based on this color wheel. If the solution is red coloured, then the green filter is used. For the green solution red filter is used (complementary colors).

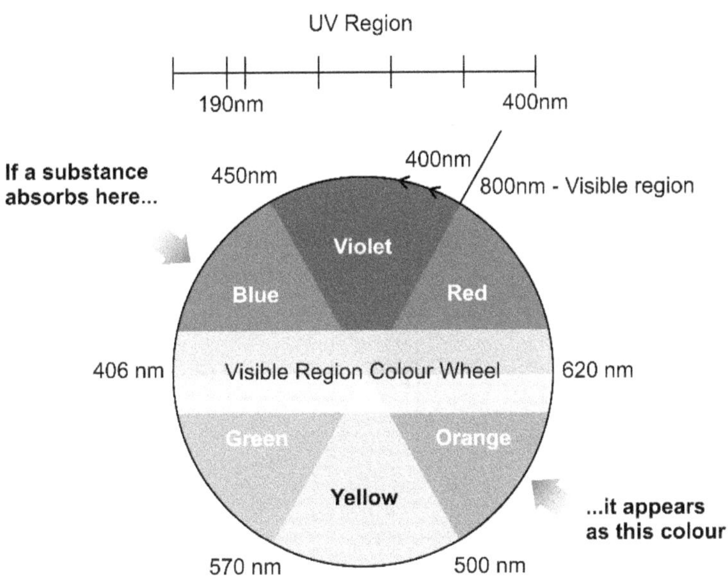

Fig. 23.9 Color wheel showing complimentary colors.

Absorption filters are further classified as **Cut off filters and band pass filters.**

Advantages:

1. Simple construction
2. Cheaper.
3. Easy Filter selection.

Disadvantages:

1. Accuracy is less because of broad band pass (± 30 nm).
2. Absorption by filters lead to less intensity of radiation

2. Interference Filters

1. This filter consists of a dielectric spacer film made up of CaF_2, MgF_2, or SiO, between two reflecting parallel silver films.
2. The thickness of the dielectric film may vary to give $1/2\lambda$ (1st order), $2\lambda/2$ (2nd order), $3\lambda/2$ (3rd order spectra), etc.
3. The principle of working is that the radiation reflected by the 2nd film and the incident radiation undergo constructive interference giving monochromatic radiation. The wavelength of the monochromatic radiation depends on the formula

$$\lambda = 2\eta b/m$$

Where λ = wavelength produced
η = dielectric constant of the film material
b = layer thickness
m = order no (1st, 2nd, 3rd, etc)

4. Band pass is 10-15 nm. Transmission is maximum 40%

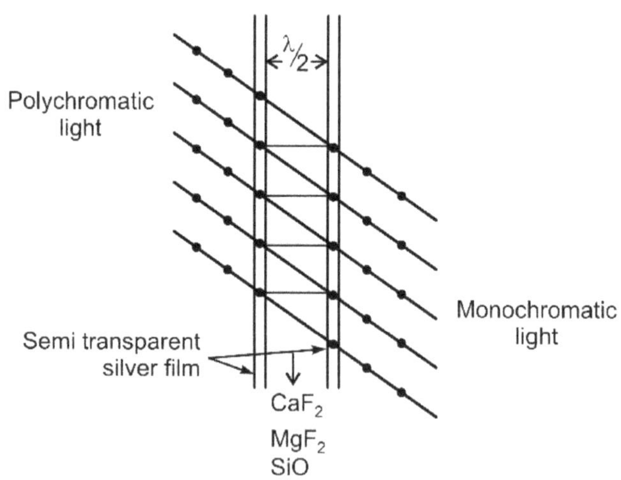

Fig. 23.10 Interference filter – FABRY PEROT.

Advantages:

1. Inexpensive
2. More accurate than absorption filters because of lower band pass.
3. Additional filters can be used to cut off undesired wavelengths.

Disadvantages:

1. Transmission is low
2. Because of the narrow band pass, higher resolution is not obtained.

(b) Monochromators: The **monochromators** are more efficient in converting the **polychromatic light to monochromatic light** when compared to filters. The parts of a monochromator are

1. Entrance slit (to get a narrow source of light)
2. Collimator (to make the light parallel)
3. Grating or prism (to disperse the light)
4. Collimator (to reform the monochromatic image of entrance slit)
5. Exit slit (to allow the light to fall on sample cell)

There are two types of monochromators

1. Prisms
2. Grating

1. Prisms: The prisms disperse the light into individual wavelengths or colors. They are made of glass and used in inexpensive instruments. Its **resolution is better than filters** because the band width is lower. The resolution of the prism is determined by the size and refractive index of the prism.

There are two types of the prism

I. Refractive type: In this type, the light from the source falls on the collimator through the entrance slit. The parallel rays of light from the collimator enter the prism, which disperses the light into component colors or wavelengths. The second collimator receives the dispersed light and reforms the images of the entrance slit. The reformed images are the colors of the VIBGYOR (Violet, Indigo, Blue, Green, Yellow, Orange, and Red). The required wavelength can be selected by rotating the prism or by moving the exit slit and the selected wavelength passes through the exit slit to the sample.

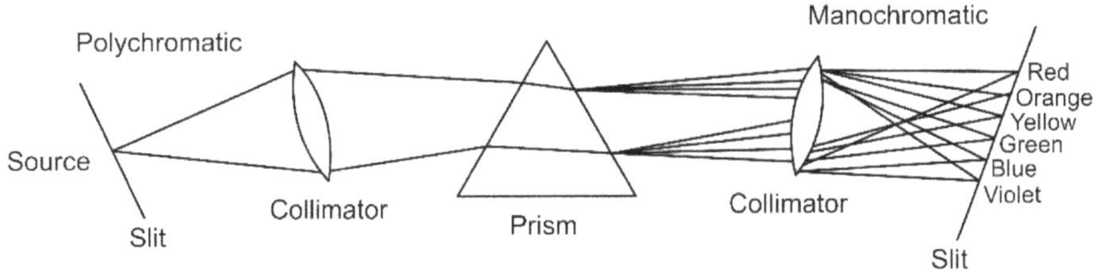

Fig. 23.11 Prism monochromator-dispersive type.

II. Reflective type (Littrow mounting): This type has a reflective surface present on one side of the prism. The dispersed radiation gets reflected on the same side of the source and is collected on the same side. The working principle is the same as the refractive type.

The advantage of prisms:

1. Dispersed wavelengths do not overlap

Disadvantages:

1. Non-linear dispersion
2. Temperature sensitive

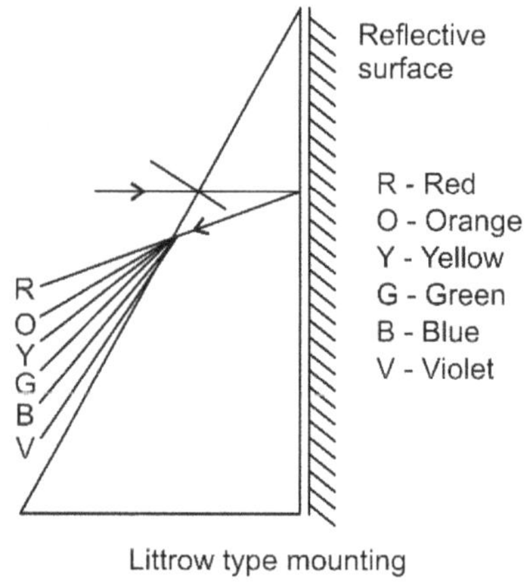

Fig. 23.12 Prism monochromator-reflective type (LITTROW MOUNTING).

2. **Gratings:** Gratings are **more efficient** in the conversion of polychromatic light to monochromatic light—a **resolution of ±0.1 nm** can be achieved with gratings, and hence they are used in spectrophotometers.

   There are two types of Gratings

   1. Diffraction grating
   2. Transmission grating

   1. **Diffraction grating:** A grating is made up of a large number of parallel lines (grooves) ruled on highly polished surfaces like glass, quartz, alumina, and alkyl halides based on the type of the instrument (visible/UV/IR spectrophotometer). Generally 3600 grooves or more per mm are drawn for ultraviolet and visible regions, and 20 grooves per mm are drawn for the IR spectrophotometer.

      These are replica gratings made from the master grating. Replica gratings are prepared by coating the original master grating with epoxy resin and removed after setting. Aluminizing its surface makes the surface of the replica grating reflective.

      The principle is **diffraction causes interference**. The incident rays on the grating, get constructive interference with the reflected rays and the resulting radiation wavelength is given by the equation

$$m\lambda = b(\sin i \pm \sin r)$$

Where λ = wavelength of produced light
b = grating spacing
i = angle of incidence
r = angle of reflection
m = order (0, 1, 2, 3, etc).

There are two different types of diffraction grating – the ruled grating and the holographic grating.

Gratings are preferred over prisms because of their efficiency.

2. **Transmission grating:** In these types of gratings, refraction takes place. The principle is **refraction produce interferences**. The radiation transmitted through the grating reinforces the partially refracted radiation leading to constructive interferences.

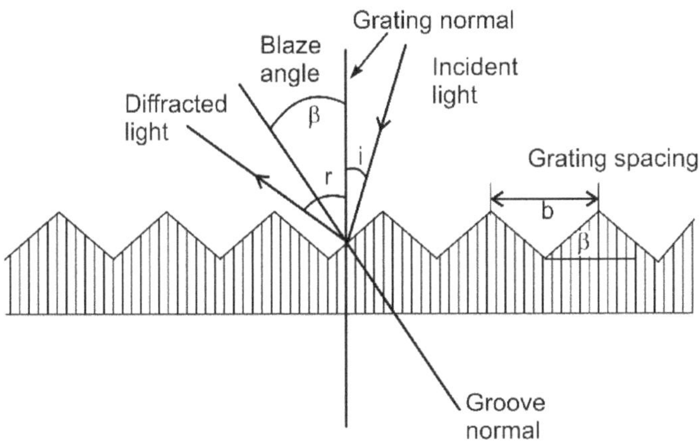

Fig. 23.13 Diffraction grating.

Transmission Grating

The wavelength produced can be calculated using the formula

$$\lambda = \frac{d \sin\theta}{m}$$

Where λ = wavelength of radiation produced.
d = 1/lines per cm
m = order no (0, 1, 2, 3, etc)
θ = angle of deflection/diffraction

Hence, the required light radiation (λ) can be produced either by moving grating and keeping the slit fixed or vice versa.

Advantage:

1. They give linear dispersion.
2. High resolution

Disadvantage:

1. Overlap of spectral orders.

Slits: The two slits are the **entrance slit and the exit slit**. The width of the monochromatic image of the entrance slit is the same as the width of the exit slit to pass through the exit slit.

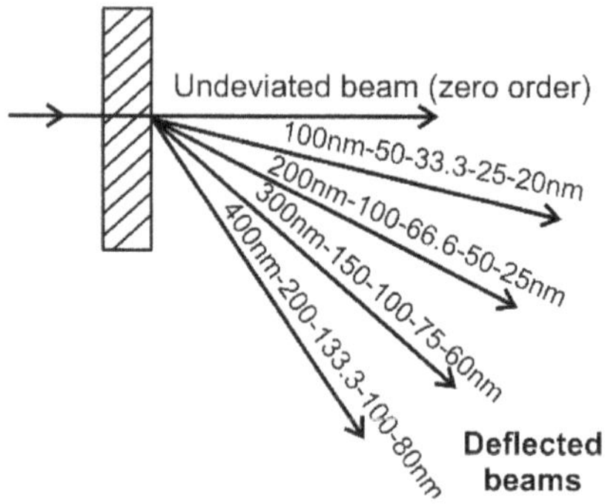

Fig. 23.14 Transmission Grating.

(c) Sample cells: The sample cells, known as cuvettes, are used to hold the sample.

The construction material of the cuvette varies with the instrument and the sample nature.

The material of the cuvette should not absorb in the working wavelength.

Material for **visible region: Color corrected fused glass.**

For aqueous solutions, Polystyrene cells are available.

For UV region: Quartz cuvettes are used because **glass absorbs UV radiation**.

The cells are available in different shapes like cylindrical or rectangle.

Small volume cells (0.5ml or less) and large volume cells (5-10ml) are available depending on their capacity to hold sample volume

The common path length (internal distance) is 1cm. Long path length cells with 10cm and short path length cells with 1 or 2mm are also available.

(d) Detectors: The radiation from the source through the monochromator passes through the sample. The sample absorbs part of the radiation, and the rest is being transmitted. This transmitted radiation falls on the detector, and the intensity of the absorbed radiation is determined by the detector and displayed.

Detectors used in UV Visible spectrophotometers are called photometric detectors. They convert the **light energy to an electrical signal** which is recorded.

Three types of detectors are

1. Barrier layer cell or Photo voltaic cell
2. Photo tubes or Photo emissive cells
3. Photomultiplier tubes.

1. **Barrier layer cell or Photo voltaic cell:** The detector consists of a metal base like iron or aluminum acting as one electrode. A thin layer of semiconductor material like selenium is deposited on its surface. The surface of the selenium is covered by a very thin layer of silver or gold which acts as a second collector electrode.

   The selenium layer separates the two electrodes, and it has extremely low electrical conductivity. When radiation falls on the selenium layer, the electrons are generated at the selenium silver interface. The silver layer collects these electrons. The collection of electrons on the silver surface creates a potential difference between the two electrodes. If the resistance in the external circuit is small, the current flows through the system. The **current produced is directly proportional to the intensity of the incident radiation** on the detector.

   Advantages:

   (i) Simple in design and rugged

   (ii) No external power supply is required.

   Disadvantages:

   (i) Less sensitive to blue region; use is limited to the visible region

   (ii) Amplification of the signal is not possible because the resistance of the external circuit should be low.

   (iii) Fatigue effects.

2. **Photo tubes or Photo emissive cells:** This detector consists of an evacuated glass tube containing a photo cathode and an anode as a collector electrode. The photo cathode is coated with a light-sensitive layer like Cesium, potassium or silver oxide.

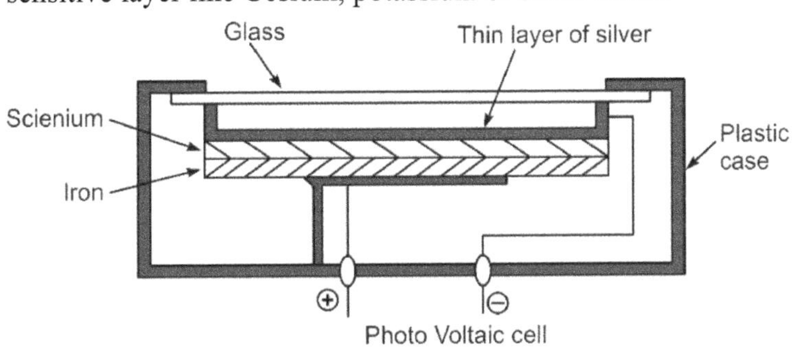

Fig. 23.15 Barrier layer cell.

When the transmitted radiation falls on the photo emissive cathode, it emits photoelectrons. The electron flow towards the anode causes the **current flow, which is proportional to the intensity of radiation falling on the detector.**

Advantages:

1. A signal from the detector can be amplified
2. More sensitive than Photovoltaic cells.
3. Composite coatings containing Cesium, cesium oxide, or silver oxide can be used on the cathode to increase the sensitivity and workable wavelength range.

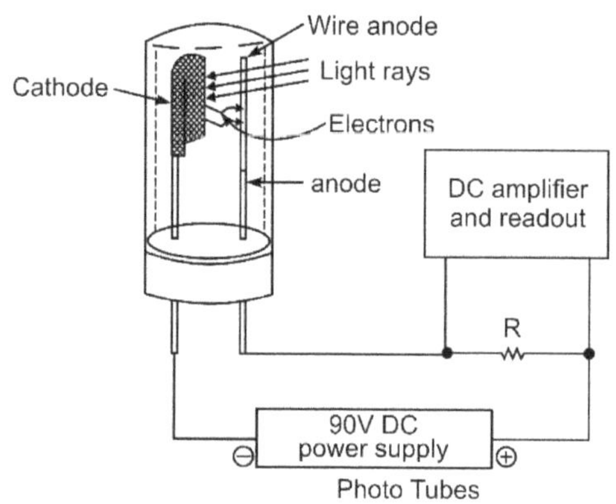

Fig. 23.16 Photo tubes.

3. **Photomultiplier tubes (PMT):** Though expensive, this detector is employed in sophisticated instruments due to its sensitivity.

   The working principle of this detector is the **multiplication of photo electrons by secondary emission of electrons.** PMT detector consists of a photo cathode and a series of anodes called dynodes. Each dynode is maintained at a successively higher potential 75-100V higher than the preceding dynode. Up to 10 dynodes are used in the series. When the radiation hits the cathode surface, electrons are emitted. When these electrons hit the dynodes, at each stage, the electrons are multiplied by a factor of 4 or 5 because of the secondary emission. An overall amplification factor of about 10^8 is achieved.

   Advantages:

   1. Most sensitive
   2. Can detect very weak signals
   3. Faster response time
   4. It can be used in fluorescence measurements

   Disadvantages:

   1. Expensive
   2. It should be shielded from stray light.

Advantages of Colorimetry

1. Specific to one chemical species.
2. Inexpensive per analysis.
3. Even non-chemistry personnel can perform the experiment.

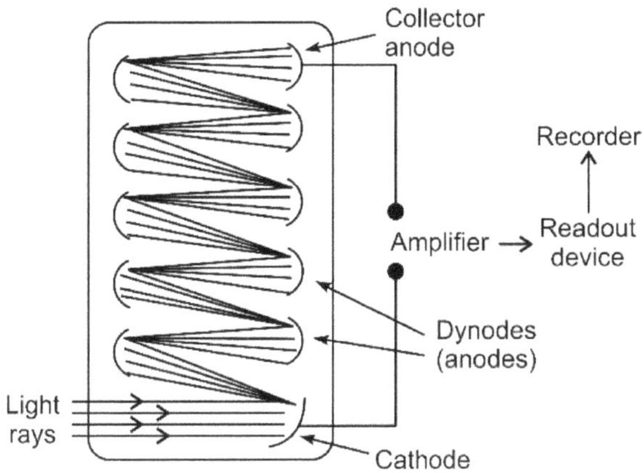

Fig. 23.17 Photo multiplier tube.

Disadvantages

1. Similar colour from interfering substances can produce errors in results
2. May not be suitable for more precise analysis.
3. Matrix interferences produce bad results in controlled conditions.

Types of instruments

The various types of instruments used in colorimetry are Colorimeters, Spectrocolorimeters, and Spectrophotometers. They differ in their construction, cost, sophistication, and automation.

Colorimeters: These instruments contain a tungsten lamp, absorption filters and photovoltaic cells. They read either transmittance or absorbance. Colorimeters are single beam instruments. Wavelength accuracy is normally ± 30nm.

Spectrocolorimeters: Contain prism monochromators instead of filters and either photovoltaic cell or phototube as a detector. These are also single beam instruments measuring either transmittance or absorbance. Wavelength accuracy usually is ± 5nm.

Spectrophotometers: These types of instruments are expensive and more sophisticated. They can read either transmittance or absorbance. They can record the absorption spectrum using a recorder. Spectrophotometers are double beam instruments, where the absorbance of sample and reference solution can be measured simultaneously. The automated devices possess various options like storage of spectrum, comparison of spectra, quantitative techniques, rapid wavelength scanning, data manipulation and derivative spectral mode. Most of them are software-driven instruments. Wavelength accuracy is normally ± 0.1 nm.

These instruments are more accurate and reliable.

The schematic diagram and the working of the instruments are given below

Single beam colorimeter

The source of light here is the tungsten lamp. A concave mirror focuses the light onto the slit. The slit allows the light to pass through the absorption filter, which selects the required wavelength and makes it fall on the sample cell containing the analyte solution. The analyte absorbs the part of the radiation, and the remaining light is transmitted. The intensity of this transmitted radiation is determined by a photo voltaic cell. The diagram of single beam colorimeter is shown in fig 23.18.

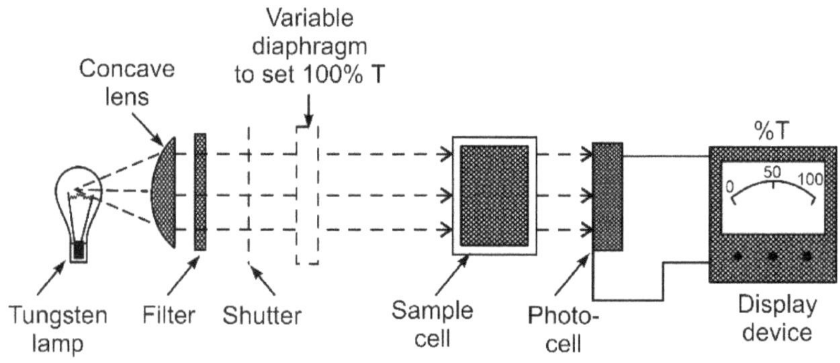

Fig. 23.18 Single beam colorimeter.

Advantages:

1. Simple in construction
2. Less cost
3. Easy operation

Disadvantages:

1. Fluctuations in the intensity of the source affect the absorbance readings.
2. Time-consuming because zero adjustment is to be done in every wavelength.
3. No recorder is available.

Double beam colorimeter: The construction of a double beam colorimeter is the same as a single beam except that the light beam, after passing through the filter or monochromator, is split into sample and reference beams by a beam splitter. Two detectors are used to detect the reference beam and the sample beam individually.

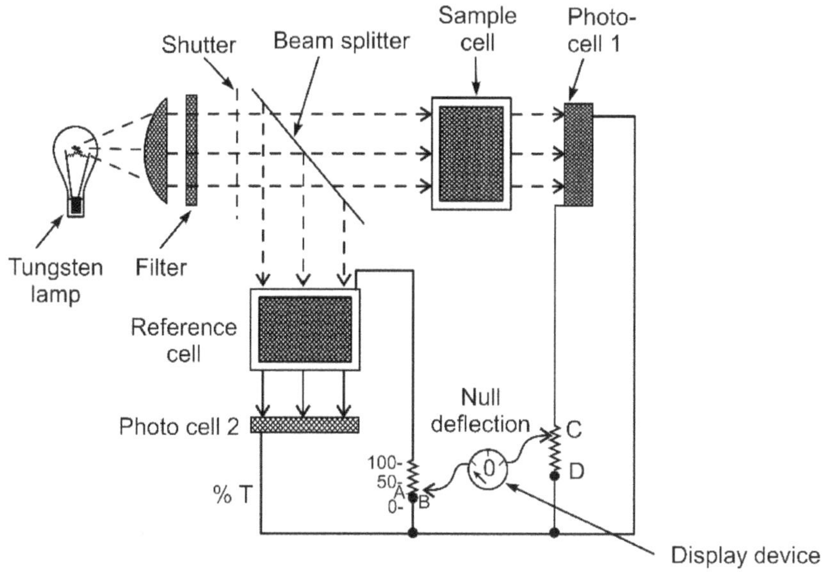

Fig. 23.19 Double beam colorimeter.

Applications of Colorimetry

1. **Purity determination:** Colorimetry is used to detect the presence of impurities in the sample. Coloured impurities absorb the radiation and give additional peaks in the spectrum.

   E.g., Vitamin B_{12} (cyano cobalamin) absorbs in three wavelengths 278,361 and 550 nm.

   The ratio of absorbances 278/361= 0.57
   550/361 = 0.3

   We can identify the presence of impurities by the change in the absorbance ratios.

2. **Quantitative analysis:** Determination of concentration and amount of the substance present in the given sample is called Quantitative estimation. Using these values, percentage purity can be determined. The quantitative estimation of drugs by colorimetry can be performed by knowing the parameters like λ_{max}, Beer's law concentration range for that substance, solvent, reagents and other conditions.

   The types of quantitative estimation are

   (a) **Using $A^{1\%}_{1cm}$ value (specific absorbance):** This method is useful in the estimations of raw material as well as formulations when the reference standard is not available.

   $A^{1\%}_{1cm}$ value can be obtained from Pharmacopoeia, Text books or Journals

(b) **Reference standard available:** If a reference standard is available, specific absorbance can be found experimentally and the above method can be used. Other methods available are

(i) **Direct comparison method (single standard):** The absorbance of a standard solution of known concentration is compared with the absorbance of the sample solution and the concentration of the sample solution is calculated. From the concentration, the amount and the % purity can be calculated.

(ii) **Calibration curve method or multiple standard method:** The calibration graph method is used to minimize the error introduced in the preparation of solutions or absorbance measurements.

In this method, a calibration curve is plotted with concentration vs. absorbance measured with five or more concentrations of the reference or standard. A straight line passing through the origin is obtained. If a straight line is not obtained, a straight line is obtained through the maximum number of points or by regression analysis leading to a line of best fit. The unknown concentration of the sample can be obtained using the absorbance of the sample and the calibration graph. The extrapolation of the graph gives the unknown concentration and amount, and the % purity of the sample can be calculated.

3. **Determination of Ligand/Metal ratio in metallic complexes:** Some organic compounds form metallic complexes with some metals, and the ratio of the metal complexes can be determined using the calibration graph method.
4. **Structural elucidation of organic compounds:** The structure of the unknown compound can be elucidated by comparing the absorption spectrum with that of the known compound. For e.g.,

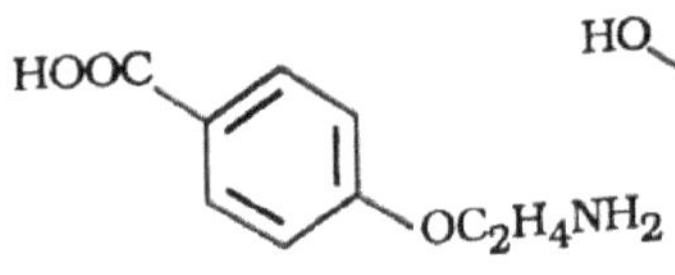

I

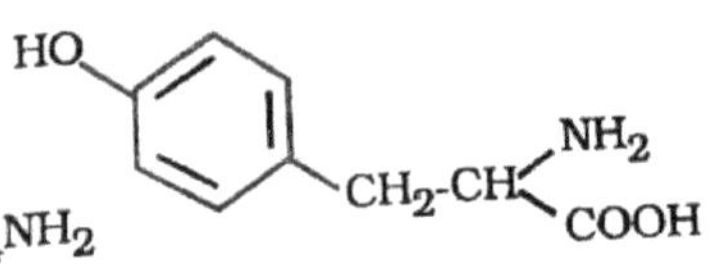

II

These are the structures proposed for Tyrosine. When the absorption spectrum of Tyrosine was obtained, it was found to be similar to the absorption spectrum of Phenol. Hence the structure II is proposed for Tyrosine.

5. **Determination of pK_a of indicators:** Determination of dissociation of acid-base indica-tors like Methyl orange, Methyl red can be determined by the formula

$$pK_a = pH - \log [ionized]/[unionized]$$

The plot of absorbance vs. concentration at different pH is recorded and pK_a is calculated using the equation.

6. **Determination of molecular weights:** Molecular weight is determined using the formula

$$Mol.\ wt = \varepsilon / a = \varepsilon \times ct/A$$

where A = absorbance, c = concentration, t = pathlength and a = absorptivity

7. **Determination of functional groups and elements:** Even low concentrations of ions, elements or functional groups can be determined by using chromogenic (colour producing) reagents.

   E.g., Determination of Iron using 1,10 phenanthroline, Ammonia using Nessler's reagent and amino acids using Ninhydrin.

8. **Determination of organic compounds and Pharmaceutical substances:** The pharmaceuticals are also determined by colorimetry using chromogenic reagents for producing colors.

   E.g., Phenols determined using Ferric chloride, Betamethasone using Phenyl hydrazine.

23.2 UV SPECTROSCOPY

INTRODUCTION

The coloured compounds absorb in the visible region, most of the colorless compounds absorb in the UV region. The UV radiation wavelength starts from the blue end of the visible light (4000Å) and extends up to 2000 Å. The UV region is divided into two regions

1. Near UV region - 2000 Å -4000 Å (200-400nm)
2. Far or vacuum UV region – below 2000 Å (200nm).

THEORY/PRINCIPLE OF UV SPECTRA

UV Spectroscopy is the study of the absorption of UV radiation by atoms or molecules. Both visible and UV radiations excite only the **valence electrons.** The molecules absorb UV radiation, and they undergo the transition from the ground state to the excited state. Thus, **electronic excitation** is the principle involved in UV spectroscopy. Because of this, UV spectroscopy is also called **Electronic spectroscopy**.

UV absorption is characteristic for each substance, and it depends on the type of electrons present in the molecule. The absorption intensity follows Beer–Lamberts law, and it is proportional to concentration and path length.

Types of electrons in molecules

Three types of electrons are present in molecules. They are

1. **σ electrons** present in saturated compounds. These electrons show absorption in **vacuum UV** region (<200nm)
2. **π electrons** present in unsaturated compounds. (e.g., double or Triple bonds).
3. **n electrons** are called non bonded electrons and are not taking part in bonding between atoms. e.g., organic compounds containing sulphur, nitrogen, oxygen, or halogens.

All molecules having π electrons, n electrons, or a combination of both electrons absorb in the characteristic wavelength region and undergo the transition from the ground state to the excited state. This characteristic absorption helps in the structural elucidation of molecules by identifying the nature of electrons present.

ELECTRONIC TRANSITIONS

When an atom or molecule **absorbs energy, electrons are promoted** from their ground state to an excited state. When a molecule is **electronically excited**, the electrons move from **bonding to antibonding orbitals**. The π electrons are excited to π* antibonding orbitals, and n electrons are excited to either σ* or π* anti bonding orbitals.

The amount of **energy** required to excite **σ electrons** is very high and hence they do not absorb in the **UV** region. The molecules which possess **π electrons (unsaturated compounds)** and **n electrons (lone pair)** absorb energy in the **UV** and **visible region** and these electrons get excited to the higher energy levels. Thus, the possible transitions are **π-π*, n-π*** transitions.

The possible electronic transitions are shown diagrammatically

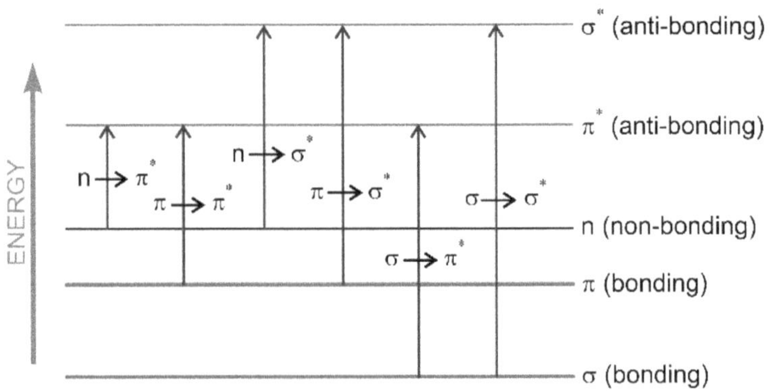

Fig. 23.20 Different types of electronic transitions.

TYPES OF ELECTRONIC TRANSITIONS

The electronic transitions are caused by the absorption of UV light by the molecules leading to the excitation of valence electrons from the ground state to the excited state. The various transitions are **π-π*, n-π*, n-σ* and σ-σ*.** The energy requirements for these transitions are given in increasing order n-π*< π-π*< n-σ*< σ-σ*.

Types of transition: It is not necessary that the exposure of the compound to UV radiation will always result in an electronic transition. The probable occurrence of the transition is dependent on the value of the molar extinction coefficient (λ_{max}) and certain other factors. Thus, the transitions can be divided into two types

(i) Allowed transitions

(ii) Forbidden transitions

(i) Allowed transitions: Transitions having ε_{max} value 10^4 or more are allowed transitions. They arise due to π-π* transitions.

E.g., In 1,3 butadiene π-π* transition has ε_{max} value of 21,000 at 217 nm. Thus, it is an allowed transition.

(ii) Forbidden transitions: Transitions having ε_{max} value less than 10^4 are forbidden transitions. They arise due to n-π* transitions.

E.g., n-π* transition of saturated aldehyde or ketone shows weak absorption near 290 nm and its ε_{max} value less than 100. So, it is a forbidden transition.

On application of selection rules, σ-σ*, n-σ*,π-π* are allowed transitions, and n-π* transition is forbidden.

DIFFERENT ELECTRONIC TRANSITIONS

1. **n-π*transitions:** This transition requires the lowest energy (longer wavelength) of all other transitions. The compounds containing n electrons (present in S, O, N, or halogens) and double or triple bonds (E.g., aldehydes and ketones, nitro compounds) exhibit these transitions. The peaks of these transitions are also called R –bands.

   Aldehydes and ketones (RCHO, RCOR) absorption peak,

   Without double or triple bonds occurs at 270-300 nm.

   With double or triple bonds separated by two or more single bonds occurs at 300-350nm

   Identification of n-π*transition can be done by recording the UV spectrum of the substance in an acid medium. The peak due to n-π* transition disappears in acid solution. The presence of other hetero atoms can be identified by comparing the spectrum of a similar compound without hetero atom.

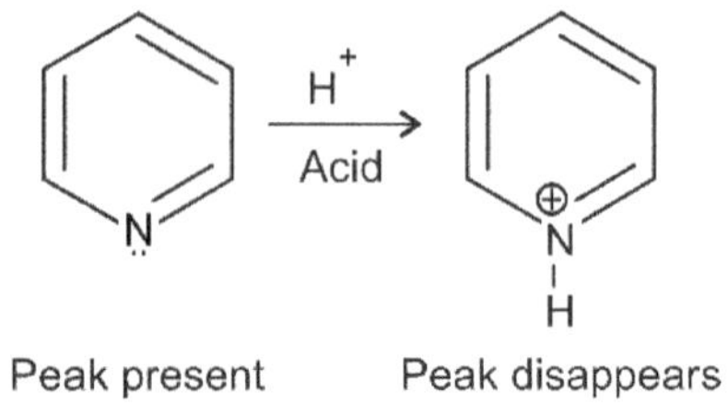

2. **π-π* transitions:** This transition gives B, E and K bands

   B bands are benzenoid bands due to aromatic and hetero aromatic systems. E bands are ethylenic bands due to aromatic systems. K bands (π-π*) are due to conjugated systems. The energy required for this transition lies between n-σ* and n-π*. **The alkyl substitutions and extended conjugations** (addition of alternate double or triple bonds) shift the λ_{max} towards longer wavelength (bathochromic shift). The trans isomer of the alkene absorbs at a longer wavelength with more intensity than the cis isomer (bathochromic shift with hyperchromic effect). Extended conjugation and alkyl substitution shift λ_{max} in such a way that the λ_{max} moves to the colorimetric region. E.g., plant pigments like β carotene, lycopene, etc.

   The λ_{max} of ethylenic (C=C) chromophore is 174nm

   The λ_{max} of acetylenic (C≡C) chromophore is 178 nm

3. **n-σ* transition:**

   Saturated compounds with nonbonding electrons (presence of heteroatoms) exhibit this transition. The energy requirement is less than σ-σ* transition. The wavelength range for this transition is 180-250nm. Transition needs more energy that is shorter wavelength because the lone pair of electrons on the hetero atoms form hydrogen bonds. **Hydrogen bonding shifts UV absorption to a lower wavelength** E.g., of compounds with n-σ* transition Methylene chloride (173nm), water (191nm), Methanol (203nm), Ethanol (204 nm), ether (215 nm) etc.

4. **σ-σ* transitions:**

   This transition requires the highest energy. This transition occurs in saturated compounds (more importantly, hydrocarbons). The absorption peaks appear in the vacuum UV region. 125-135nm. E.g., Methane (122nm), Ethane (135 nm). The commercial UV spectrophotometers operate above 200nm, saturated hydrocarbons like cyclohexane (195 nm) can be used as nonpolar solvents because the solvent peak does not appear.

Laws of absorption

The two laws related to UV Visible spectroscopy are

1. Beer's law (concentration-dependent)
2. Lambert's law (Thickness/path length dependent absorbance)

Lambert's law states that when a beam of monochromatic light is allowed to pass through a transparent medium, the rate of **decrease of intensity** with the **thickness** of the medium is **directly proportional** to the intensity of incident light.

Beer's law: Beer observed a similar relationship between transmittance and the concentration of a solution. Beer's law states that the intensity of a beam of monochromatic light decreases exponentially with an increase in the concentration of absorbing species arithmetically.

$$A = act$$

$$\mathbf{Log\ I_0/I_t = act}$$

is the mathematical expression of Beer Lambert's law,

Where A = absorbance, a = absorption coefficient or absorptivity, c = concentration of the substance and t = path length in cm.

The derivation of Beer lambert's law is given in colorimetry (chapter 23 pg. no. 282-285).

CHROMOPHORES

Any group which exhibits absorption of electromagnetic radiation in the visible or UV region is called as chromophore. It may or may not impart colour to the compound. Example of important chromophores is ethylene, acetylene, carbonyls, acids, esters, and nitrile group.

Eg: NO_2, N=N, C=O, C=C, N=O, C=N, C=C, C=S

Types of Chromophores

1. **Chromophores with π electrons**

   These chromophores undergo **π → π*** transitions. E.g., ethylenes and acetylenes.

2. **Chromophores with both π electrons and n (non-bonding) electrons**

   These chromophores undergo two types of transitions.

π → π* and n → π*, E.g., carbonyls, nitriles, azo compounds and nitro compounds

Examples of some chromophores

1. Nonconjugated alkenes show intense absorption below 200 nm and are inaccessible to UV spectrophotometer. (π → π*)

2. Non-conjugated carbonyl group compounds give a weak absorption band in the 200-300nm region. ($n \rightarrow \pi^*$).
3. Conjugation of C=C and C=O groups shifts the λ_{max} of both groups to longer wavelengths.

Some simple chromophore groups are given in the Table 23.3.

Table 23.3 Some simple examples of chromophores.

Chromophore	Transition	λ_{max}
C=C	$\pi \rightarrow \pi^*$	175
C≡C	$\pi \rightarrow \pi^*$	175
C=O	$n \rightarrow \pi^*$. $\pi \rightarrow \pi^*$	285 180
N=O	$n \rightarrow \pi^*$. $\pi \rightarrow \pi^*$	275 200
C-X X=BR,I	$n \rightarrow \sigma^*$ $n \rightarrow \sigma^*$	205 255

AUXOCHROME

It is a group that itself **does not act as a chromophore. Still,** when **attached to** a chromophore, it shifts the **absorption maximum towards a longer wavelength with an increase in the intensity of absorption**.

Ex: The auxochrome NH_2, when attached to a benzene ring, shifts its absorption maximum (λ_{max}) from 255 to 280nm.

Other Eg: OH, NH_2, OR, NHR and NR_2

All auxochromes have one or more nonbonding pair of electrons.

The auxochrome, when attached to a chromophore, extends the conjugation of chromophores by sharing nonbonding pair of electrons. Ex: $CH_2=CH\text{-}:NR_2 \leftrightarrow :^{-}CH_2 - CH=NR_2^{+}$

SPECTRAL SHIFTS

Isolated chromophores such as >C=C < and C≡C absorb in the far UV region, which cannot be observed in normal spectrophotometers. The position of absorption maximum and the intensity of absorption can be modified by some structural changes or changes of solvent. These kind of changes of λ_{max} and intensity of absorption are called spectral shifts. The different kinds of spectral shifts are explained below.

BATHOCHROMIC SHIFT OR RED SHIFT

It is the shift of absorption maximum **(λ_{max}) towards longer wavelength** because of the presence of groups like OH and NH_2 (auxochrome) or by change of solvent.

Decreasing the polarity of the solvent causes a redshift in the carbonyl compounds (n-π* transitions)

When two or more chromophores are present in conjugation in a molecule, redshift is observed.

Eg: ethylene π-π* transitions – 170nm

1, 3 butadiene (two double bonds in conjugation) – 217nm

HYPSOCHROMIC SHIFT OR BLUE SHIFT

It is the shift of absorption maximum towards **shorter wavelength**. This may be caused due to the removal of conjugation in a system or by the change of the solvent. The absorption shift towards a shorter wavelength is also called a **blue shift**.

E.g., Aniline absorption is maximum at 280 nm because the pair of electrons on the nitrogen atom is in conjugation with π bond system of the benzene ring.

In acidic solutions, the absorption shifts to a shorter wavelength (blue shift 200nm). Anilinium ion is formed in acidic solution, and the electron pair is no longer present, and hence conjugation is removed.

HYPER CHROMIC EFFECT

It is the **increase in the intensity of absorption** and is brought about by the introduction of an auxochrome.

E.g.: Introduction of methyl group in 2nd position of Pyridine increases ε_{max} (λ_{max} 262nm) from 2750 to 3560 (λ_{max} 262nm) for π-π*.

HYPO CHROMIC EFFECT

It is the **decrease in the intensity of absorption** and is brought about by groups that are able to distort the geometry of the molecule.

E.g., When a methyl group is introduced in position 2 of the biphenyl group, there is a decrease in intensity because of distortion caused by the methyl group.

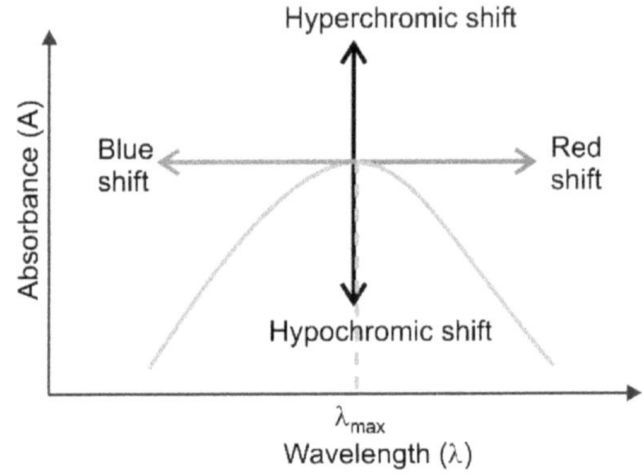

Fig. 23.21 Different types of spectral shifts.

SOLVENT EFFECT ON ABSORPTION SPECTRA

The most commonly used solvent is 95% ethanol. Other solvents which can be used in UV spectroscopy are n-hexane, methyl alcohol, cyclohexane, acetonitrile, diethyl ether, water, etc.

The λ_{max} and the intensity of absorption get shifted for a chromophore by changing the polarity of the solvent. In general, the absorption maximum for the nonpolar compounds is usually shifted with the change in polarity of the solvents.

1. **Effect of solvent on n-π* transitions:** The absorption **shifts to a shorter wavelength** (blue shift) when the **polarity of solvent is increased**. In n-π* transitions, (e.g., carbonyl), the ground state is more polar than the excited state. When the polarity of the solvent is increased, the nonbonding electrons in the ground state are more stabilized than the excited state by hydrogen bonding. So, more energy is required to cause excitation, and thus absorption shifts to a shorter wavelength. E.g., absorption maximum of acetone is 279 nm in hexane but it is 264 nm in water.

   Thus, an increase in polarity of solvent generally shifts n-π* and n-σ* transitions to a shorter wavelength.
2. **Effect of solvent on π-π*transitions:** The absorption shifts to a **longer wavelength (red shift)** when the **polarity of solvent is increased.** The π*orbitals get more stabilized by hydrogen bonding with polar solvents like ethanol and water. The polarity of π* orbital is more than the π orbital. When the polarity of the solvent is increased, the dipole-dipole interactions with the solvent molecules lower the energy of the excited state than the ground state. Thus, the energy required for π-π* transitions decreases, leading to shifting of absorption maximum to longer wavelength (red shift).

Thus, an increase in polarity of solvent generally shifts π-π*transitions to longer wavelength.

Generally,

1. The absorption maximum will be shifted to a shorter wavelength for a group which is more polar (carbonyl) in the ground state than the excited state (n-π*)
2. The absorption maximum will be shifted to a longer wavelength for a group which is more polar in the excited state than the ground state (π-π*).

CHOICE OF SOLVENT

The solvent for the UV spectroscopy should have the following requirements

(i) It should not absorb in the region of absorbance measurement of the sample (should be transparent). It should not affect the absorption of the sample.

(ii) It should be less polar so that its interaction with the solute molecules is minimum.

A commonly used solvent is 95% ethanol. It is cheap, has good solvating power, and is transparent above 210nm.

Example of other solvents transparent above 210 nm is n-hexane, cyclohexane, methanol, water, and ether. The other solvents like benzene, chloroform, and carbon tetrachloride cannot be used because they absorb in the 240-280 nm range.

The solvents like hexane and other hydrocarbons are preferred to polar solvents due to their minimum interactions with the solute molecules.

Some common solvents used in UV spectroscopy and their absorption wavelengths are given in the following Table 23.4.

Table 23.4 Common UV solvents and their absorption wavelengths.

Solvent	Wavelength
Water	205nm
Methanol	210nm
ethanol	210nm
Ether	210nm
Chloroform	245nm
Carbon tetra chloride	265nm
Cyclohexene	210nm
Dichloroethane	220nm

INSTRUMENTATION

The common instruments used for measuring the emission or absorption of radiant energy in the UV region are UV spectrophotometers.

Table 23.5 Summary of Instrumentation in UV spectrophotometers.

Source of light	Filters and Monochromators	Sample cells	Detectors
Hydrogen discharge lamp Deuterium lamp Xenon Discharge lamp Mercury arc lamp	Absorption filters. Interference filters **Prisms** Refractive type Reflective type **Grating** Diffraction grating Transmission grating	Quartz cuvettes are used because **glass absorbs UV radiation**.	1. Barrier layer cell or Photovoltaic cell 2. Photo tubes or Photo emissive cells 3. Photomultiplier tubes. 4. Photo diode array detector

The essential components of instrument are

(a) Source of light
(b) Filters or monochromators
(c) Sample cells
(d) Detectors
(e) Display or readout devices
(f) Computers and recorders

Now we will discuss these components

(a) Source of light /radiation sources: The Ultraviolet (UV) region extends from 200-400nm

The requirements of the radiation sources are

1. It must be stable, and no fluctuations should be there.
2. It should provide continuous radiation from 200-400nm.
3. Its intensity should be adequate.

(i) **Hydrogen discharge lamp:** Hydrogen gas is stored under high pressure in these lamps. When an electric discharge is passed through the gas, excited hydrogen molecules are produced, which emit UV radiations. The high pressure of hydrogen gives a continuous spectrum. Hydrogen lamp gives radiation from 120 -350 nm.

Advantages:

1. Stable, robust and widely used
2. Emits broadband (continuous spectrum)

(ii) **Deuterium lamp:** In this lamp, deuterium is used in the place of hydrogen, leading to 3 to 5 times increase in the intensity of emitted radiation.

Advantages:

1. More intensity

Disadvantage

1. Expensive

(iii) **Xenon Discharge lamp:** Xenon gas is stored under 10-30 atmosphere pressure in this lamp. It has got two tungsten electrodes separated by a distance of 8 mm. When a low voltage is applied, an intense arc is produced between the electrodes producing UV radiation. The intensity produced is greater than the hydrogen discharge lamp.

(iv) **Mercury arc lamp:** In this lamp, mercury vapour is used under high pressure, and the mercury atoms are excited by electrical discharge. The spectrum produced is not continuous and hence not used widely.

(b) **Filters and Monochromators:** The source emits continuous spectra from 200-400nm. This is called polychromatic light consisting of several wavelengths. A colorimeter or spectrophotometer works only with a monochromatic light consisting of a single wavelength. A filter or a monochromator is used in these instruments to convert the polychromatic light into monochromatic light.

(i) **Filters:** There are two types of filters

1. Absorption filters.
2. Interference filters

1. Absorption filters: These filters are made of a solid sheet of glass coloured by dissolved or dispersed pigments. Dyed gelatin is also used as an absorption filter.

Absorption filters are further classified as Cut off filters and bandpass filters.

Advantages:

1. Simple construction
2. Cheaper.
3. Easy Filter selection.

Disadvantages:

1. Accuracy is less because of broad bandpass (± 30 nm).
2. Absorption by filters lead to less intensity of radiation

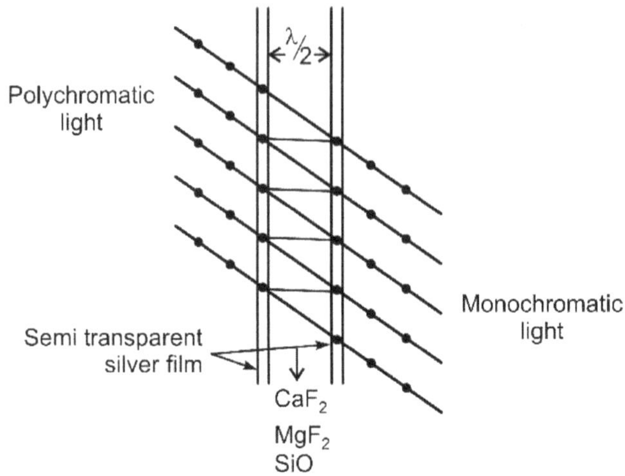

Fig. 23.22 Interference filter FABRY PEROT.

2. **Interference Filters**
   1. This filter consists of a dielectric spacer film made up of CaF_2, MgF_2, or SiO, between two reflecting parallel silver films.
   2. The thickness of the dielectric film may vary to give $1/2\lambda$ (1st order), $2\lambda/2$ (2nd order), $3\lambda/2$ (3rd order), etc.

      The principle of working is that the radiation reflected by the 2nd film and the incident radiation undergo constructive interference to give monochromatic radiation. The wavelength of the monochromatic radiation depends on the formula

      $$\lambda = 2\eta b/m$$

      Where λ = wavelength produced

      η = dielectric constant of the film material

      b = layer thickness

      m = order no(1st, 2nd, 3rd, etc)
   3. Bandpass is 10-15 nm. Transmission is maximum 40%

Advantages:

1. Inexpensive
2. More accurate than absorption filters because of the lower bandpass.
3. Additional filters can be used to cut off undesired wavelengths.

Disadvantages:

1. Transmission is low
2. Because of the narrow bandpass, higher resolution is not obtained.

(ii) **Monochromators:** The **monochromators** are more efficient in converting the **polychromatic light to monochromatic light** when compared to filters. The parts of a monochromator are

1. Entrance slit (to get a narrow source of light)
2. Collimator (to make the light parallel)
3. Grating or prism (to disperse the light)
4. Collimator (to reform the monochromatic image of entrance slit)
5. Exit slit (to allow the light to fall on sample cell)

There are two types of monochromators

1. Prisms
2. Grating

1. Prisms: The prisms disperse the light into individual wavelengths or colours. They are made of glass and used in inexpensive instruments. Its resolution is better than filters because the bandwidth is lower. The resolution of the prism is determined by the size and refractive index of the prism.

There are two types of the prism

I. Refractive type: In this type, the light from the source falls on the collimator through the entrance slit. The parallel rays of light from the collimator enter the prism, which disperses the light into component colours or wavelengths. The second collimator receives the dispersed light and reforms the images of the entrance slit. The reformed images are the colours of the VIBGYOR (Violet, Indigo, Blue, Green, Yellow, Orange, and Red). The required wavelength can be selected by rotating the prism or by moving the exit slit and the selected wavelength passes through the exit slit to the sample.

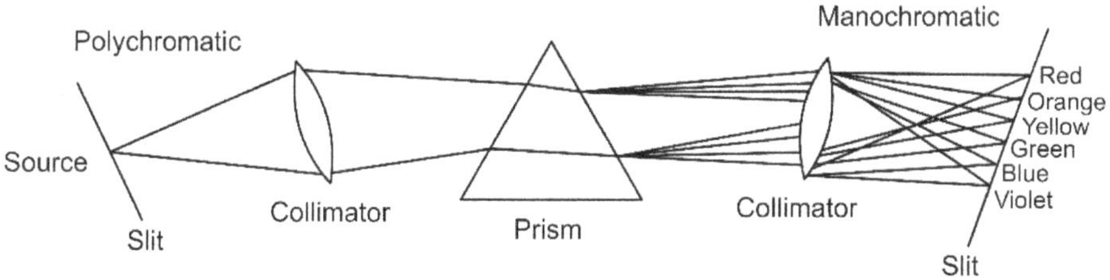

Fig. 23.23 Prism monochromator-Dispersive type.

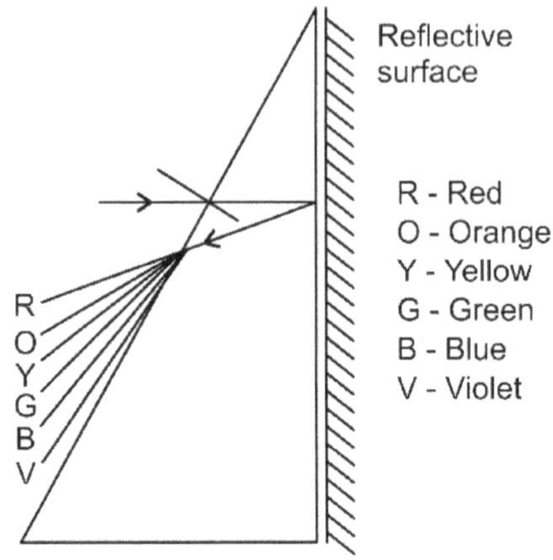

Fig. 23.24 Prism monochromator-Reflective type (Littrow mounting).

II. Reflective type (Littrow mounting): This type has a reflective surface present on one side of the prism. The dispersed radiation gets reflected on the same side of the source and is collected on the same side. The working principle is the same as the refractive type.

The advantage of prisms:

1. Dispersed wavelengths do not overlap

Disadvantages:

1. Non-linear dispersion
2. Temperature sensitive

2. **Gratings:** Gratings are more efficient in the conversion of polychromatic light to monochromatic light. A resolution of ±0.1 nm can be achieved with gratings, and hence they are used in spectrophotometers.

There are two types of Gratings

I. Diffraction grating

II. Transmission grating

I. Diffraction grating: A grating is made up of a large number of parallel lines(grooves) ruled on highly polished surfaces like glass, quartz, alumina and alkyl halides based on the type of the instrument (visible/UV/IR spectrophotometer. Generally, 3600 grooves or more per mm are drawn for ultraviolet and visible regions, and 20 grooves per mm are drawn for the IR spectrophotometer.

These are replica gratings made from the master grating. These are prepared by coating the original master grating with epoxy resin and removed after setting. Aluminizing its surface makes the surface of the replica grating reflective.

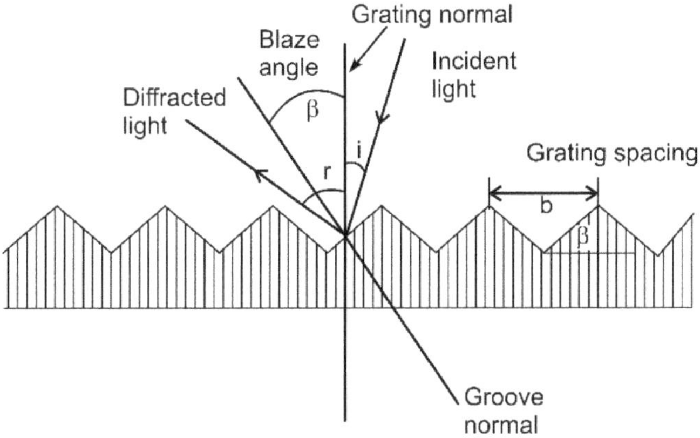

Fig. 23.25 Diffraction grating.

The principle is diffraction causing reinforcement. The incident rays on the grating, get reinforced with the reflected rays and the resulting radiation wavelength is given by the equation

$$m\lambda = b\,(\sin i \pm \sin r)$$

Where λ = wavelength of produced light
b = grating spacing
i = angle of incidence
r = angle of reflection
m = order (0, 1, 2, 3, etc).

Gratings are preferred over prisms because of their efficiency.

II. **Transmission grating:** In these types of gratings, refraction takes place. The principle is refraction produces reinforcement. The radiation transmitted through the grating reinforces with the partially refracted radiation leading to reinforcements.

Transmission grating: The wavelength produced can be calculated using the formula

$$\lambda = \frac{d\,\sin\theta}{m}$$

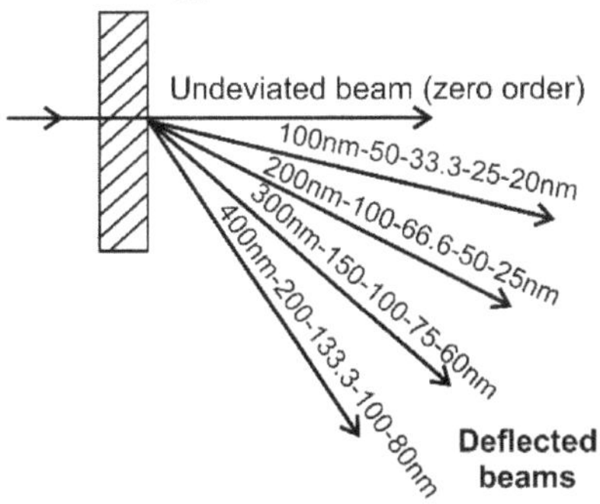

Fig. 23.26 Transmission grating.

Where λ = wavelength of radiation produced.
d = 1/lines per cm
m = order no (0, 1, 2, 3, etc)
θ = angle of deflection/diffraction

Hence, the required light radiation (λ) can be produced either by moving grating and keeping the slit fixed or vice versa.

Advantage:

1. They give linear dispersion.
2. High resolution

Disadvantage:

1. Overlap of spectral orders.

Slits: The two slits are the **entrance slit and the exit slit**. The width of the monochromatic image of the entrance slit is the same as the width of the exit slit so that it can pass through the exit slit.

(c) **Sample cells:**

- The sample cells, known as cuvettes, are used to hold the sample.
- The construction material of the cuvette varies with the instrument and the sample nature.
- The material of the cuvette should not absorb in the working wavelength.
- Material for **visible region**:

  Colour corrected fused glass.

  For aqueous solutions, Polystyrene cells are available.

  For UV region: Quartz cuvettes are used because **glass absorbs UV radiation**.
- The cells are available in different shapes like cylindrical or rectangle.
- Small volume cells (0.5ml or less) and large volume cells (5-10ml) are available depending on their capacity to hold sample volume
- The common path length (internal distance) is 1cm. Long path length cells with 10cm and short path length cells with 1 or 2mm are also available.

(d) **Detectors:** The radiation from the source through the monochromator passes through the sample. The sample absorbs part of the radiation, and the rest is being transmitted. This transmitted radiation falls on the detector, and the intensity of the absorbed radiation is determined by the detector and displayed.

Detectors used in UV Visible spectrophotometers are called as photometric detectors. They convert the **light energy to an electrical signal** which is recorded.

Three types of detectors are

1. Barrier layer cell or Photovoltaic cell
2. Photo tubes or Photo emissive cells
3. Photomultiplier tubes.

1. **Barrier layer cell or Photo voltaic cell:** The detector consists of a metal base like iron or aluminium acting as one electrode. A thin layer of semiconductor material like selenium is deposited on its surface. The surface of the selenium is covered by a very thin layer of silver or gold which acts as a second collector electrode.

   The selenium layer separates the two electrodes, and it has extremely low electrical conductivity. When radiation falls on the selenium layer, the electrons are generated at the selenium silver interface. The silver layer collects these electrons. The collection of electrons on the silver surface creates a potential difference between the two electrodes. If the resistance in the external circuit is small, the current flows through the system. The **current produced is directly proportional to the intensity of the incident radiation** on the detector.

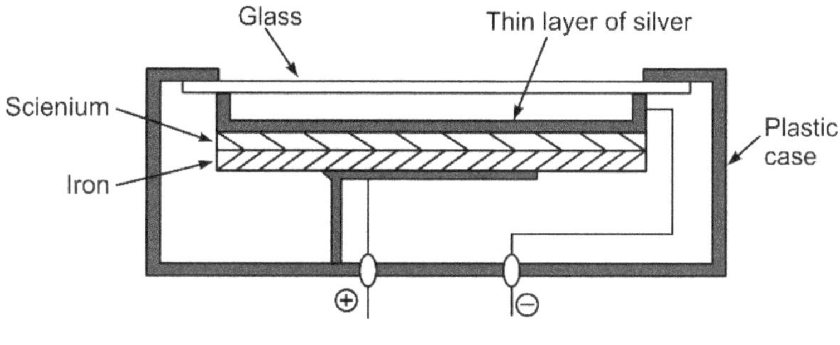

Fig. 23.27 Barrier layer cell.

Advantages:

1. Simple in design and rugged
2. No external power supply is required.

Disadvantages:

1. Less sensitive to blue region. use is limited to the visible region
2. Amplification of the signal is not possible because the resistance of the external circuit should be low.
3. Fatigue effects.

2. **Photo tubes or Photo emissive cells:** This detector consists of an evacuated glass tube containing a photocathode and an anode which acts as a collector electrode. The photocathode is coated with a light-sensitive layer like Cesium, potassium, or silver oxide. When the transmitted radiation falls on the photoemissive cathode, it emits photoelectrons. The electron flow towards the anode causes the **flow of the current, which is proportional to the intensity of radiation falling on the detector.**

   Advantages:

   1. The signal from the detector can be amplified
   2. More sensitive than Photovoltaic cells.
   3. Composite coatings containing Cesium, caesium oxide, or silver oxide can be used as the cathode to increase the sensitivity and workable wavelength range.

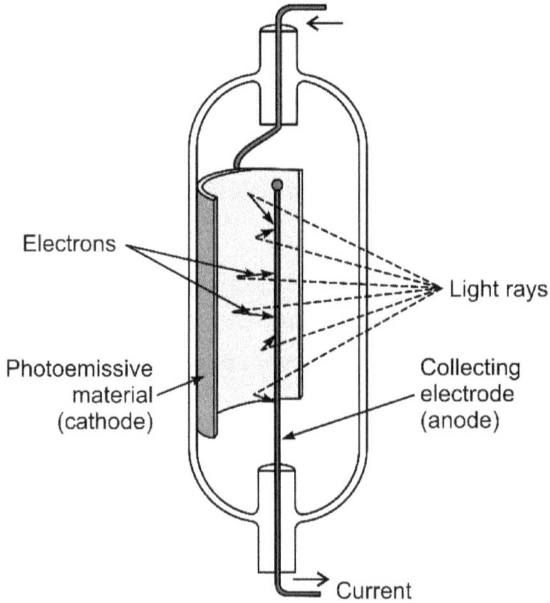

Fig. 23.28 Photo tube.

3. **Photomultiplier tubes (PMT):** Though expensive, this detector is employed in sophisticated instruments due to its sensitivity.

   The working principle of this detector is the **multiplication of photoelectrons by secondary emission of electrons.** PMT detector consists of a photocathode and a series of anodes called dynodes. Each dynode is maintained at a successively higher potential 75-100v higher than the preceding dynode. Up to 10 dynodes are used in the series.

When the radiation hits the cathode surface, electrons are emitted. When these electrons hit the dynodes, at each stage, the electrons are multiplied by a factor of 4 or 5 because of the secondary emission. An overall amplification factor of about 10^8 is achieved.

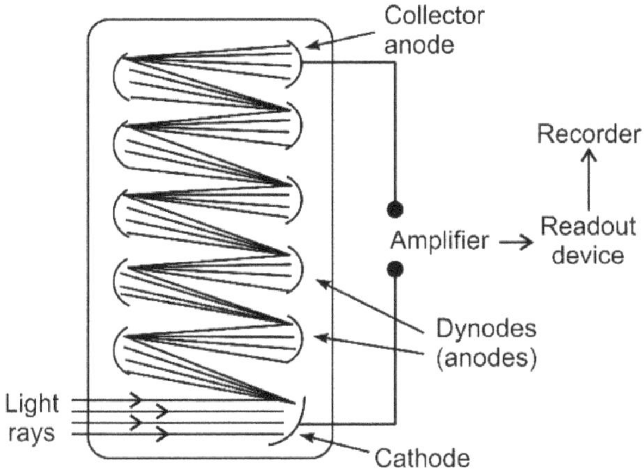

Fig. 23.29 Photo multiplier tube (PMT).

Advantages:

1. Most sensitive
2. Can detect very weak signals
3. Faster response time
4. It can be used in fluorescence measurements

Disadvantages:

1. Expensive
2. It should be shielded from stray light.

3. Silicone photodiode detector: (PDA detector):

Photodiodes are made up of photosensitive semiconductor materials like silicon, gallium, arsenide, etc. They absorb light in the wavelength range 250 to 1100 nm, characteristic of silicon. These detectors can measure light at different wavelengths simultaneously.

A photodiode is one type of light detector used to convert the light into current.

It comprises of optical filters, built-in lenses and also surface areas. These diodes have a slow response time when the surface area of the photodiode increases.

But they are less sensitive than PMTs.

Working of Photodiode

The working principle of a photodiode is, when a photon of ample energy strikes the diode, it makes a couple of electron-hole. This mechanism is also called the inner photoelectric effect. If the absorption arises in the depletion region (junction), then the carriers are removed from the junction by the inbuilt electric field of the depletion region. Therefore, holes (positive charge where the electrons are removed) in the region move toward the anode, electrons move toward the cathode, and a photocurrent will be generated.

A photodiode continually operates in a reverse bias mode. The current produced is directly proportional to light incident on the Photodiode layer

PDA detector/Diode Array Detectors (DAD)

It is an assembly of individual photodiodes on a chip.

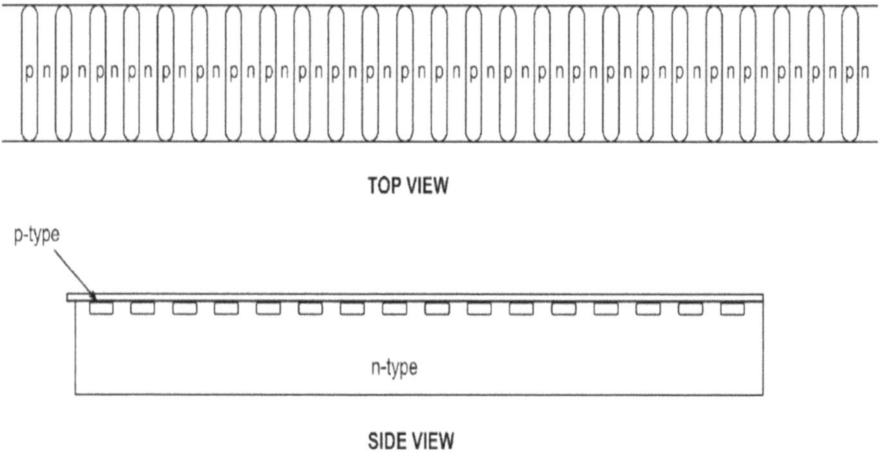

Fig. 23.30(a) Assembly of individual photodiodes on a chip.

Each diode can be addressed individually

Monochromator disperses light across PDA, with a small no of diodes /wavelength.

Allow simultaneous collection of all wavelengths.

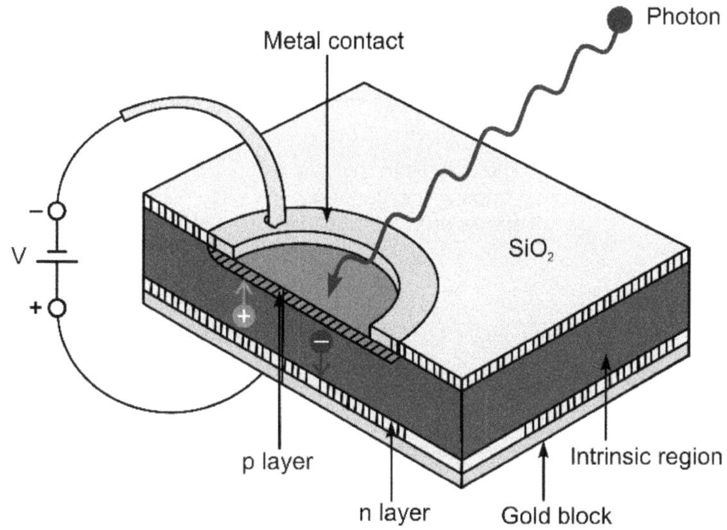

Fig. 23.30(b) Photo diode array (PDA) detector.

DADs differ from UV-VIS detectors in that **light from the lamps is shone directly onto the flow** cell, light that passes through the flow cell is **dispersed by the diffraction grating**, and the amount of the dispersed light is estimated for each wavelength in the photodiode arrays

Advantages of PDA detector

1. Determination of absorbance in all wavelengths in one run.
2. Absorbance maximum can be calculated for each peak
3. Peak purity can be determined
4. Rapid scanning.
5. Used for kinetic studies
6. Used as a detector in LC

Disadvantages

1. Large noise because the amount of light is small
2. Lamp fluctuations

(e) **Display or Readout Devices:** The electrical energy from the detector is displayed in a read-out system such as LCD. They have faster responses and are easier to read.

(f) **Computers and Recorders:** Computers are helpful in storing and processing of the data received from the detector. The recorders are for recording the absorption spectrum or absorbance of the analyte of interest.

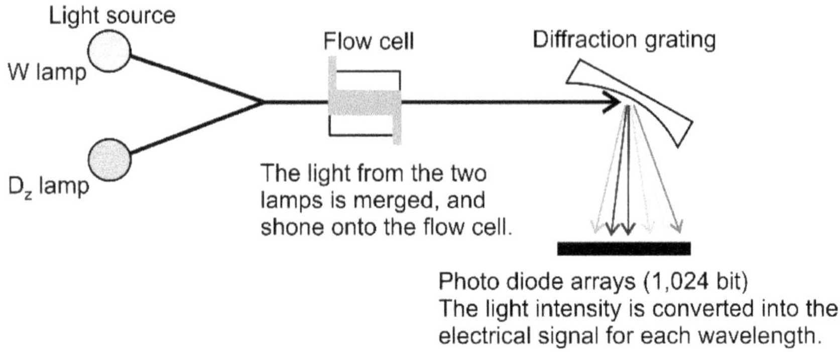

Fig. 23.31 Working of photo diode array (PDA) detector.

The different types of instruments used in UV spectroscopy are

1. Single Beam UV spectrophotometer
2. Double beam UV spectrophotometer

1. **Single beam spectrophotometer:** The construction and working of a single-beam spectrophotometer are the same as a single beam colorimeter, except the source and the detectors used are different here. The schematic diagram is given below

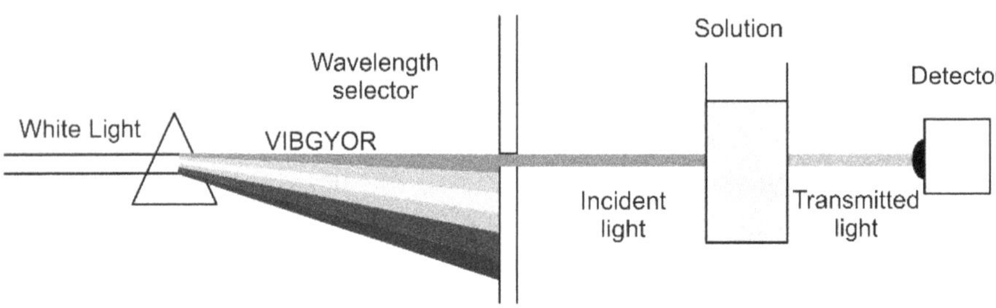

Fig. 23.32 Single beam spectrophotometer.

2. **Double beam UV Spectrophotometer:** The construction and working of the double beam are the same as that of the double beam colourimeter. The difference is that instead of a filter or prism, here grating monochromator is used, and photomultiplier detectors are used in the place of photo tube detectors. These are the widely used instruments.

   Working:

   1. The radiation from the source passes via the mirror system to the monochromator.
   2. The monochromator allows a narrow range of wavelengths to pass through the exit slit.
   3. The radiation from the monochromator through the exit slit is received by the optical chopper, which divides the beam into

two beams; one passes through the reference and the other through the sample cell.

4. The beams, after passing through reference and sample cells, are passed to the detector.
5. The output of the detector is connected to the amplifier, which responds to the change in transmission through the sample and reference.
6. Then the signal is transferred to the recorder, where the absorbance or transmittance is recorded as a function of wavelength.

Advantages:

1. Zero adjusting can be done for all wavelengths simultaneously and need not be repeated for every wavelength.
2. In double beam spectrophotometers, the ratio of sample and reference beams is used for measurement, minimizing the errors due to variation in the intensity of the source and detector fluctuation.
3. Rapid scanning over a wide wavelength region.
4. High accuracy, sensitivity, reliability, and repeatability.

Disadvantages:

1. Complicated
2. Expensive

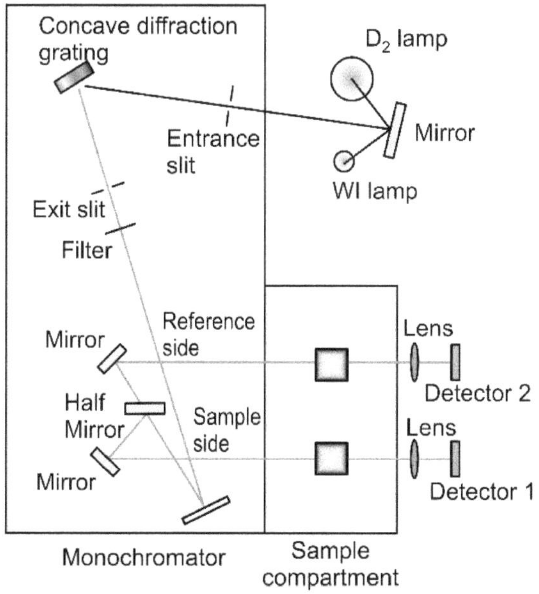

Fig. 23.33 Double beam UV Visible spectrophotometer.

APPLICATIONS

1. **Spectrophotometric titrations:** In these titrations, the absorbance of the solution is measured after each addition of the titrant, and the **absorbance is plotted against the volume of the titrant**. The endpoint is determined from the graph. The titrant or the titrated substance can be the absorbing species. The endpoint is determined by the intersection of lines of the titration curve. If there is a curvature without intersection due to incomplete reaction, the lines can be extrapolated to give the endpoint

   The first curve (a) is the example where the **titrant only absorbs**. In this titration, only the titrant that is bromine is absorbing, and its absorption is plotted against the volume of the titrant. So, the absorbance will not change till all the arsenic is consumed. Once all the arsenic is consumed by the titrant, only bromine will be there, causing an increase in absorption.

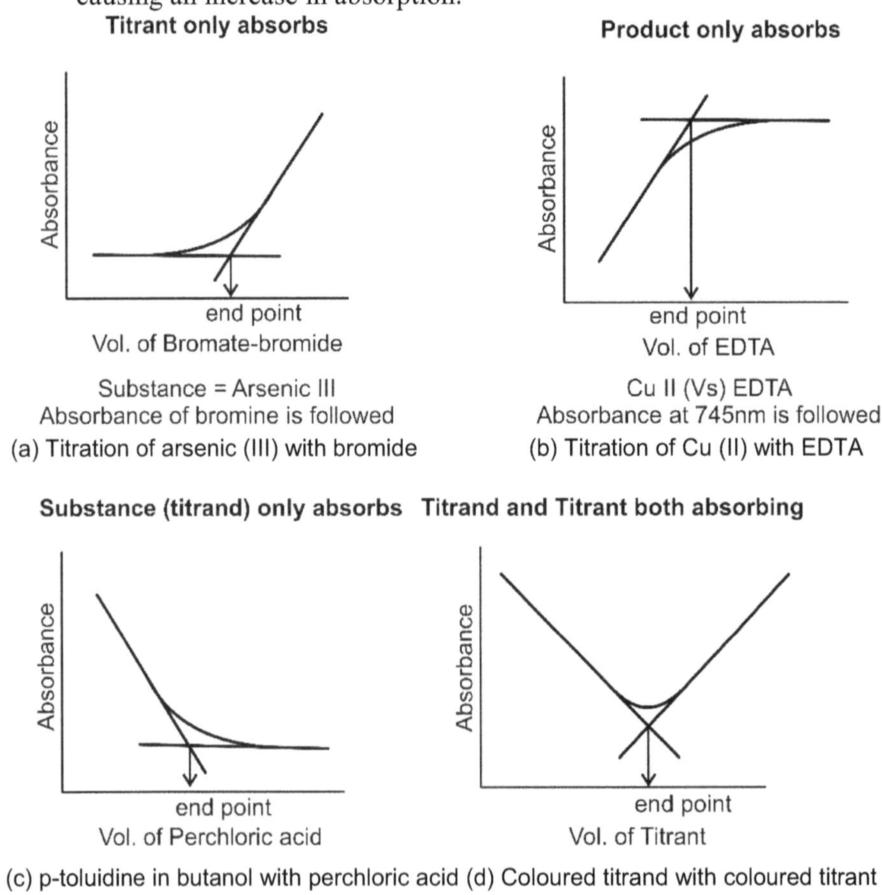

Fig. 23.34 Types of spectrophotometric titrations.

The second curve (b) is the example of the case where **only the product is absorbing**. E.g., is the titration of Cu II ions with Ethylene diamine tetracetic acid (EDTA). There is an increase in absorbance as the product is formed, and once the reaction is complete, no new product is formed, and the absorbance becomes constant with no further increase.

In the third case, (c) **only the substance titrated (titrand) absorbs.** Eg is the titration of p-toluidine in butanol with perchloric acid. As p-toluidine is being consumed by the perchloric acid, there is a decrease in absorbance, and once all the p-toluidine is consumed, there is no change in absorbance. The graph becomes horizontal with no further change in absorbance.

In the fourth case (d), coloured substance reacts with coloured titrant to give a colourless product. So, **both the titrand and the titrant will be absorbing and the product is not absorbing**. Initially, there is a sharp decrease in absorbance due to the formation of non-absorbing product formation. After the endpoint, the concentration of the absorbing titrant increases, leading to an increase in absorbance.

Conditions to be followed:

(a) Titrand, titrant, or product should absorb in the selected wavelength.

(b) The concentration should be in the Beer's law range

(c) Titrant must be stronger so that dilution error can be minimized (absorbance is proportional to concentration).

Applications

1. **Acid-base titrations:** Eg: titration of phenols with sodium hydroxide. Absorbance due to phenolate ion is recorded.
2. **Oxidation-reduction titrations:** Eg: Ce (III) titration with Co (III).Ce(IV) formation is followed.
3. **Complexometric Titrations:** Eg: Cu (II) is titrated with EDTA. Cu-EDTA complex formation is followed.
4. **Precipitation Titrations:** Eg: SO_4^{2-} ions titrated with Ba (II) ions, and the turbidity appearance is followed.

Advantages

1. As only one absorbing species is needed, these titrations can be applied to a large no. of non –absorbing substances.
2. No interference from other absorbing species, as only the change in absorbance is important
3. The method is applicable to highly coloured solutions where visual indicators cannot be used.
4. The endpoint can be determined even if the reaction is incomplete
5. Accurate and precise.

6. No need to work only at the absorption maximum (λ_{max}). So wavelength choice is there.
7. Dissociation constants can be determined from these graphs.
8. Convenient, rapid.

2. **Single component analysis:** Determination of concentration and amount of the substance present in the given sample is called Quantitative estimation. Using these values, percentage purity can be determined. The quantitative estimation of drugs by UV-visible spectrophotometry can be performed by knowing the parameters like λ_{max}, Beer's law concentration range for that substance, solvent, reagents and other conditions.

   The types of quantitative estimation are

   1. **Using $A^{1\%}_{1cm}$ value (specific absorbance):** This method is useful in the estimations of raw material as well as formulations when the reference standard is not available. $A^{1\%}_{1cm}$ value can be obtained from Pharmacopoeia, Textbooks or Journals
   2. **Reference standard available:** If reference standard is available, specific absorbance can be found experimentally and the above method can be used.
   3. **Direct comparison method (single standard):** The absorbance of the standard solution of known concentration is compared with the absorbance of sample solution and the concentration of sample solution is calculated. From the concentration, the amount and the % purity can be calculated.
   4. **Calibration curve method or multiple standard Method:** The calibration graph method is used to minimize the error introduced in the preparation of solutions or absorbance measurements.

      In this method, a calibration curve is plotted with concentration vs. absorbance measured with five or more concentrations of the reference or standard. A straight line passing through the origin is obtained. If a straight line is not obtained, a straight line is obtained through the maximum no of points or by regression analysis leading to a line of best fit. The unknown concentration of the sample can be obtained using the absorbance of the sample and the calibration graph. The extrapolation of the graph gives the unknown concentration and amount and the % purity of the sample can be calculated.
   5. **Measurement of equilibrium constant and rate constant by spectroscopy**

      Spectroscopy can indeed be utilized to measure equilibrium constants and rate constants, particularly in reactions involving changes in absorbance, fluorescence, or emission spectra over time.

Measurement of Equilibrium Constant: For reactions that involve changes in absorbance due to formation or consumption of certain species, one can monitor the absorption spectra at different stages of the reaction. By plotting absorbance vs. concentration of reactants and products, one can determine the equilibrium constant using Beer-Lambert law.

Measurement of Rate Constant:

UV-Vis Spectroscopy: By monitoring absorbance changes over time at specific wavelengths, one can determine the rate of reaction. The rate constant can then be derived from the slope of concentration vs. time plots, typically using methods like the pseudo-first-order approximation for fast reactions.

6. **Multi-component analysis:** Simultaneous analysis of numerous components in a sample is called multi-component analysis. Several methods are available in UV spectroscopy for multi-component analysis. In these methods, the absorption spectra is recorded and mathematically processed.

The basis of all the Spectrophotometric techniques for multi-component samples is

"At all wavelengths, the absorbance of a solution is the sum of absorbance of the individual components"

or

The measured absorbance is the difference between the total absorbance of the solution in the sample cell and that of the solution in the reference cell.

The excipients present in the formulation should not be absorbed at the wavelength of the experiment.

The different UV spectrophotometric multi component analysis methods are

1. Simultaneous equation method (Vierdott's method)
2. Absorbance ratio method (Q-Absorbance method)
3. Derivative Spectrophotometric method
4. Multi wavelength UV-spectrophotometry
5. Dual wavelength method
6. Difference spectroscopy
7. Geometric correction method
8. Orthogonal poly nominal method
9. Solvent extraction method
10. H-point standard addition method
11. Least square approximation method

1. **Simultaneous equation method (Vierdott's method):** If a sample contains two absorbing drugs (X & Y) with λ_{max} at λ_1 and λ_2 respectively, then it is possible to determine the concentration of both the drugs by simultaneous equation method if certain criteria are satisfied.

   Criteria for using the simultaneous equation method are

   The criteria are that the ratios,

   $$\frac{A_2 / A_1}{ax_2 / ax_1} \quad \text{and} \quad \frac{ay_2 / ay_1}{A_2 / A_1}$$

   should lie outside the range of 0.1-2

   This criteria is satisfied only when the λ_{max} of the two components are reasonably dissimilar.

   The second criterion is that the two components should not interact chemically with each other.

   Example: Validated spectrophotometric methods for simultaneous′ estimation of Telmisartan and Indapamide in the pharmaceutical dosage form. λ_{max}: TEL 296 nm IND 242 nm

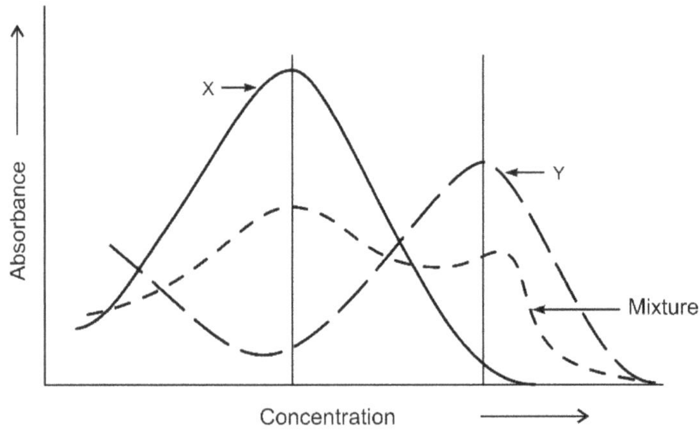

Fig. 23.35 Simultaneous estimation of Telmisartan and Indapamide in pharmaceutical dosage forms.

At λ_1 and λ_2, the absorbance of the mixture is the sum of the individual absorbance of X & Y. Two equations are constructed using this fact.

At λ_1, $A_1 = a_{x1}\, bc_x + ay_1\, bc_y$ .....(1)

At λ_2, $A_2 = a_{x2}\, bc_x + ay_2\, bc_y$ .....(2)

Where,

The absorptivity of X at λ_1 is ax_1, and the absorptivity of X at λ_2 is ax_2

The absorptivity of Y at λ_1 is ay_1 and at λ_2 is ay_2.

The absorbance of the diluted sample at λ_1 and λ_2, A_1 and A_2 respectively.

The concentration of X & Y are C_x & C_y respectively, in the diluted sample.

Rearrange eq. (2).

$$c_y = A_2 - ax_2cx / ay_2$$

Substituting for c_y in eq. (1). and rearranging gives

$$\mathbf{C_x = A_2ay_1 - A_1ay_2 / ax_2ay_1 - ax_1ay_2}$$

$$\mathbf{C_y = A_1ax_2 - A_2ax_1 / ax_2ay_1 - ax_1ay_2}$$

2. **Absorbance ratio method:** The absorbance ratio method is a modification of the simultaneous equations method. It depends on the property that, for a substance, which obeys Beer's law at all wavelengths, the ratio of absorbances at any two wavelengths is a constant value and is independent of concentration or path length.

   In the quantitative estimation of two components in a mixture by the absorbance ratio method, absorbance is measured at two wavelengths, λ_{max} one of the components (λ_2) and wavelength of equal absorptivity of two components (λ_1), i.e. an iso-absorptive point.

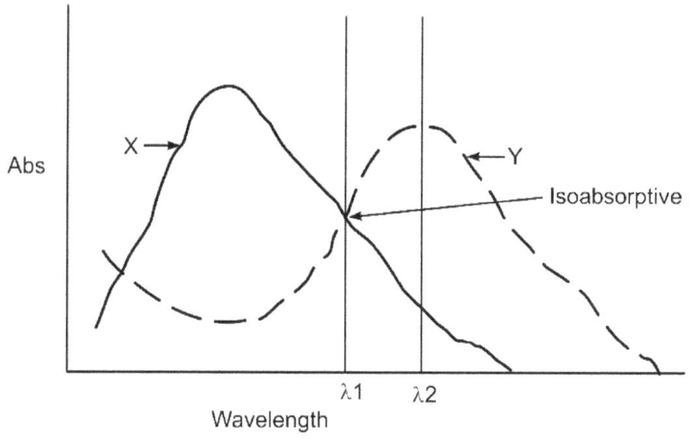

Fig. 23.36 Absorbance ratio method of Atrovastatin and Niacin in tablet dosage forms.

The concentration of the components x and y can be determined by the equation

$$C_X = (Q_m-Q_y).\ A_1 / (Q_x-Q_y).\ ax_1$$

$$C_Y = (Q_m-Q_x).\ A_1 / (Q_y-Q_x).\ ay_1$$

Where $Q_m = A_2/ A_1$ $\quad Q_x = ax_2/ ax_1$ $\quad Q_y = ay_2/ay_1$

A_2 =Absorbance at λ_2; A_1 =Absorbance at λ_1

ax_1 = Absorptivity of Drug X at λ_1

ay_1 = Absorptivity of Drug Y at λ_1
ax_2 = Absorptivity of Drug X at λ_2
ay_2 = Absorptivity of Drug Y at λ_2

E.g., Spectrophotometric method for absorbance ratio method of Atorvastatin and Niacin in the tablet dosage form. λ_{max}: ATR: 246nm NIA: 262nm. The iso-absorptive point at 258nm in Methanol.

3. **Derivative spectrophotometric method:** When the mixture has got interfering absorption, the derivative spectroscopy method is employed.

   Derivative spectroscopy involves the conversion of a normal spectrum to its first, second or higher derivative spectrum.

   The normal spectrum is known as fundamental, zero-order, or D^0 spectra. The plot of the rate of change of absorbance with wavelength against wavelength is called the first derivative spectrum (D1)

   i.e. plot of $\Delta A/\Delta\lambda$ vs λ

   The second derivative spectrum is a plot of Δ2A/ Δλ2 vs λ

   The quantitative estimations in derivative spectroscopy give accurate results with second derivative spectroscopy.

   For the quantitative estimation of binary mixtures(A&B) using the derivative spectroscopy, the Zero Crossing Points (ZCP) for both the components (A and B) are noted.

   The ZCP for A and B is selected in such a way that at that particular ZCP, the other component shows remarkable absorbance.

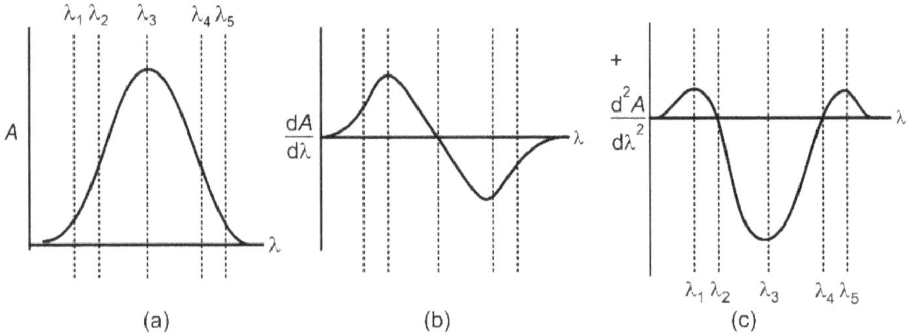

Fig. 23.37 Zeroth (a), First (b), Second (c) derivative spectra

The calibration curve of A is constructed at the ZCP of B and B at the ZCP of A. Unknown concentrations can be found from the calibration graph by extrapolation.

E.g., Simultaneous Spectrophotometric estimation of Ofloxacin and Satranidazole in the tablet dosage form.

4. **Multi wavelength UV-spectrophotometry:** This method helps in the determination of the composition of a binary mixture with overlapping spectra without determining molar absorptivities. The method requires standard solution absorbance of each component and the unknown mixture absorbance
   All the standard solutions can be scanned over the range of 200-400nm in the multi-component mode, using two sampling wavelengths. The overlay spectra of standard solutions can be used to determine the concentrations of the drugs in a sample solution.
   E.g., Simultaneous Estimation & Validation of Paracetamol, Phenylephrine Hydrochloride and Chlorpheniramine Maleate in Tablets by Spectrophotometric Method:
5. **Dual wavelength method:** The dual-wavelength method is also known as the two wavelengths method. In this method, one of the drugs is considered as analyte and the other drug is considered as an interfering component and vice-versa. The two wavelengths are selected in such a way, that in one wavelength, the interfering component shows the same absorbance (ΔA equals zero), and the analyte shows a significant difference in absorbance with a concentration in the other wavelength. The difference in absorbance (ΔA) between two points on the mixture sample spectra is directly proportional to the concentration of the analyte independent of the interfering component
   E.g., Simultaneous determination of atenolol and indapamide
6. **Difference spectroscopy:** Quantitative estimation of the substance in the presence of absorbing interferents can be carried out by this method. The essential feature of this method is that the measured value is the absorbance difference (ΔA) between two equimolar solutions in the same wavelength.
   Two equimolar solutions of the analyte in different chemical forms will exhibit different spectral characteristics. The difference in absorption in the selected wavelength is measured.
   The alteration in the spectral properties of the analyte is mainly done by the adjustment of the pH using acids, alkalies, or buffers.
   Eg: Difference in absorbance of Ibuprofen in 0.1N HCl and 0.1 N NaOH is used in determination of ibuprofen
7. **Geometric correction method:** It is the three-point geometric procedure, the simplest of mathematical correction procedures and it is applied if the interfering absorption is linear at the three wavelengths selected.
   If the wavelengths λ_1, λ_2 and λ_3 are selected to that the background absorbances B_1, B_2 and B_3 are linear, then the corrected absorbance D

of the drug may be calculated from the three absorbances A_1, A_2 and A_3 of the sample solution at λ_1, λ_2 and λ_3 respectively as follows

The general formula is

$$D = y(A_2 - A_3) + z(A_2 - A_1) / y\ (1 - w) + z(1 - v)$$

Where

A_1, A_2 and A_3 – three absorbances of the sample

y and z –wave length intervals $(\lambda_2 - \lambda_1)$ and $(\lambda_3 - \lambda_2)$

v and w - absorbance ratios vD/D and wD/D respectively

Let vD and wD be the absorbance of the drug alone in the sample solution at λ_1 and λ_3 respectively,

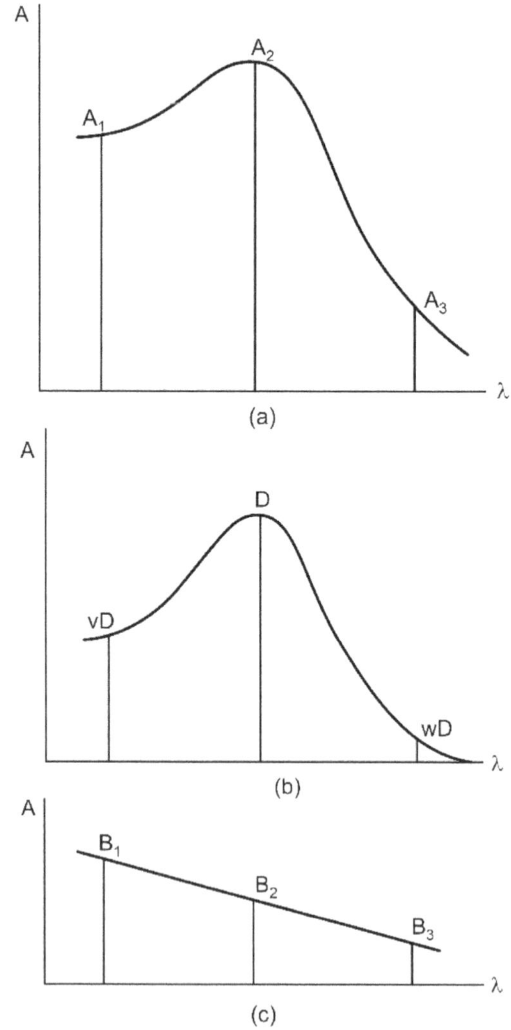

Fig. 23.38 An absorption spectrum (a), the spectrum of analyte (b), background absorption (c).

8. **Orthogonal polynomial method:** It is another mathematical correction procedure, which involves more complex calculations.
   In this method, an absorption spectrum is represented in terms of orthogonal functions like
   $$A(\lambda) = p\,P(\lambda) + p1\,P1(\lambda) + p2\,P2(\lambda) \ldots\ldots pn\,Pn(\lambda)$$
   Where A denotes the absorbance at wavelength λ. A set of n+1 equally spaced wavelengths are used at which the orthogonal polynomials, P (λ), P1 (λ), P2 (λ) ….. Pn (λ) are defined
9. **Solvent extraction method:** In this method, different solvents are selected based on the solubility of the components of the mixture and the components are extracted individually. Then the extracted components are analyzed separately.
10. **H-point standard addition method:** The H-point standard addition method (HPSAM) is a modification of the standard addition method. The method is used for resolving strongly overlapping spectra of two analytes and errors produced by the matrix of the sample can also be corrected directly. The technique is a combination of dual-wavelength spectrophotometry and the standard addition method.
11. **Least square approximation method:** Experimental measurements are always subject to random errors. To correct these errors and to obtain an accurate result, more number of experimental data is used. That is, the analysis of a binary mixture is carried out in three or four wavelengths instead of at two wavelengths,
    The method of least squares is a standard approach to the approximate solution of overdetermined systems, i.e., sets of equations in which there are more equations than unknowns. "Least squares" means that the overall solution minimizes the sum of the squares of the errors made in the results of every single equation.

Other Applications of UV spectroscopy

1. **Qualitative analysis:** Identification of the compounds is done by comparing the absorption spectrum with the spectra of standard known compounds.
2. **Detection of Impurities:** UV spectroscopy is one of the best methods for the detection of impurities in organic compounds. When comparing the absorption spectrum of the sample with a standard absorption spectrum, the presence of additional peaks indicates the presence of impurities. Impurities can also be detected by measuring in specific wavelengths characteristic for them
   E.g., The impurity, cyclohexane, in benzene can be detected by measuring the absorption at 255nm.
3. **Structural elucidation of Organic compounds:** Structural elucidation like the presence/absence of unsaturation, presence of heteroatoms like S, O, N, or halogens can be determined using UV

spectroscopy. The general absorptions of these features are given E.g. Saturated compound σ - σ^* appears below 200nm (vacuum uv) The other three possibilities are given below, and they appear between 200-400 nm.

Presence of heteroatoms (S, N, O) with saturation n - σ^*

Unsaturated compounds π - π^*

Hetero atom and double bond n-π^*

Thus the location of peaks in the absorption spectrum gives an idea about the structural features.

4. **Structural analysis of organic compounds:** The effect of conjugation, cross conjugation, and alkyl substitution are discussed here
   (i) **Detection of conjugation:** It helps to know the presence of different groups with respect to conjugation, e.g., The conjugation maybe

   Between two or more C=C (or triple) bonds
   Between C=C and C=O
   Between double bonds and aromatic rings.

   The presence of aromatic rings can be identified and the no and positions of attachment to the carbons of the conjugated system can also be identified.

   Extension of the conjugation gives **bathochromic** shift or redshift by shifting the λ_{max} to longer wavelength.

   Reduction or saturation of double bonds leads to **hypsochromic** shift or blue shift by shifting the λ_{max} to the shorter wavelength.

   (ii) **Detection of Geometrical Isomerism:** The **trans isomer** of the geometrical isomers absorb at a **longer wavelength** and have a **larger extinction coefficient** than cis isomers.

   Eg: Calciferol- λ_{max} 265 nm (cis)
   Iso vitD_2-λ_{max} 287 nm (trans)

   Conversion of Cis – trans-isomer shows Bathochromic shift &
   Hyperchromic effect
   Conversion of Trans to cis exhibits
   Hyposochromic shift and
   Hypochromic effect

   (iii) **Cross conjugation:** The cross conjugation has got no effect on λ_{max}.

   (iv) **Alkyl substitution:** Bathochromic shift occurs with alkyl substitution. More the no of alkyl substitution more is the shift.

   (v) **No of rings:** Bathochromic shift occurs with the addition of rings.

CHAPTER 24

IR Spectroscopy

IR spectroscopy is a valuable tool used for the structural determination of organic compounds in conjunction with other techniques like NMR and Mass spectroscopy. The absorption of infrared radiation by a molecule causes changes in their vibrational and rotational energy levels, and hence IR-spectroscopy is also known as vibrational-rotational spectroscopy. IR spectroscopy provides a spectrum with a large number of absorption bands and hence provide plenty of information about the structure of a compound. Different bonds in the spectra correspond to various functional groups and bonds present in the molecule.

IR spectroscopy is the study of changes in vibration of the molecule when there is absorption of IR radiation by the molecule. Certain functional groups in the molecule give rise to bands at the same wavelength range irrespective of the structure of the molecule. This characteristic band gives useful structural information about the compounds when compared with the generalised charts of characteristic group absorbance bands. IR spectrum is characteristic of the molecule.

After absorbing IR radiation, the molecules of the compounds vibrate at many rates of vibration, giving rise to closely appearing bands in the IR spectrum, which is the fingerprint for the identification of the molecule. The characteristic functional groups and bonds of the compounds give rise to these bands, making it the fingerprint of the molecule.

THEORY

The IR absorption by the molecules causes excitation of both vibrational and rotational energies, and the spectrum appears as bands. The IR spectrum is otherwise called **vibrational spectroscopy**. Each vibrational energy change is accompanied by a number of rotational energy changes. These vibrational-rotational energy bands occurring between 4000 – 400cm^{-1} are studied in IR spectroscopy.

Range of IR Radiation

IR range is divided into three regions.

Near IR (0.8 – 2.5μm) : 13000 – 4000cm^{-1}
Far IR (25 – 1000μm) : 400-10 cm^{-1}
Mid IR (2.5- 25 μm) : 400cm^{-1} to 4000cm^{-1}

In pharmaceutical analysis, the mid-IR region is used, which gives useful information about the vibration of molecules and the functional group present.

Bands in IR spectra are presented in wave numbers, and its unit is cm^{-1}. Wave numbers are reciprocal of the wavelength.

$$cm^{-1} = 10^4 / \text{wavelength in } \mu m$$

The band intensity expressed in the wave number unit is easy to handle than the wavelength, either as absorbance or transmittance, because wave numbers are larger values, easy to handle and wavelengths show only small differences between functional group bands.

The mid-infrared spectrum extends from 4000 to 400 cm^{-1} and results from vibrational and rotational transitions. This region is most useful for the organic chemist since most organic molecules absorb in this region.

The mid-infrared can be divided into two regions, viz

- Functional group region (4000-1300cm^{-1})
- Fingerprint region (1300-600cm^{-1}).

Functional group region (4000-1300cm^{-1}): Most of the functional groups present in organic molecules exhibit absorption bands in the region **4000-1300 cm^{-1}**; hence this is known as the functional group region. In this region, each band can be assigned to a particular **deformation (bending)** of the molecule, the movement of a group of atoms, or the bending or **stretching** of a particular bond.

Fingerprint region (1300-600cm^{-1}): The region from **1300 cm^{-1} to 600 cm^{-1}** usually contains a very complicated series of absorptions. These are mainly due to molecular vibrations, usually bending motions that are characteristic of the entire molecule or large fragments of the molecule. Except for enantiomers, any two different compounds cannot have precisely the same absorption pattern in this region. Thus, **absorption patterns** in this region are unique for any particular compound; that is why this is known as the fingerprint region.

It is very difficult to assign individual bands in this region.

A typical IR spectrum is shown in figure 24.1.

Two molecules having the same functional group may show similar spectra in the functional group region, but their spectra differ in the fingerprint region. Therefore, both regions are very useful for confirming the identity of a chemical substance. This is generally accomplished by comparing the spectrum of an authentic sample. When two compounds show a good match between the IR spectra in all frequency ranges, mainly in the fingerprint region, it strongly indicates that they have the same molecular structures.

To understand the importance of fingerprint region to identify a compound, the example of propan-1-ol and propan-2-ol is given in Fig. 24.2 and 24.3.

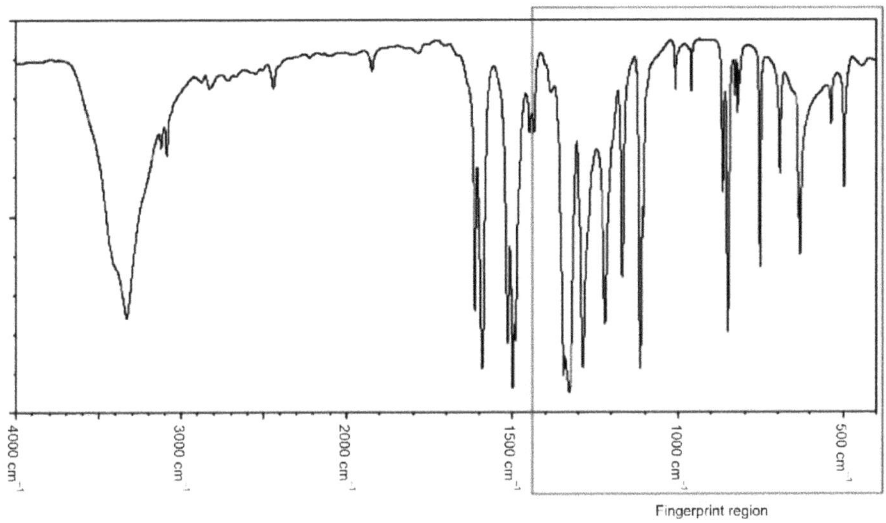

Fig. 24.1 A typical IR Spectrum.

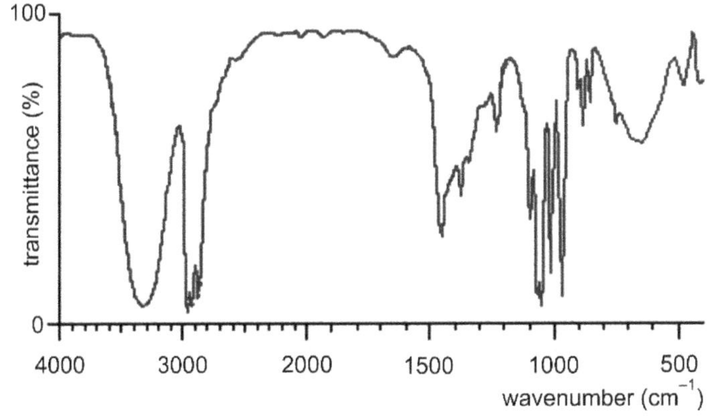

Fig. 24.2 IR spectra of Propane-1-ol – $CH_3CH_2CH_2OH$.

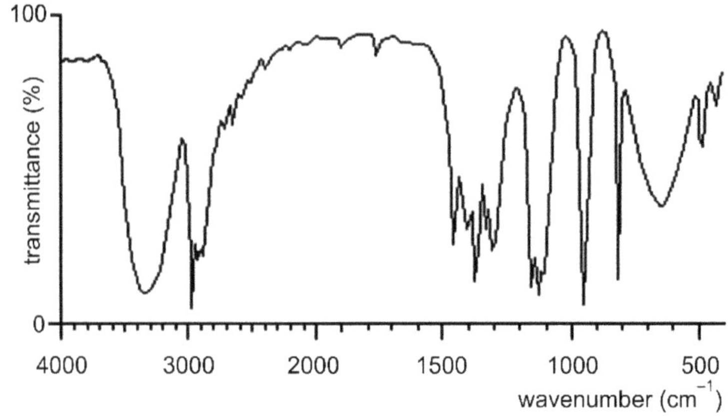

Fig. 24.3 IR spectra of Propane-2-ol. $CH_3CH(OH)CH_3$

Both the compounds are alcohols and contain precisely the same bonds. Now, if you compare the infra-red spectra of these compounds, the functional group region is very similar for both the compounds, but the fingerprint region is different like a fingerprint. Therefore, the fingerprint region can play a crucial role in identifying the compound.

CRITERIA FOR THE COMPOUND TO ABSORB IN IR REGION

(i) The functional groups in a molecule absorb IR radiation only when the **applied IR frequency** is **equal** to the **natural frequency** of vibration of the groups in the molecule

(ii) The IR radiation absorbed should cause a change in the dipole moment of the molecule

PRINCIPLE

The atoms or groups of atoms in a molecule are connected by bonds. These bonds are not rigid in nature, and the structure of the molecule acts like balls connected by a spring. Balls represent atoms, and the springs represent bonds. There are some vibrations of some frequency in the molecule, which is characteristic of the functional groups or bonds present in the molecule. These vibrational frequencies are called the natural frequency of vibration for that molecules. The applied IR radiation is absorbed when

Applied IR frequency = natural frequency of vibration of the molecule

As soon as the radiation is absorbed, a band appears in the spectrum.

The different functional groups or bonds in the molecules absorb different frequencies of IR radiation. Thus, for every functional group or bond, a characteristic band is observed.

Hence IR spectrum becomes the fingerprint of a molecule.

There are two types of molecular vibrations: stretching and bending.

Stretching is the change in bond length.

Bending is the change in bond angle.

Hooke's law can be used in the assignments of stretching frequencies of groups in molecules. The vibrating bond is compared to a physical model of a vibrating spring system. In application of Hooke's law, a bond and the connected atoms are considered to be a spring with two masses attached (Simple harmonic oscillator). The Hooke's law equation

$$\bar{\nu} = 1/2\pi c \times [f/(M_xM_y)/(M_x + M_y)]^{1/2}$$

Where $\bar{\nu}$ = vibrational frequency in cm^{-1}, C = velocity of light, f = force constant of bond (dynes/cm) and M_x and M_y = masses of (g) atom x and atom y respectively.

The equation indicates how the frequency $\bar{\nu}$, of the absorption changes as the properties of the system change.

An example of a molecule absorbing IR radiation is shown in figure 24.4. E.g., Methanol CH_3OH

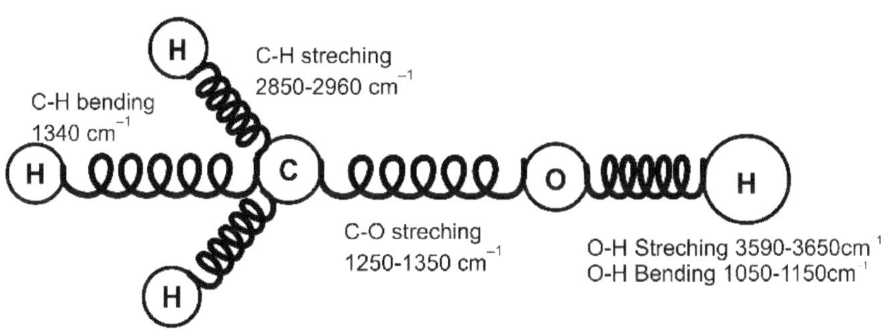

Fig. 24.4 Vibrations of a molecule after absorbing IR radiation.

Dipole Moment: The electrical dipole present in the molecule interacts with the electrical component of IR radiation. This interaction causes the change in the dipole moment of the molecule. The symmetrical diatomic molecules like O_2 and N_2 do not possess electric dipole, and they do not absorb IR radiation.

FUNDAMENTAL MODES OF VIBRATIONS IN POLYATOMIC MOLECULES

Molecular vibrations can be broadly classified into fundamental vibrations and non-fundamental vibrations. Under non-fundamental vibrations, we have overtones, combinations and Fermi resonance. The fundamental vibrations are further divided into **stretching and bending** vibrations. The **stretching vibrations** are further classified as **symmetric and asymmetric** stretching vibrations. The **bending vibrations** are classified as **in-plane** and **out of plane bending**, which are further divided into scissoring, rocking, wagging and twisting.

In fundamental vibrations, there is no change in the centre of gravity of the molecule. The principal fundamental vibrations are stretching and bending vibrations.

1. **Stretching vibration:** In these vibrations, the atoms move along the bond axis, and there will be changes in the **bond length** (increased/decreased) at regular intervals. These are two types of stretching vibrations
   - Symmetrical
   - Asymmetrical

   Symmetrical stretching: In this stretching, there is symmetrical increase or decrease of bond length occurs.

   Asymmetrical stretching: In this stretching, one bond length increases and the other bond length decreases.
2. **Bending vibrations:** A change in **bond angle** occurs in these vibrations. Bending vibrations are otherwise called **deformation vibrations** which are further classified as **in-plane bending and out of plane bending.**

   In-plane bending: Change in **bond angle** (bending) occurs in the **same plane**. Two types of in-plane bending are possible.

   (i) **Scissoring:** In this type of bending, bond angle decreases

   (ii) **Rocking:** Both bonds are moving, but the bond angle is maintained.

   Out of plane bending: Bending of the bonds (bond angle change) occurs outside the plane of the molecule. The types are

   (i) **Wagging:** Both the atoms move to the same side of the plane

   (ii) **Twisting:** In this type of bending, one atom moves above the plane and the other atom moves below the plane.

   The different types of vibrations are shown diagrammatically in Fig. 24.5.

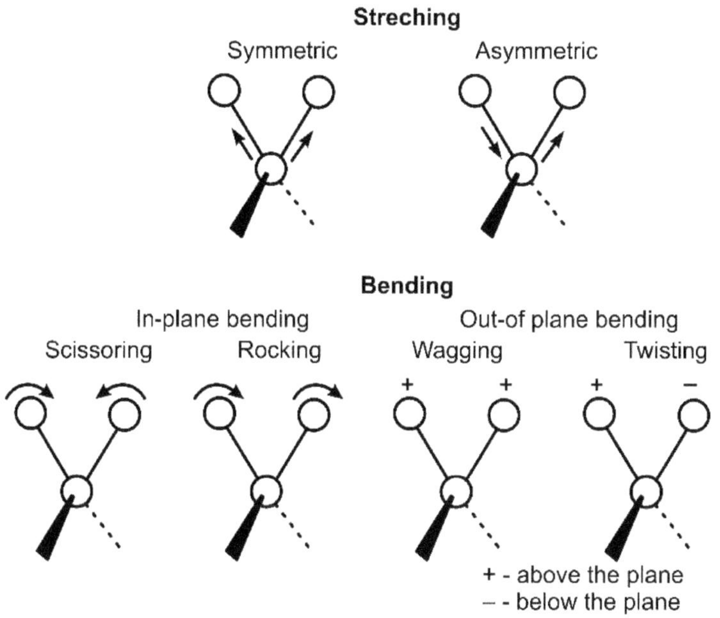

Fig. 24.5 Fundamental modes of vibrations of a molecule.

NUMBER OF VIBRATIONS IN A MOLECULE

A compound's IR spectrum may show more than one vibrational absorption band. The number of these bands corresponds to the number of fundamental vibrations in the molecule, which can be calculated from the molecule's degree of freedom (DOF). Each atom in the molecule has three degrees of freedom (translational, rotational and vibrational). To describe the position of an atom in relation to other atoms in the molecule, the three Cartesian coordinates (x,y,z) are necessary. These three coordinates correspond to three degrees of freedom of the atom. Thus, there are 3n degrees of freedom for a molecule containing n atoms.

To find the number of vibrational degrees of freedom, the number of rotational and translational degrees of freedom should be deducted from total number of degrees of freedom.

For nonlinear molecules like H_2O

Total number of degrees of freedom = 3n = 3× 3 = 9 (n represents number of atoms)

3 degrees of freedom --⟶ rotational changes

3 degrees of freedom -⟶ translational changes

So vibrational degrees of freedom = 3n – (3 + 3) = 3n – 6 = 9 – 6 = 3

Thus 3 vibrational changes are possible in a non-linear molecule.

For a linear molecule

For a linear molecule like CO_2

Total number of degrees of freedom = $3n = 3 \times 3 = 9$ (n represents number of atoms)

For rotational changes → 2 degrees of freedom

For translational changes → 3 degrees of freedom.

Therefore, vibrational degrees of freedom or fundamental vibrations = $3n - (3 + 2) = 9 - 5 = 4$

Thus four vibrational changes are possible in a linear molecule.

In the actual IR spectrum, the number of theoretical fundamental bands is rarely observed because some of the factors like overlapping of the spectrum, low resolution and weak peaks **may increase or decrease the number of bands**

Example CO_2 is linear molecule so expected to have 4 fundamental vibrations.

But actual spectrum shows only 2 vibrations ($666 cm^{-1}$ and $2350 cm^{-1}$).

Reasons

1. Symmetrical stretching of CO_2 is inactive in IR (no change in dipole moment)
2. Two scissoring/ bending vibrations are equivalent, and they appear at ($666 cm^{-1}$) same frequency (degenerate)
3. Asymmetrical stretch appears as strong band at $2350\ cm^{-1}$

Thus, only two bands appear for CO_2 in the IR spectrum.

FACTORS INFLUENCING VIBRATIONAL FREQUENCIES

The value of vibrational frequency of a functional group calculated by Hooke's Law is not always equal to their observed value. The vibrational frequency of the group gets changed with the electronic and steric effects caused by other groups present in the surroundings. Following are some important factors affecting the vibrational frequency of a bond.

1. Effect of Bond order
2. Electronic effects
3. Effect of Resonance
4. Degree of Conjugation
5. Hydrogen bonding
6. Coupled vibrations and Fermi resonance

1. **Effect of Bond Order:** Bond order affects the position of absorption bands.
   The higher the bond order **larger** is the band frequency.
   The frequency decreases with increasing atomic weight.
   Frequency increases with increasing bond energy.

Table 24.1 Effect of bond energy and atomic masses on stretching frequencies.

Bond		Bond Energy [kcal (kJ)]		Stretching Frequency (cm^{-1})	
		Frequency dependence on atomic masses			
C—H	heavier atoms ↓	100 (420)		3000	$\bar{\nu}$ decreases ↓
C—D		100 (420)		2100	
C—C		83 (350)		1200	
		Frequency dependence on bond energies			
C—C		83 (350)	stronger bond ↓	1200	$\bar{\nu}$ increases ↓
C=C		146 (611)		1660	
C≡C		200 (840)		2200	

2. **Electronic Effects:** The frequency shift of the functional groups occurs due to electronic effects like **inductive effect, mesomeric effect and field effects**. Changes in the force constant or the bond strength are caused by these electronic effects leading to frequency shifts in absorption.

- **The +I effect of the alkyl groups** causes lengthening or weakening of the bond, and the absorption shifts to a **lower wave number**.
  E.g., Absorption wave number of Carbonyl group (C=O)
  (i) Formaldehyde, HCHO — 1750 cm^{-1}
  (ii) Acetaldehyde, CH_3CHO — 1745 cm^{-1}
  (iii) Acetone, CH_3COCH_3 — 1715 cm^{-1}
- Substitution of electronegative atoms or groups with **–1 effect** shifts the absorption frequency to a **higher wave number**.
  (i) Acetone, CH_3COCH_3 — 1715 cm^{-1}
  (ii) Chloro acetone, $ClCH_2COCH_2$ — 1725 cm^{-1}
  (iii) Dichloroacetone, $Cl_2CHCOCH_3$ — 1740 cm^{-1}
- Mesomeric effect also works along with inductive effect.
- The mesomeric effect involves the electrons in the **pie and nonbonding orbitals,** and it operates in general opposite to the inductive effect. These effects cannot be isolated from one another, and only one of them can be applied to determine approximate results.

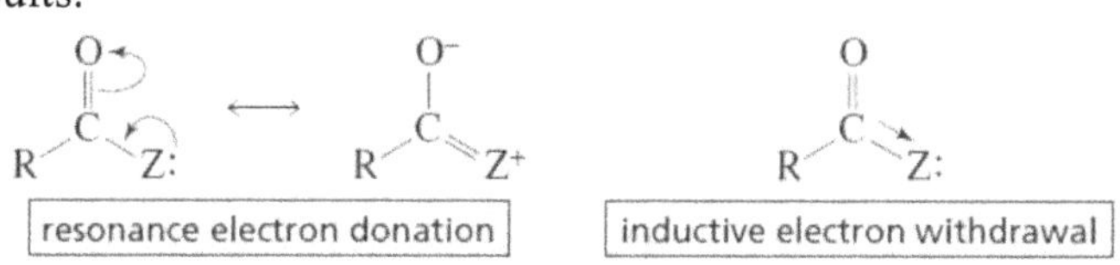

3. Effect of Resonance

- Resonance also plays an essential role in frequency shifting.
- The C-O stretching frequency appears in the range of 1250-1050 cm^{-1}.
- If the C-O bond is in alcohol or ether, the stretching frequency will appear towards the lower end of the range.
- If this C-O bond is a part of a carboxylic group, the stretching frequency will occur at the higher end of the range.
- The position of the absorption varies because the bond in alcohol is a pure single bond, whereas the bond in a carboxylic acid has the partial double bond character that is due to resonance electron donation by the OH group in acids.
- Esters show stretches at both ends of the range because esters have two single bonds, one that is a pure single bond and the other bond has partial double-bond character.

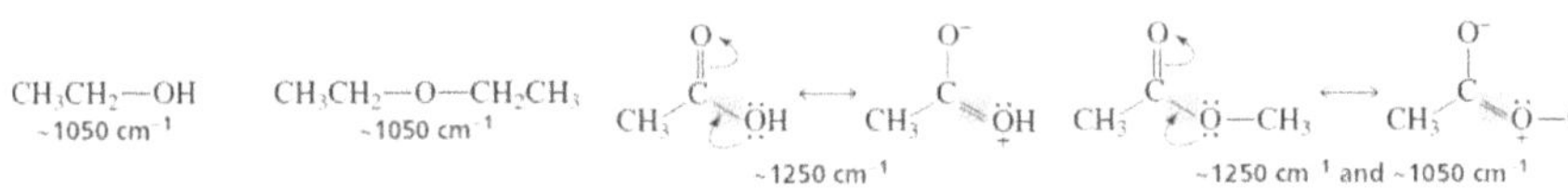

Fig. 24.6 Effect of resonance on Stretching.

4. Degree of conjugation

Conjugation shifts the absorption frequency to lower wave number

The presence of a greater degree of conjugation shifts the carbonyl absorption frequency to a relatively lower range than esters.

E.g., Benzamide and Phenylacetate.

The nitrogen atom is less electronegative than the oxygen atom in amide; It is more labile and participates to a greater extent in conjugation. So, Benzamide absorbs at a lower frequency than an ester.

5. Hydrogen Bonding

The presence of hydrogen bonding changes the position and shape of an infrared absorption band in both stretching as well as bending vibrations

The X-H stretching bands move to a lower frequency, usually increasing intensity and band widening.

The X-H bending vibration usually shifts to higher frequencies.

The stronger the hydrogen bonding, the greater is the absorption shift from the normal values.

The use of infrared spectroscopy can differentiate the two types of hydrogen bonding (intramolecular and intermolecular).

The more concentrated the solution, the more likely it is for the OH-containing molecules to form intermolecular hydrogen bonds.

It is easier to stretch an O-H bond if it is hydrogen-bonded because the hydrogen is attracted to the oxygen of the neighbouring molecule. Therefore, the O-H stretching of a concentrated (hydrogen-bonded) solution of alcohol occurs at about 3550 cm^{-1}, whereas the O-H stretching band of a dilute solution (with little or no hydrogen bonding) appears at 3650 cm^{-1}. (Fig 24.7)

Hydrogen-bonded OH groups also have broader absorption bands, whereas the absorption bands of non-hydrogen–bonded OH groups are sharper.

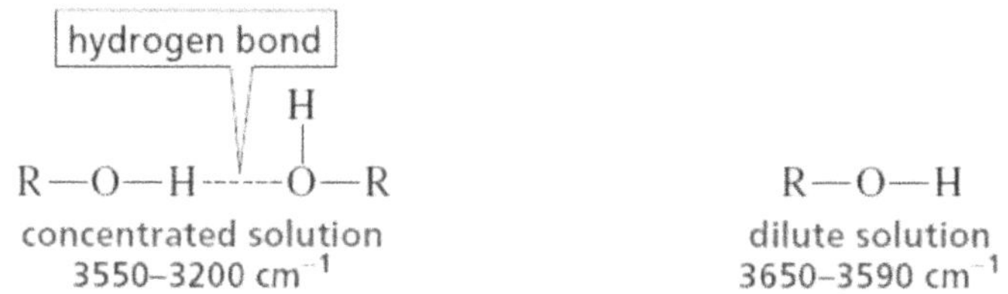
hydrogen bond
concentrated solution
3550–3200 cm⁻¹
dilute solution
3650–3590 cm⁻¹

Fig. 24.7 Effect of hydrogen bonding on Stretching.

6. **Coupled vibrations and Fermi resonance**

   For an isolated C-H bond, there is only one absorption frequency. But two absorptions occur for the CH_2 group corresponding to symmetric and asymmetric stretching vibrations. Asymmetric vibrations occur at a higher wave number when compared to symmetric vibrations. These vibrations are coupled vibrations because they occur at a different frequency than the isolated C-H vibrations. Because of these coupled vibrations, CH_3 also has stretching vibrations in different frequencies. Fermi resonance is a phenomenon that accounts for the shifting of the energies and intensities of absorption bands in infrared spectroscopy. Sometimes, it happens that two different vibrational levels have nearly the same energy. If such vibrations belong to the same species of molecules, then a mutual perturbation of energy may occur, resulting in the shift towards a lower frequency and the other towards a higher frequency. It is also accompanied by a substantial increase in the intensity of the respective bands. Fermi resonance was first discovered in carbon dioxide by Fermi, and it is also found in the vibrational spectra of aldehydes, where the fundamental stretching vibration of the C-H bond in the CHO group interacts with the second harmonic level(overtone) of the deformation vibration of the CHO group (2×1400 cm^{-1}). The result is a Fermi doublet with branches around 2830 cm^{-1} and 2730 cm^{-1}. It is essential for Fermi resonance that the vibrations connected with the two interacting levels be localized in the same part of the molecule.

INSTRUMENTATION

Common optical materials like glass or quartz absorb in the IR region. So, these materials are not used in the construction of an IR Spectrophotometer

The components of the IR spectrophotometer are

1. Radiation sources
2. Monochromators
3. Sample cells
4. Detectors

Table 24.2 Components of IR spectrophotometer.

Radiation source	Monochromators	Sample	Detectors
Nernst Glower	Alkali halides	Solid	Thermocouple
Incandescent lamp	Prisms	Liquid	Bolometer
Mercury arc	Gratings	Gas	Thermistor
Tungsten lamp	Filters		Golay cell
Globar source			Pyroelectric
Nichrome wire			Photoconductor

1. **Radiation sources**

   (a) Incandescent lamps

   1. It is made up of nichrome wire.
   2. They are used in near IR instruments.
   3. Has a low spectral emissivity.
   4. It is heated up to 1100K.
   5. Used to detect complex organic molecules
   6. It fails in far IR because it is enclosed in glass.

   (b) Nernst Glower

   1. It consists of a hollow rod about 2mm in diameter and 30 mm in length.
   2. They are made up of rare earth oxides of Zirconia, Thoria, Yttria etc.
   3. At room temperature, it is a non-conductor, and it is heated by external ways to bring it to conducting state.
   4. Heated up to 1000 to 1800°C
   5. Maximum radiation is provided at 7100 cm^{-1}

   Advantages:

   1. IR radiation emitted over a wide wavelength range
   2. Steady emission of radiation intensity.
   3. Constant over a longer period of time.

Disadvantages:

1. Frequent mechanical failure.
2. Energy emitted in visible and near IR region

(c) **Globar source**

1. It is made up of sintered silicon carbide rod of 50mm in length and 4mm in diameter.
2. On heating up to a temperature between 1300 and 1700°C, it emits radiation in the IR region.
3. Maximum radiation is provided at 5200 cm^{-1}

Advantages:

1. It is self-starting
2. It can be controlled with a variable transformer as it's the temperature coefficient is positive.
3. More satisfactory for wavelengths longer than 650cm^{-1}

Disadvantages:

1. Less intense

(d) **Mercury Arc**

1. These lamps are used in the wave number region, less than 200 cm^{-1}(far IR region).
2. High pressures are used
3. In quartz mercury lamps, the quartz envelope emits radiation at shorter wavelengths, and the longer wavelengths are emitted by mercury plasma.

2. Monochromators

1. They convert polychromatic light into monochromatic light.
2. They must be constructed of materials which transmit the IR.

They are of 3 types.

(a) Metal halide prisms
(b) Sodium Chloride (NaCl) prisms
(c) Gratings

(a) **Metal halide prisms**

1. Prisms that are made up of Potassium bromide (KBr) are used in the wavelength region from 12-25μm.
2. Lithium Fluoride (LiF) prisms are used in the wavelength region from 0.2-6μm.
3. Caesium bromide (CeBr) prisms used in the wavelength region from 15-38μm.
4. Caesium bromide and Thallium Bromoiodide prisms are also used.

(b) Sodium chloride (NaCl) prisms

1. They are used in the whole wavelength region from 4000-650 cm^{-1}.
2. They have to be protected above 20°C because of their hygroscopic nature.

(c) Gratings

1. They offer better resolution at a low frequency than prisms.
2. Diffraction gratings of alkyl halides undergo etching in atmospheric moisture.

3. Sample cells

1. Sample cells made up of alkali halides like NaCl or KBr are used.
2. Aqueous solvents cannot be used as they dissolve alkali halides.
3. Only organic solvents like chloroform are used.
4. IR spectroscopy has been used to characterize solid, liquid, gas samples.

4. Detectors: The various detectors used in IR spectrophotometers are Bolometers, thermocouple, Thermistors, Golay cell and pyroelectric detectors

Bolometer

1. The principle of operation is that the electrical resistance of a metal increases with an increase in temperature.
2. It consists of a thin metal wire
3. When radiation falls on this conductor, its temperature changes.
4. The change in resistance measures the radiation falling on the bolometer.
5. Bolometer is used as one arm of Wheatstone bridge with a similar metal strip in balancing arm.
6. The bridge remains balanced till no radiation falls on the bolometer
7. When IR radiation falls on the bolometer, the bridge is unbalanced, with a change in resistance leading to current flow indicated by the galvanometer.
8. The intensity of radiation falling on the detector is measured by the current flowing through the galvanometer.
9. The bolometer response time is 4 msec

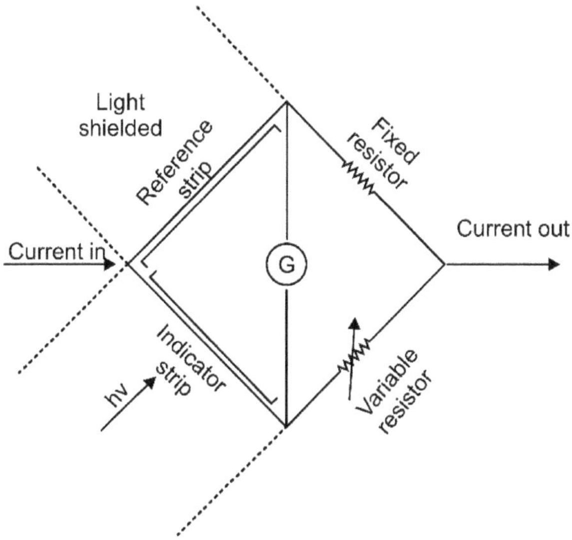

Fig. 24.8 Schematic diagram of the bolometer-Wheatstone bridge.

Thermocouple

1. Two dissimilar metal wires are joined head to tail.
2. One end is exposed to IR radiation (hot junction), and the other junction is insulated(cold junction)
3. The hot junction which is exposed to IR radiation increases in temperature, and the cold junction is maintained at a constant temperature
4. The temperature difference between the two junctions creates a potential difference that is directly proportional to the radiation falling on the hot junction
5. The response time is about 60msec

This detector is based on the principle that the difference in temperature between the junctions is directly proportional to the current flowing through the system, which in turn depends on the intensity of radiation.

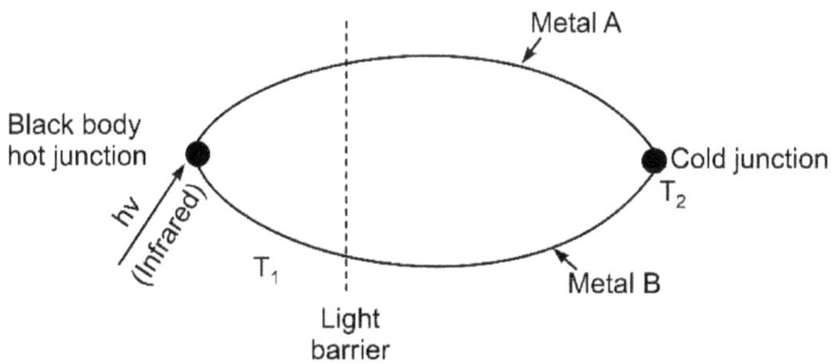

Fig. 24.9 Schematic diagram of a thermocouple.

Thermistors

1. These detectors are made up of sintered oxides of Mn, Co and Ni.
2. The principle here is as the temperature of the mixture increases, the resistance decreases
3. Response time is 4 seconds.

Golay cell

1. Used in commercial spectrophotometers
2. It consists of a metal cylinder with a blackened metal plate at one end and a flexible metallised diaphragm at the other end.
3. The cylinder is filled with Xenon gas.
4. IR radiation falling on the metal plate heats up the gas and expands it. The resulting pressure increase deforms the diaphragm.
5. When light falls on the diaphragm from the source, it reflects the light to a photocell.
6. The motion of the diaphragm results in changes in the output of the cell, which is recorded as a signal.
7. Response time 0.01 sec

Advantages:

1. Wide wavelength range
2. Linear response

Disadvantages:

1. Bulky
2. Expensive

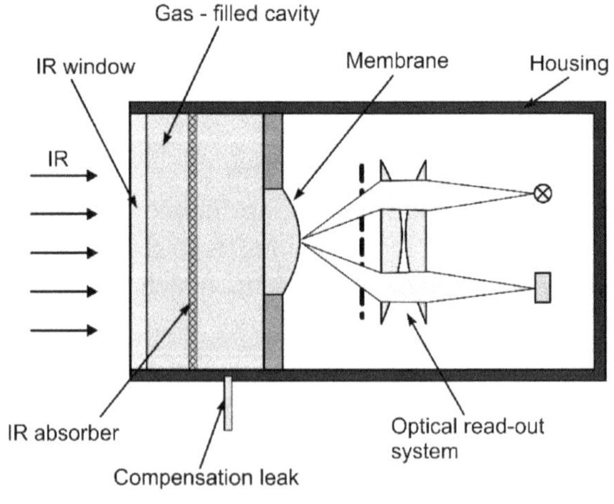

Fig. 24.10 Golay cell.

Photoconductivity cell

1. It is a non-thermal detector.
2. It comprises a thin layer of lead sulphide or lead telluride deposited on glass sealed in an evacuated glass envelope.

3. The conductance of semiconductors increases when IR radiation falls on it, leading to the flow of currents.
4. Its response time – 0.5 msec

Advantages:

1. Greater sensitivity
2. Faster response.

Disadvantages

1. Range limited to near IR radiation at room temperature.

Pyroelectric Detectors

A dielectric material, when placed in an electrostatic field, is polarized and this polarization depends on the dielectric constant of the material. If the polarization persists even after the removal of the electric field, then the material is said to be pyroelectric. This residual polarization is temperature-dependent.

1. These detectors are made by sandwiching the pyroelectric material between two electrodes to give a temperature-dependent capacitor.
2. The incident IR radiation causes temperature changes leading to a change in capacitance of the material, which can be measured.
3. Commonly used pyroelectric material is Triglycerine Sulphate (TGS)
4. Deuterated TGS can be used at room temperature, and it is used in FTIR.

Advantages:

1. Fast response
2. Multiple scanning
3. Used in FTIR

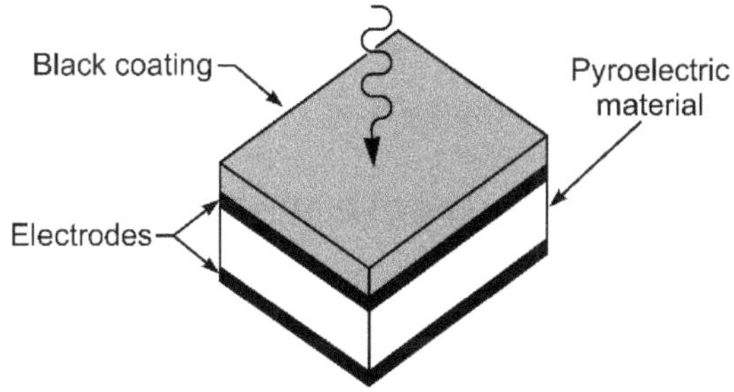

Fig. 24.11 Pyroelectric detectors.

Semiconductor detectors: Semiconductors are insulators, and they become conductors when exposed to radiation, which causes a change in electrical resistance.

Materials like telluride, indium antimonide and copper or mercury doped with germanium are used as semiconductor detectors.

5. **Recorder:** A recorder is used for recording the spectrum.

TYPES OF INSTRUMENTS

SINGLE BEAM IR SPECTROPHOTOMETER

In a single beam instrument, the radiation source passes through the sample and then through the fixed prism and Littrow mirror to select the desired wavelength. Finally, the radiation falls on the detector.

Thus, in IR instrumentation, the intensity of radiation is measured after it passes through the sample and monochromator.

Sample cells are present before monochromators to diminish stray/scattered light problems.

Disadvantages:

1. The intensity of emitted radiations is not uniform.
2. Solvent bands appear in the spectrum.

DOUBLE BEAM SPECTROPHOTOMETER

The light energy is split into a reference beam and sample beam. They pass through the respective cells and reach the detector through the monochromator. When there is no sample in the sample cell, there is no absorption, and a steady signal reaches the detector. When there is absorption, there is a decrease in the intensity of light reaching the detector producing a signal.

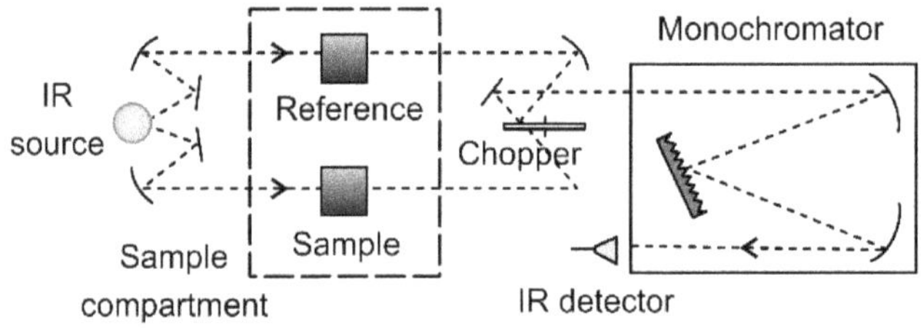

Fig. 24.12 Schematic diagram of Dispersive IR spectrophotometer.

FOURIER TRANSFORM IR SPECTROPHOTOMETER

This instrument depends upon the interferences of various frequencies of radiation to produce a spectrum.

FTIR spectrophotometer consists of an interferometer which consists of four optical arms at right angles to each other. It consists of a beam splitter at the centre. Radiation from the source passes through the first arm, split by the beam splitter into two perpendicular beams of equal intensity. These split beams enter into the other two arms of an interferometer. In these arms, one arm has a fixed mirror, and the other arm has a movable mirror. The motion of the moving mirror makes the total path length variable from the pathlength taken by the fixed mirror beam. These two beams meet again at the beam splitter, they recombine, and their difference in path length causes constructive and destructive interference to give the interferogram.

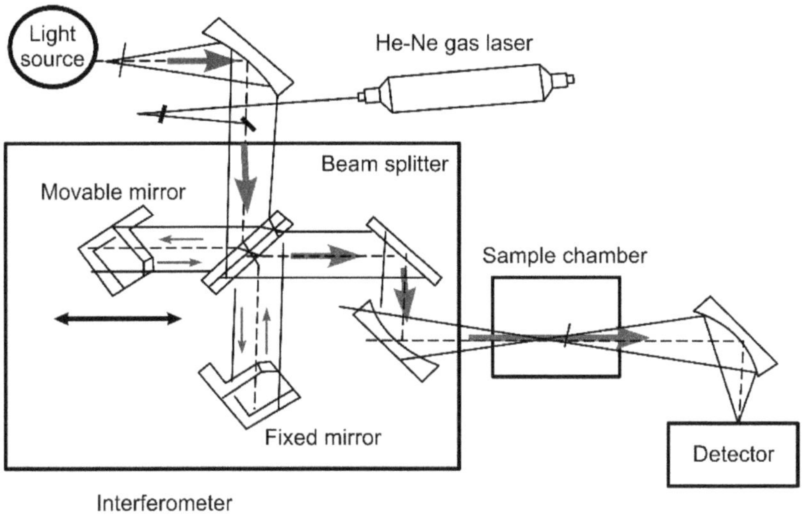

Fig. 24.13 Schematic diagram of FTIR spectrophotometer.

The recombined beam passes through the sample. The sample absorbs its characteristic wavelengths, and the detector detects the variation in the intensity of the transmitted light. The spectrum is recorded as intensity versus time for all wavelengths simultaneously.

A mathematical function called Fourier Transform is used to convert the intensity versus time spectrum into intensity versus frequency spectrum.

In practice, it is difficult to control the speed of the moving mirror and hence it is controlled by a laser beam. The laser beam serves as a reference for the operation of the instrument.

Table 24.3 Difference between FT IR and dispersive IR.

DISPERSIVE IR	FTIR
1. Many moving parts lead to wear and tear.	Only one mirror moves during the experiment.
2. Calibration against reference spectra is required to measure frequency.	The laser provides high-frequency accuracy.
3. Stray light causes errors in the readings.	Stray light does not affect the detector.
4. To improve resolution, only a small amount of IR radiation is allowed to pass through the slits	A larger beam is used. (internal calibration). Data collection is clear.
5. Only radiation of narrow frequency falls on the detector at a given time.	All frequencies of radiation fall on the detector simultaneously.
6. The scan speed is slow.	Rapid scan
7. Sample shows the thermal effect	No thermal effect.
8. Lesser accuracy.	More accuracy
9. Sensitivity is less.	Sensitivity is more.

SAMPLE HANDLING TECHNIQUES IN IR

There are no good solvents that are transparent throughout the IR region. Because of this, sample handling or preparation becomes a tedious and time-consuming part of IR analysis. Sample handling of different types of samples are given below

Sampling of solids

Four techniques are employed for preparing solid samples.

1. Solids run in solution
2. Solid films
3. Mull technique
4. Pressed Pellet technique
5. ATR crystal technique. (evanescent wave)

1. **Solids run in solutions:** If the sample can be dissolved in a suitable solvent, then the cells for liquids can be used. The drawback of this method is the limited number of solvents that do not absorb in the IR region. Examples of solvents: chloroform, carbon tetrachloride, acetone and cyclohexane.

   Disadvantages:

   1. There is no solvent available which do not absorb throughout the IR region.
   2. Interaction of solvent with the solute should be monitored (H-bonding compounds).
   3. The solvent should not absorb in the working IR range.

2. **Solid film:** The sample is dissolved in a non-aqueous solvent, non-reacting, IR transparent in the working IR range. A drop of this solution is placed on an alkali metal plate (e.g., NaCl/ KCl plate), and the solvent is evaporated to dryness, leaving a thin sample film. This technique is suitable for polymer resin and amorphous solids. For non-crystalline solids, a thin homogenous film is deposited on the plate, which can be directly mounted and scanned directly.

   Advantages: This technique is useful for qualitative analysis.

   Disadvantages: Not suitable for quantitative analysis.

3. **Mull technique:** A small quantity of sample (2-4mg) is thoroughly ground in a clean mortar until the powder is very fine. The mulling agent (mineral oil or Nujol) is introduced in small quantities, just sufficient to make a mixture approximating the consistency of toothpaste.

   Then the mixture is transferred to the mull plates & the plates are squeezed together to get the desired thickness of the sample between IR transmitting windows which is mounted in the path of the IR beam, and the spectrum is obtained.

Disadvantages

1. Although Nujol is transparent throughout the IR region, yet it has an absorption maxima at 2915, 1462, 1376 & 719 cm^{-1}.
2. So, when the IR spectrum of a solid sample is taken in Nujol mull, absorption bands of a solid sample that happen to coincide with the absorption bands of the Nujol mull will be hidden (but others will be clearly seen in the IR spectrum)
3. This method is good for qualitative analysis but not for quantitative analysis.
4. If hydrocarbon bands interfere, Fluorolube, a halogenated polymer, can be used.

4. **Pressed pellet technique:** In this technique, a small amount of finely ground solid sample is intimately mixed with about 100 times the weight of powdered Potassium bromide in a vibrating ball mill. This finely ground mixture is then pressed under very high pressure (25000 p sig) in an evacuable die or Minipress to form a small pellet (about 1-2 mm thick and 1cm in diameter). (10,000 -15,000 pounds). The resulting pellet is transparent to IR radiation and is used as such to record the spectrum.

   The powder (KBr + sample) is introduced in between the two bolts, and the upper screw A is tightened until the powder is compressed to a thin disc. After compressing the sample bolts, A & A′ are removed, and a steel cylinder with a pellet inside it is placed in the path of the beam of IR spectrometer, and a blank KBr pellet of identical thickness is kept in the path of the reference beam.

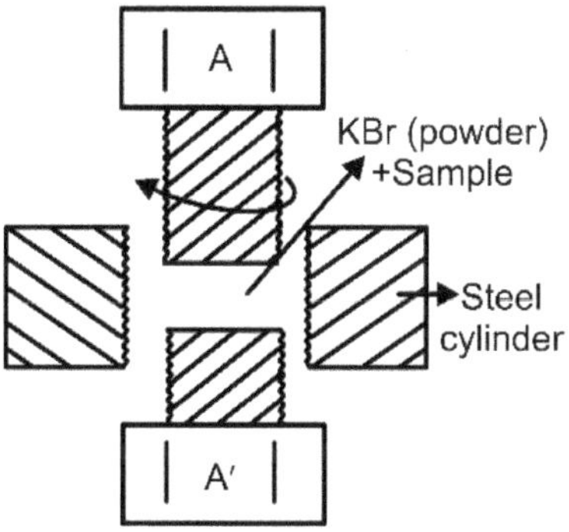

Fig. 24.14 Device used for potassium bromide discs.

Advantages of this technique over mull technique

1. The bands due to mulling agent in mull technique are not present in the KBR pellet technique
2. KBr pellets can be stored for longer periods of time.

3. It can be used for quantitative analysis, as the concentration of the sample can be adjusted in pellets
4. The spectrum resolution in KBr is superior to that obtained with mulls.

Disadvantages

1. The –OH group of moisture present in the sample gives a band at 3450 cm^{-1}.
2. The high pressure used in pellet formation may bring about polymorphic changes in crystallinity in the samples (Especially inorganic complexes), which may cause complications in the IR spectrum. Even substitution of the ligand by bromide may be possible in inorganic complexes.
3. This method is not applicable for some polymers which are difficult to grind with KBr.

5. **ATR (Attenuated Total Reflection) crystal technique:** Without further preparation, samples can be analysed directly in a solid or liquid state. The sample is in contact with the surface of an ATR crystal, which is made up of a material with a higher refractive index. E.g., silver chloride, zinc selenide, zinc sulphide, germanium silicon and diamond. Liquid samples are simply poured over the crystal, and solid samples are clamped onto it. When IR radiation passes through the sample, an evanescent wave is formed, and this absorption is detected by the detector.

Sampling of liquids: Liquid samples are taken in sample cells made up of NaCl, KBr or ThBr and the IR spectra is measured directly.

A thin layer of the sample with a thickness of about 0.01 - 0.05 mm is used.

For double beam instruments, are matched cells with the same thickness used for reference and sample.

The cells should be protected from moisture.

Sampling of gases: In the gas sample cell, the light path is made of KBr or NaCl.

They are larger cells with longer pathlength about 10cm to 1m long to compensate for the small number of molecules in the sample gas. Multiple reflection pathlengths are used to make the pathlengths as long as 40 cm as shown in figure 24.15.

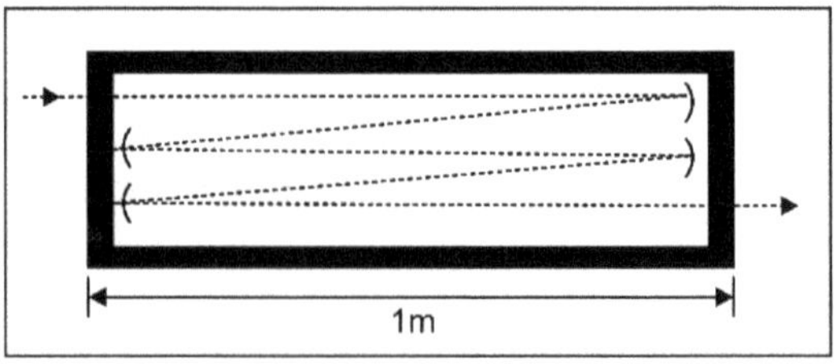

Fig. 24.15 Gas absorption cell.

The gas sample cell is a cylinder of glass or metal. Both ends of the cylinder are closed with IR transparent materials like NaCl/KBr.

They are equipped with valves or stopcocks for the introduction of a sample.

SOLVENTS

1. No single solvent is transparent throughout the mid-IR region.
2. Water and alcohol are rarely employed because they absorb strongly and attack the sample cells, which are made up of alkali metal halides.

Table 24.4 IR Absorption of Some Common Functional Groups.

Functional Groups	Range (cm^{-1})
C-H stretching (alkane) C-H bending	2960-2850 1340
C-H stretching (alkene)	3040-3010
C-H stretching (aromatic) C-H bending	3030 700-850
C=C stretching (alkene)	1680-1620
C≡C stretching (alkyne)	2100-2200
C=C stretching (aromatic)	1450-1600
C=O stretching (ketone)	1705-1725
C=O stretching (aldehyde)	1720-1740
C=O stretching (ester)	1735-1750
C=O stretching (acid)	1700-1725
C=O stretching (amide)	1650-1700
O-H stretching (Free)	3590-3650
O-H bending(alcohols) C-O stretching	1050-1150 1250-1350
O-H bending(Phenols) C-O stretching	1200 1310-1410
N-H stretching N-H bending	3400-3500 1500-1650
C-N vibrations	1000-1400
C≡N stretching	2240-2260
C=N stretching	1630-1690

APPLICATIONS

1. **Identification of functional group and structural elucidation:** The peaks corresponding to every functional group in the sample appears in the group frequency region – 4000-1500 cm^{-1} which is useful in structural elucidation. The fingerprint region is useful in identifying the sample, including the isomer.
2. **Qualitative estimation:** The structure of the sample can be confirmed if the IR spectrum of the sample and standard are identical (spectral matching).
3. **Identification of impurities in a drug sample:** Impurities give extra peaks in the spectrum when compared with the spectrum of the pure drug thus presence of impurities can be confirmed.
4. **To study the progress of reaction:** The disappearance of a characteristic absorption frequency of a reactant shows the progress of the reaction. Spectra of samples taken at different time intervals can be used in studying the progress of the reaction.
5. To identify and find the ratio of geometrical isomers (cis, trans) in a mixture
6. Identification of tautomers.
7. To find the shape of symmetry of a molecule.
8. The presence of water in a sample can be identified using the IR spectrum, which shows characteristic absorption of water in 3 regions 3600-3200 cm^{-1}, 1650cm^{-1}, 600-300 cm^{-1}.
9. **Quantitative analysis:** The quantitative estimation of the substance can be determined in pure form or as a mixture of two or more components.

Two methods are used: 1. Cell in cell-out method. 2. Baseline method.

In the cell-in-cell-out method, the unknown concentration of sample is determined using calibration curve of the standard or using beers law by comparing log I_0/I_t (absorbance) of the standard and sample.

In the baseline method, tangents are drawn, I_0 and I_t are measured, absorbance is plotted against concentration, and unknown concentration is determined.

CHAPTER 25

Fluorimetry

INTRODUCTION

A large number of substances absorb ultraviolet or visible radiation. Some of these substances lose a part of their excess energy as electromagnetic radiation in a longer wavelength than the absorbed wavelength. This process of emitting radiation is known as **luminescence**. In luminescence, the light is produced at low temperatures. The types of luminescence are

(a) Photoluminescence
(b) Chemiluminescence
(c) Bio luminescence
(d) Electroluminescence
(e) Radio luminescence
(f) Thermo luminescence.

Photoluminescence is caused by moving electrons to energetically higher levels through the absorption of photons. It is further subdivided into

(i) Fluorescence - When a beam of light is incident on certain substances, they **emit visible light or radiations**. This phenomenon is known as **fluorescence** and the substances showing this phenomenon are called **Fluorescent substances**.

Fluorescence is **instantaneous** and starts immediately after the absorption of light and stops as soon as the incident light is cut off.

Materials exhibiting fluorescence emit radiation within $\mathbf{10^{-6}}$ **to** $\mathbf{10^{-4}}$ seconds of absorption.

(ii) Phosphorescence - When light radiation is incident on certain substances, they emit radiation continuously **even after the incident light is cut off.** This type of **delayed fluorescence** is called phosphorescence. Substances showing this phenomenon are called **phosphorescent substances**.

Materials exhibiting phosphorescence emit radiation within $\mathbf{10^{-4}}$ **to 20** seconds or more.

The lifetime of phosphorescence is much longer than fluorescence.

Most of the molecules in their ground state do not have unpaired electrons (singlet state). When such a molecule absorbs UV or Visible radiation, the electrons (π electrons) get raised to an excited singlet state where there is no change in the spin of the electrons. If one set of electron spins undergo unpairing (change in spin), the resulting electrons will make an excited Triplet state.

From the excited singlet state, the molecule will return to the ground state by any one of the following possibilities.

1. Returning to the ground state by **collisional deactivation** without emitting any radiation.
2. The molecule in the excited singlet state may **emit UV or Visible light** photons. This is known as **fluorescence.**
3. The molecule in the excited singlet state may undergo transition to **metastable triplet state (intersystem crossing)** and then return to the ground state by **emitting UV or Visible light** photons. This is known as **phosphorescence.**

Principle

International Union of Pure and Applied Chemistry (IUPAC) define fluorescence as spontaneous emission of radiation (luminescence) from an excited molecular entity with the formation of a molecular entity of the same spin multiplicity.

When a beam of light is incident upon certain substances, they emit visible light or UV radiation. This phenomenon is called **fluorescence** and the substances exhibiting this property are called Fluorescent substances. It is instantaneous. It starts as soon as the substance absorbs the light and stops immediately after the incident radiation is cut off.

Absorption of UV or visible radiation causes the transition of electrons in the molecules from the singlet ground state to the excited singlet state. As the excited state is not stable, the electrons return to the ground state by losing energy in the form of UV/visible radiation. Thus the principle of fluorimetry is the study or measurement of the emitted radiation when the electrons return from the **excited singlet state to ground singlet state** after absorbing light.

Electronic states

The different electronic states are

1. Singlet ground state
2. Doublet state
3. Triplet state
4. Singlet excited state.

These terms tell us the **number of unpaired electrons in the absence of a magnetic field**. There will be n+1 number of degeneracy states (equal energy) associated with the electron spin if there are n number of unpaired electrons. For no unpaired electrons (n=0), there is only one spin state. (n+1 =1).This state is called as singlet state. Thus,

Singlet ground state is a state where there are no unpaired electrons in a molecule. i.e. all electrons are paired. ↑↓

In **Doublet state** one unpaired electron is present (n + 1 = 1 + 1 = 2) ↑ or ↓

In the **Triplet state,** two unpaired electrons are present. Both electrons have the same spin

↑↑

In the **singlet excited state** also there are **no unpaired electrons**. Though the electrons are in an excited state still they are paired **(No change in spin)**

Excitation states

Pauli's Exclusion Principle states that no two electron in an atom can have the same set of 4 quantum numbers, i.e. principal, azimuthal, magnetic and spin quantum number. This restriction requires that no more than 2 electrons can occupy an orbital and further that the two must-have opposite spin states. Under these circumstances, the spin is said to be paired. Because of spin pairing, most molecules exhibit no net magnetic field and are thus said to be diamagnetic, i.e. they are neither attracted nor repelled by the static magnetic field.

Singlet excited state. A molecular electronic state in which all electron spin are paired even in the excited state is called a singlet excited state. No splitting of electronic levels occurs when the molecules are exposed to a magnetic field. Electrons are unpaired, but the **net spin is zero**.

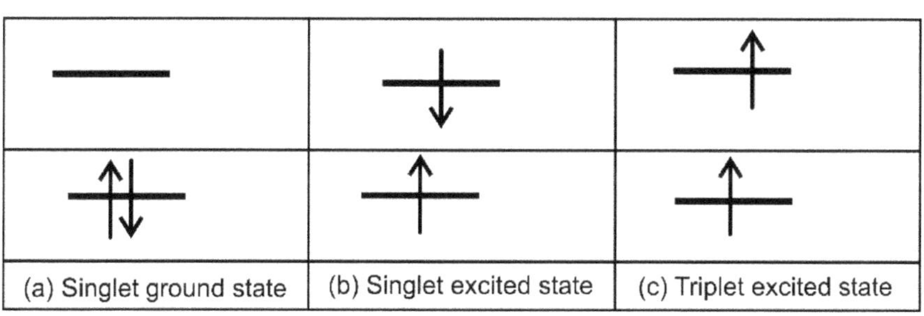

Fig. 25.1 Different electronic states of a molecule after the absorption of light.

A Triplet state is a state when one of the paired electrons of the molecule is excited to a higher energy level, it forms an excited singlet state, and when the spin of the excited electron changes and becomes unpaired, the state is termed as triplet state. The property of molecule differs in triplet state than in the singlet-excited state, for example, paramagnetic and diamagnetic. Singlet excited to triplet transition, which involves a change in the spin of electron, is significantly less probable event than singlet ground to singlet excited state transition.

Singlet excited state is the state where one of the paired electrons absorbs light and goes to the excited state resulting in unpairing, but there is no change in the spin of the electron.

Fluorescence process can be broken down into three phases

1. **Excitation** – Excitation is the absorption of light of an appropriate wavelength by a fluorophore and the transition of an electron from ground level to an excited level. Chromophores which exhibit the phenomenon of fluorescence are called fluors or fluorophores. Fluorophores are organic molecules of 20-100 Daltons.
2. **Excited-state** – After the absorption of a photon of appropriate energy, fluorophore undergoes vibrational and conformational changes
3. **Emission** – Release of excess energy in the form of a photon of light is emission phase. The fluorescence process is cyclical; therefore, a fluorophore can be excited repeatedly. Absorption of UV or visible radiation causes transition of electrons in the molecules from the singlet ground state to the excited singlet state. As the excited state is not stable, the electrons return to the ground state by losing energy

   Loss of energy can occur by these ways:

   1. Vibrational relaxation/ Collisional deactivation
   2. Internal conversion (Radiationless transititions)
   3. External conversion
   4. Intersystem crossing
   5. Fluorescence
   6. Phosphorescence

   1. **Vibrational relaxation/Collisional deactivation:** Vibrational energy is the energy used to lengthen or shorten bonds or widen or squeeze bond angles. An electron in a molecule may be promoted to any of the several vibrational levels during the electronic excitation process. In solution, the excess of vibrational energy is immediately lost as a consequence of the collision between the molecule of the excited species and those of solvent. The result is an energy transfer and a minuscule increase in the temperature of the solvent. This relaxation process is so efficient that the average

lifetime of a vibrationally excited molecule is 10-12 sec or less (a period significantly shorter than the average lifetime of an electronically excited state. As a result, fluorescence from solution when it occurs involves a transition from the lowest vibrational level of an excited state). This also results in the displacement of fluorescence band towards a longer wavelength than the absorbed one; this is called **Stokes shift.**

Vibration relaxation of an excited electron from the highest vibrational level in singlet excited state to lowest vibrational level results in stokes shift which is shown in figure.

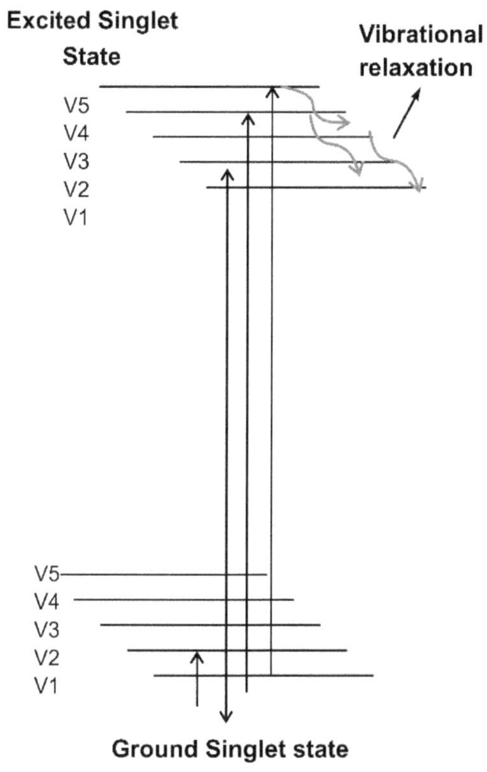

Fig. 25.2 Vibrational relaxation.

2. **Internal conversion (Radiationless Transitions):** Electrons tend to avoid giving off a giant photon if they can get to a lower energy state by giving off small packets of energy at a time, by simple hopping down to lower and lower vibrational levels. They may relax all the way down to the ground state via vibrational relaxation if any of the excited state's lower vibrational levels have energy that overlaps with some of the higher vibrational levels of the ground state.

Internal conversion is a process by which a molecule passes to a lower electronic state without the emission of radiation. Internal conversions are efficient when two electronic energy levels are significantly close for the existence of overlap in vibrational energy level, i.e. the potential energies of the two excited states are identical. This equality permits efficient transition through overlapping, which is usually more probable than the loss of energy by fluorescence from a higher excited state.

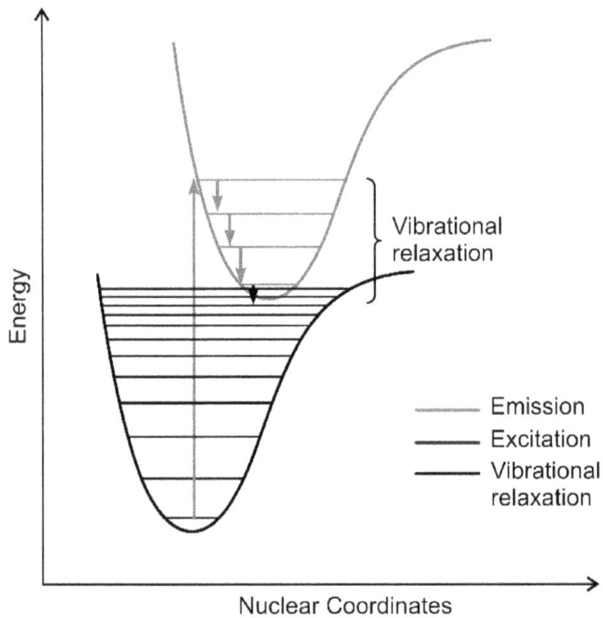

Fig. 25.3 Internal conversion.

3. **External conversion:** External conversion involves interaction and energy transfer between the excited molecule and the solvent or other solute. This markedly affects the fluorescence intensity. Conditions which tend to reduce the number of collisions between particles (low temperature, high viscosity) generally lead to enhanced fluorescence. Radiationless transition to ground state from the lowest excited singlet state and triplet state probably involve external conversion as well as internal conversion.
4. **Intersystem crossing:** An organic molecule with no unpaired electrons in its ground state is said to be in a singlet state. According to one of the selection rules for electronic excitation, the excited state must also have no unpaired electrons. In other words, the spin of the electron that gets excited is the same after excitation as it was before excitation.

The intersystem crossing is a process in which there is a change in multiplicity of the molecule, and the spin of an excited electron is reversed from + 1/2 to -1/2 or vice versa. This results in an electronic state of lower energy (single electrons in different orbitals prefer to have parallel spin) with a multiplicity (possible orientations of the spin) M= 3, which is thus designated as a triplet state, T1. (multiplicity is $2S+1 = 3$, so that the total spin $S = 1$. This spin is due to two unpaired electrons based on Hund's rule, favouring degenerate orbitals' single filling. The triplet consists of three states with spin components +1, 0 and –1). This is enhanced if the vibrational level of the two states overlaps. The intersystem crossing is most common in the molecule that contains heavy atoms, i.e., iodine, bromine and is also known as the heavy atom effect. The interaction between the spin and orbital motion becomes large in the presence of such an atom. The presence of paramagnetic species such as molecular oxygen in solution also enhances intersystem crossing and as a result, decreases fluorescence.

5. **Fluorescence**: The molecule in the excited state emits UV or visible radiation of a longer wavelength to lose energy. **The emission of radiation occurs at a longer wavelength** because the energy of emitted radiation is lesser than the energy of absorbed radiation. This happens because some amount of the absorbed energy is lost by vibrational or collisional deactivation.

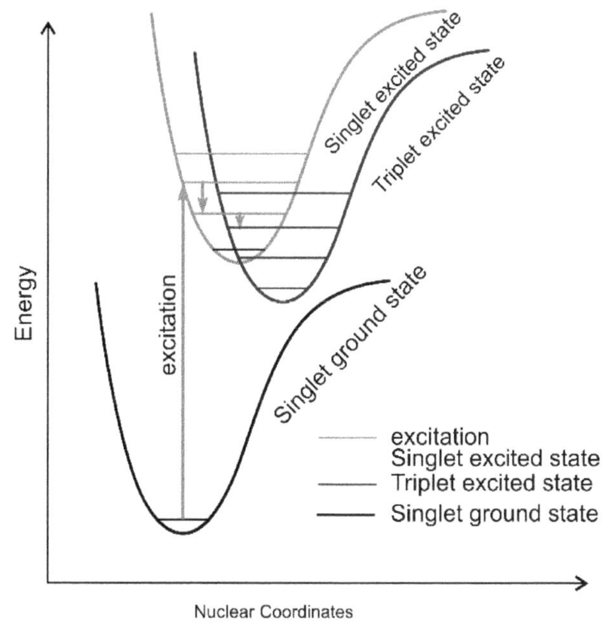

Fig. 25.4 Intersystem crossing.

Thus, fluorescence is the phenomenon of emission of radiation from singlet excited state to singlet ground state. The absorption wavelength is called excitation wavelength, and that of the emitted radiation is called emission wavelength. These two wavelengths are characteristic for a given substance under given conditions.

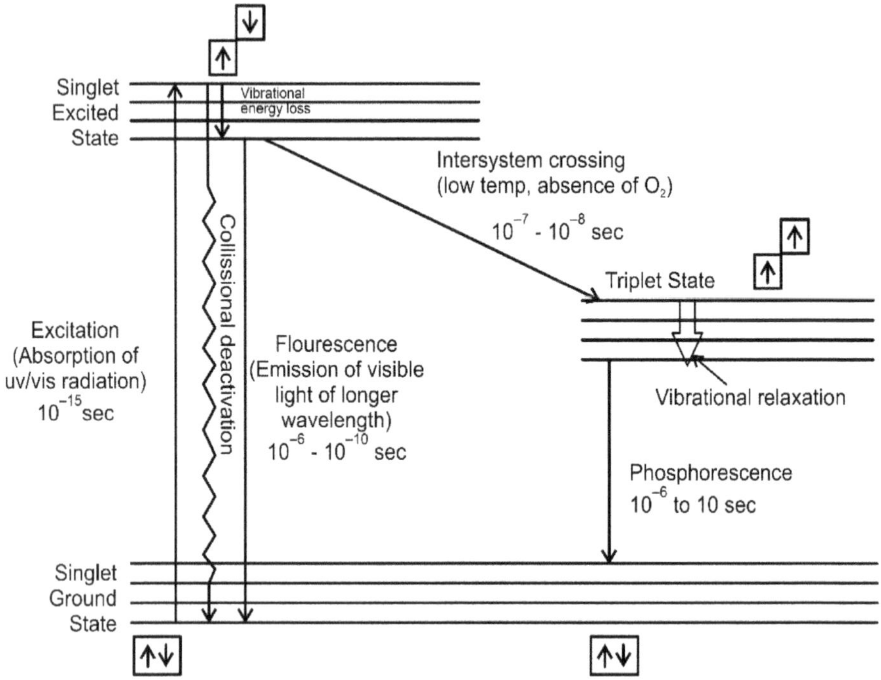

Fig. 25.5 Jablonski diagram.

6. **Phosphorescence:** The molecule in the unstable excited singlet state may undergo transition to a metastable triplet state and from there returns to the ground state by emitting UV/Visible radiation. This is called phosphorescence. **The process of transition from excited singlet state to excited triplet state is called intersystem crossing**. It occurs at favourable conditions like **low temperature** and the **absence of oxygen**. The energy of the excited triplet state is lower than the excited singlet state, and the emission occurs at a longer wavelength. The lifetime of phosphorescence is longer, and it continues even after the incident radiation is cut off. It is also called **delayed fluorescence**.

FACTORS AFFECTING FLUORESCENCE

The factors affecting fluorescence can be classified as two types

1. Structural factors
2. Non-structural factors

1. Structural factors

- (i) Nature of molecules
- (ii) Nature of substituent groups
- (iii) Rigidity of structures
- (iv) Effect of pH

2. Non -structural factors

- (i) Effect of concentration
- (ii) Adsorption
- (iii) Light
- (iv) Effect of Temperature and viscosity
- (v) Effect of oxygen
- (vi) Photo-decomposition

(i) Nature of molecules: All molecules which absorb radiation cannot show the phenomenon of fluorescence and phosphorescence. The molecules must possess conjugated double bonds (π electrons) so that the UV/visible radiation can be absorbed and fluorescence can be observed.

(ii) Nature of substituent groups: Electron donating groups like amino (NH_2) and hydroxyl (OH) groups enhance fluorescence intensity. Groups like SO_3H,NH_4^+ and alkyl groups do not have much effect on fluorescence and phosphorescence.

Electron withdrawing groups like -COOH,-NO_2,-N=N- and halides reduce or sometimes even destroy the fluorescence intensity.

If an atom with a high atomic number is introduced in the π electron system, this enhances phosphorescence and decreases the Fluorescence intensity.

(iii) Effect of concentration: Fluorescence **is proportional to concentration,** but this relationship holds only when the **concentration of the substance is low** (μg or ng/ml). **Higher concentration** leads to a **decrease** in fluorescence intensity

(iv) Adsorption: Only dilute solutions should be used in fluorimetry. Concentrated solutions lead to the adsorption of fluorescent substances on the container walls of sample cell leading to decreased fluorescence. E.g., Quinine.

Table 25.1 Effect of substituent on fluorescence intensity.

Substituent	Effect on λ	Effect on intensity
Alkyl	Not affected	Not much effect
COOH,CHO,COOR,COR	Shifts to Longer	Decrease in intensity
OH, OMe, OEt	Shifts to Longer	Increase in intensity
CN	Not affected	Increase in intensity
NH_2,NHR,NR_2	Shifts to Longer	Increase in intensity
NO_2,NO	Shifts to Longer	Quenching
SH	Shifts to Longer	Decrease in intensity
SO_3H	Not affected	Not affected
F, Cl, Br, I	Shifts to Longer	Decrease in intensity

(v) **Light:** Monochromatic light is essential for quantitative fluorescent analysis because the intensity varies with wavelength.

(vi) **Rigidity of structures:** Rigid structures give **more** fluorescence intensity, and the **flexible structures** provide **less intensity.**

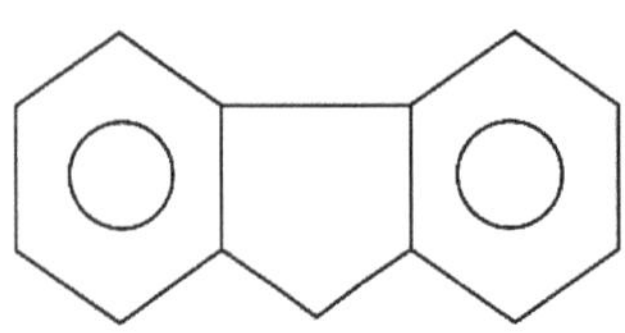

Fig. 25.6 Rigid structure Fluorene.

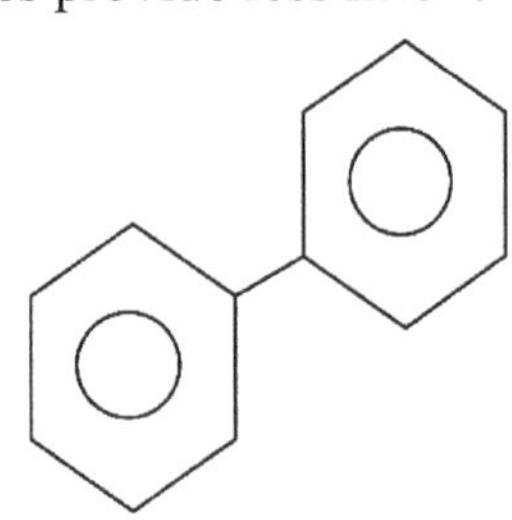

Fig. 25.7 Flexible structure Biphenyl.

(vii) **Effect of Temperature and viscosity:** An increase in temperature leads to a decrease in viscosity which results in decreased fluorescence. This is because the excited molecules get deactivated by collision. A decrease in temperature gives increased fluorescence due to decreased collisions (increase in solvent viscosity).

(viii) **Effect of Oxygen:** The presence of oxygen decreases the fluorescence intensity. It can happen in two ways

1. It can oxidize the fluorescent substance to a non-fluorescent substance.
2. Because of its paramagnetic properties (triplet ground state), oxygen quenches fluorescence.

(ix) **Effect of pH:** A change in pH will change the ionic state of the molecule. Thus, the pH effect is dependent on the chemical nature of the molecule.

E.g.,

1. Aniline in an acid medium (ionized) gives fluorescence in the UV region, whereas in a neutral and alkaline medium (unionized) gives visible fluorescence.
2. Phenols are undissociated in acid medium and don't exhibit fluorescence, but in the alkaline condition, they are in an ionic state giving fluorescence.

(x) **Photodecomposition:** The magnitude of photodecomposition depends upon the intensity of the light source. Spectrofluorimetry requires a high intensity of radiation to enhance the sensitivity of the instrument, thus leading to photochemical decomposition. Hence the wavelength which is not strongly absorbed should be chosen to eliminate such decompositions. If not error of upto 20% is possible in the measurements.

TYPES OF FLUORESCENCE

Fluorescence and phosphorescence come under the classification of photoluminescence.

Based on the emitted radiation wavelength, fluorescence can be classified as

(a) **Stokes fluorescence:** In this type of fluorescence, the wavelength of the emitted radiation occurs at a longer wavelength. This is the conventional fluorimetric experiment.

(b) **Anti-stoke's fluorescence:** The wavelength of emitted radiation is shorter than the absorbed radiation. This type of fluorescence occurs in thermally assisted fluorescence.

(c) **Resonance fluorescence:** This is the fluorescence in which both the emitted radiation and the absorbed radiation are equal. E.g., Mercury vapour at 254 nm.

QUENCHING AND ITS TYPES

QUENCHING

Quenching is any process that reduces the fluorescence intensity of a given substance.

This may occur due to various factors like pH, concentration, temperature, viscosity, presence of oxygen, heavy metals, specific chemical substances, etc. Example of **quenching agents: Thiocyanate, Chloride, Iodide, Disulfide, Nitric oxide.**

TYPES OF QUENCHING

1. Collisional Quenching
2. Static Quenching
3. Chemical Quenching
4. Concentration Quenching/Self-Quenching

1. **Collisional Quenching:** Collisional quenching occurs by the increased collision of quencher molecules with excited molecules of the fluorescing substance. Halides ions such as chlorides or iodides, increased temperature and decreased viscosity are well-known collisional quenchers. For example, quenching of quinine drug by chloride ion or tryptophan by iodide ion follow the collisional quenching process.
2. **Static Quenching:** A complex formation occurs between the fluorescing molecule at the ground state and the quencher molecule through a strong coupling. Such complex may not undergo excitation or may be excited to a little extent reducing the fluorescence intensity of the molecule. Caffeine and related xanthenes and purines reduce the intensity of riboflavin by static mechanism. Quenching that occurs due to oxygen also follows this mechanism.
3. **Chemical Quenching:** Chemical quenching is due to various factors like - change in pH, presence of oxygen, halides, electron-withdrawing groups and heavy metals, etc.
   (a) **Change in pH:** Aniline at pH (5-13) gives blue fluorescence when excited at 290 nm. But in pH <5(occurs as a cation) or pH >13(occurs as an anion) does not show any fluorescence.
   (b) **Oxygen:** Oxygen leads to the oxidation of fluorescent substances to non-fluorescent substances and thus causes quenching due to its paramagnetic property (triplet ground state).
   (c) **Halides and electron-withdrawing groups:** Halides like chloride ions, iodide ions and electron-withdrawing groups like -NO, -COOH, -CHO groups lead to quenching.
   (d) **Heavy metals:** The presence of heavy metals also leads to quenching because of collision and complex formation.
4. **Concentration Quenching / Self-Quenching:** Concentration quenching is a kind of self-quenching. It occurs when the concentration of the fluorescing molecule increases in a sample solution. The fluorescence intensity is reduced in a highly concentrated solution (>50 μg/ml).At high concentrations, there is no proportional increase in fluorescence intensity with an increase in concentration. There is a decrease in fluorescence intensity with an increase in concentration. This phenomenon is called concentration quenching or self-quenching.

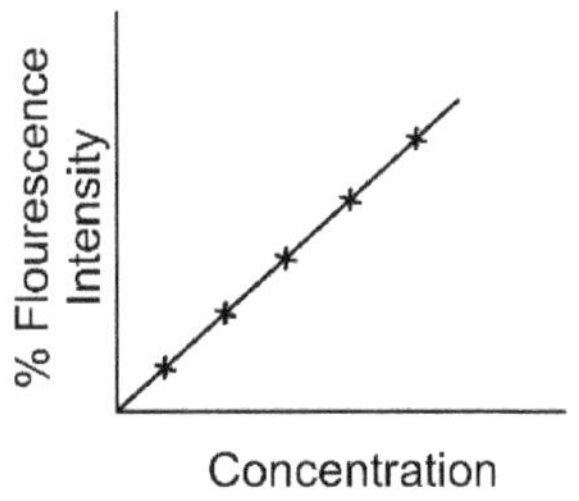

Fig. 25.8(a) Calibration curve in low concentration.

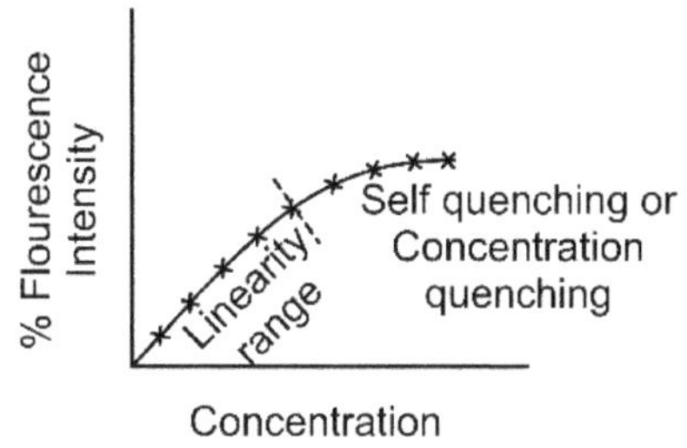

Fig. 25.8(b) Calibration curve in high concentration.

At higher concentrations, there is a deviation from linearity. i.e., there is no proportional increase in fluorescence with an increase in concentration, but there is a decrease in fluorescence. **This is called self-quenching or concentration quenching.** This phenomenon occurs because of the internal circulation of energy(radiation) caused by the absorption and re-emission of radiation by adjacent molecules before falling on the detector. The concentration used for the fluorescence measurement should be in the beer's law range.

Effect of concentration on fluorescence intensity

Fluorescence intensity = Q × I_a

where Q- fluorescence efficiency

$$\text{Fluorescence efficiency} = \frac{\text{Fluorescence intensity emitted}}{\text{Electromagnetic radiation intensity absorbed}}$$

I_a = Intensity of absorbed light

$I_a = I_o - I_t$ since emission is proportional to absorption. .....(25.1)

where I_o = intensity of incident light and

I_t = intensity of transmitted light

By Beer-Lambert's law $I_t = I_0 e^{-act}$

Substituting this for I_t in equation 1

$$I_a = I_o - I_0 e^{-act}$$
$$I_a = I_o (1 - e^{-act})$$
$$I_a = I_o [1 - (1 - act)]$$
$$I_a = I_o [1 - 1 + act]$$
$$I_a = I_o \times act$$

Therefore, Fluorescence intensity = Q × I_a = QI_0act

i.e., $F = QI_0act$

where Q = constant for the given substance

I_0 = constant for the instrument

a = molar extinction coefficient and it is constant for the substance t = pathlength (constant for the given cell)

c = Concentration of the substance

∴ F = KC where K = QI_0a and t

Or in other words, **fluorescence is directly proportional to Concentration.**

But this relationship holds good only in dilute solutions in the range of μg or ng/ml.

In high concentrations (mg/ml), it does not obey beers law (No linearity observed).

INSTRUMENTATION

The instruments used for fluorimetric analysis are called **fluorimeters or fluoro photometers.** In these instruments, **filters** arc used for spectral wavelength isolation.

Spectrofluorimeters employ **two monochromators** to isolate the required wavelength. These instruments are used for scanning the spectrum of wavelength continuously and automatically.

Table 25.2 Summary of instrument components.

Light Source	Filters and Monochromators	Sample cells	Detectors
Mercury vapour lamp Xenon arc lamp Tungsten lamp	Primary filter secondary filter excitation and emission monochromators (gratings)	Cylindrical glass cuvettes Pathlength 1cm All sides polished	Photomultiplier tubes, Photovoltaic cell, Photo tubes placed at 90° angle to incident radiation

CONSTRUCTION OF FLUORIMETERS

1. **Light Source:** The light source should emit radiation continuously over the required wavelength region. It should be stable and provide intense radiation.
   (a) **Mercury vapour lamp:** High pressure (8 atmospheres) mercury vapour gives intense lines in a continuous background above 350 nm. Lines are obtained at 365, 398, 436, 546, 579, 690 and 734 nm. An additional line at 254 nm is obtained with a low-pressure mercury lamp which is used as a source in filter type fluorimeters
   (b) **Xenon arc lamp:** The radiation is intense when compared to mercury vapour lamps. They are used in Spectrofluorimeters.

(c) **Tungsten lamp:** This lamp is used if the excitation wavelength is in the visible region. This lamp cannot work in the UV region. The intensity of this lamp is very low.

2. **Filters and Monochromators:** In fluorimetry, the excitation wavelength and the emission wavelengths are different. A filter or monochromator is used for the selection of these wavelengths. In photofluorimeters, **primary filters and secondary filters** are used for this purpose.

   Primary filter absorbs visible radiation and transmits UV radiation.

   Secondary filter absorbs UV radiation and allows the visible radiation to pass through.

   Spectrofluorimeters contain excitation and emission monochromators with gratings.

   Excitation monochromator selectively allows only the wavelength absorbed by the sample (excitation wavelength).

   Emission monochromator isolates and allows only the **radiation emitted** by the fluorescent molecule (emission wavelength).

   Filters and monochromators are explained in UV spectroscopy.

3. **Sample cells:** The sample cells, known as cuvettes, are used to hold the sample.

   The cells are made of colour corrected fused glass.

   The cells are available in different shapes like cylindrical or rectangle.

   Small volume cells (0.5ml or less) and large volume cells (5-10ml) are available depending on their capacity to hold sample volume. The common pathlength (internal distance) is 1cm.Long path length cells with 10cm and short pathlength cells with 1 or 2mm are also available.

   In colorimetry, one set of opposite sides of the cells are polished (for transmission of light), and the other set of opposite sides are ground (for handling).But in fluorimetry, all surfaces are polished so that the **fluorescence measurements** can be made at **90° angle to the incident radiation.**

4. **Detectors:** As the **emitted** radiation is mostly **visible** radiation and sometimes UV radiation, the detectors used are **Photovoltaic cells, Photo tubes, or Photomultiplier tubes.**

   Photomultiplier tubes are more **accurate and best** because when low concentration of the substance is used, only weak radiation is emitted.

Detectors are explained in the UV chapter.

The common types of instruments are

(i) Single beam filter fluorimeters

(ii) Double beam filter fluorimeters

(iii) Double beam Spectrofluorimeters

(i) Single beam filter fluorimeters: These are inexpensive instruments containing tungsten lamps as the source. The optical system consists of a primary filter that absorbs visible radiation and transmits the UV radiation for the excitation of the molecules of the sample in the sample cell. The emitted fluorescence is measured at 90° using the secondary filter, which absorbs UV radiation and allows the visible radiation to pass through to the detector. If the detector is used at 180° as in colourimetry, both the emitted radiation and the transmitted radiation will produce detector response leading to error in measurements.

Advantages:

1. Simple in construction
2. Cheaper
3. Easy to use

Disadvantages:

1. Sample and reference solutions cannot be measured simultaneously.
2. Rapid scanning is not possible

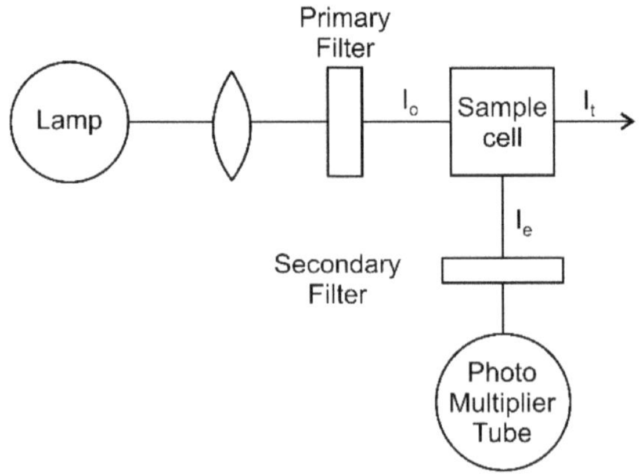

Fig. 25.9 Single beam filter fluorimeter.

(ii) **Double beam filter fluorimeters:** The construction is the same as a single beam except that from a single light source, two incident beams pass through two primary filters separately and fall on the sample and reference standard. The emitted radiation from the sample and reference pass separately through two secondary filters to the detector, and a combined response is obtained from the detector.

Advantage:

Sample and reference can be analyzed simultaneously.

Disadvantage:

Sensitivity and accuracy is less due to the use of filters

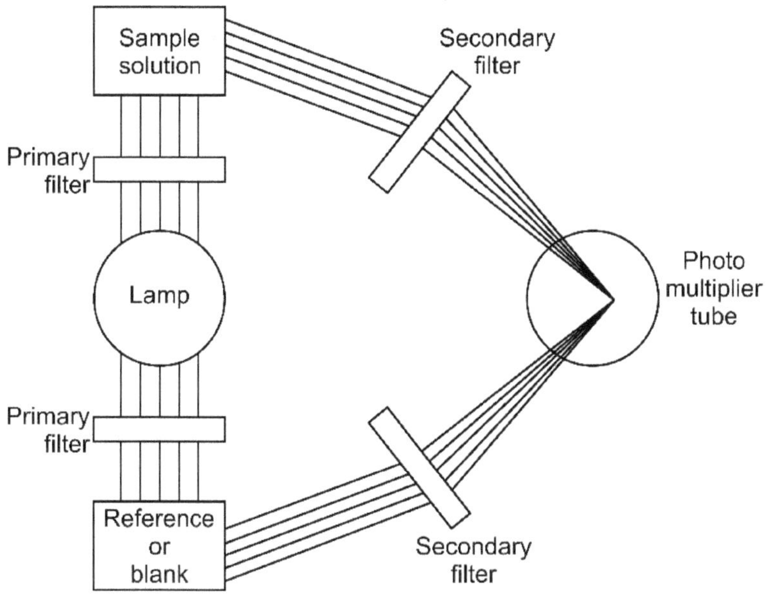

Fig. 25.10 Double beam filter fluorimeter.

(iii) **Double beam Spectrofluorimeters:** In Spectrofluorimeters, the excitation and emission monochromators are used instead of primary and secondary filters of double beam filter fluorimeter. A beam splitter is used to split the incident beam into a sample and reference beam. A **Photomultiplier tube** is used as a detector.

Advantages:

1. Rapid scanning
2. More sensitive and accurate.

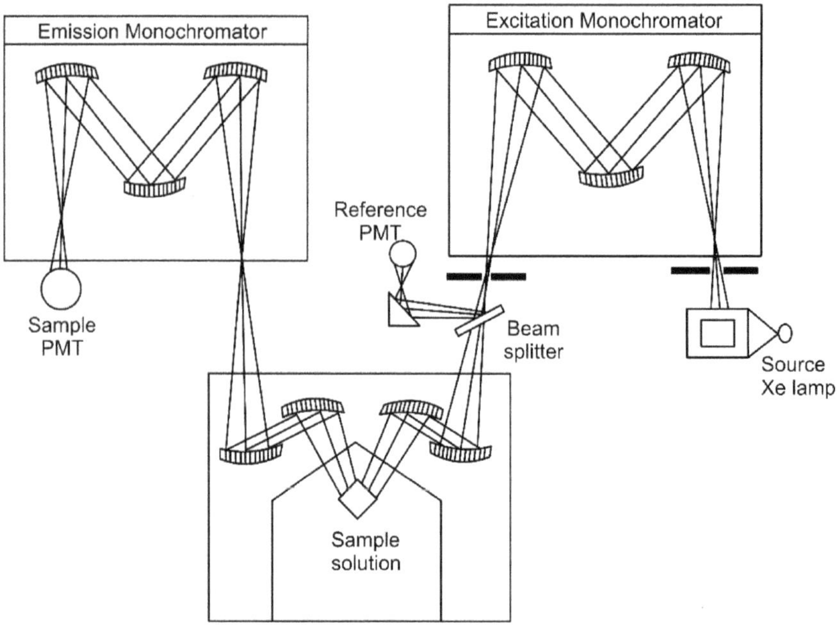

Fig. 25.11 Double beam spectrofluorimeter.

ADVANTAGES OF FLUORIMETRY

1. **Sensitivity** is more compared to other absorption techniques because concentrations like μg or ng /ml can be analyzed by fluorimetry.
2. **Accurate:** The accuracy of fluorescence is approximately 100 times more than that of an absorption procedure.
3. **Specific:** Excitation and the emission wavelengths are characteristic for the substance, making fluorescence more specific than the absorption methods.
4. **Application range:** Using chemical reactions, even non-fluorescent compounds can be converted to fluorescent compounds.

Limitations:

1. Variation in pH affects fluorescence intensity.
2. The presence of oxygen affects fluorescence intensity.
3. The presence of Heavy metals, halides affect fluorescence intensity.
4. All substances are not fluorescent in nature.
5. UV absorption may cause chemical changes in some substances.

APPLICATIONS

1. **Determination of inorganic compounds**
   (a) Generally, inorganic ions do not possess fluorescence. But they form fluorescent chelates with non-fluorescent organic substances.
      (i) E.g., a. Determination of ruthenium ion in the presence of platinum by forming a complex with 5- methyl-1,10-phenanthroline
   (b) Determination of aluminium III in alloys with Pontachrome blue-black RM
   (c) Estimation of traces of boron in steel by complexation with benzoin.
   (d) Quantification of calcium with calcein by fluorimetry.
2. **Fluorescent indicators**

   In fluorimetry, a wide range of compounds can be used as indicators, depending on the specific application and desired characteristics. Some common indicators used in fluorimetry include:

   Fluorescein: A synthetic organic compound commonly used as a fluorescent tracer in various applications, including biological labeling, flow cytometry, and pH measurement.

   Rhodamine: Another synthetic organic compound with strong fluorescence properties, often used in microscopy, flow cytometry, and fluorescence imaging.

   GFP (Green Fluorescent Protein): GFP is a protein separated from the jellyfish, Aequorea Victoria. It exhibits strong green fluorescence when exposed to UV or blue light. GFP and its variants are widely used as genetic markers and protein tags in molecular and cell biology.

   Fluorescent Dyes: Various fluorescent dyes are available with different spectral properties, such as Alexa Fluor dyes, Cy dyes, and DAPI (4',6-diamidino-2-phenylindole). These dyes are used for labeling biomolecules, staining cells and tissues, and detecting specific targets in assays.

   These are just a few examples of compounds used as indicators in fluorimetry. The choice of indicator depends on factors such as the specific application, desired fluorescence properties, compatibility with the sample matrix, and available detection instrumentation.

   Fluorescent indicators are substances whose **intensity and colour depend on pH range.** These are used in acid-base titrations. Examples with pH range are given below.

E.g., Eosin(3-4), Fluorescein (4-6), Quinine sulphate(3-5), 2-Naphthaquinone (4.4-6.3), Acridine (5.2-6.6)

3. **Fluorometric reagent:** They are used **for cation analysis.** They form chelates with metal ions**.** E.g.,
   (a) Alizarin garnet B for Al^{3+} determination
   (b) 8-Hydroxy quinoline in Li^{+} determination
   (c) Flavanol in Sn^{4+} determination.
   (d) Benzoin in Zn^{2+} determination
4. **Determination of vitamin B**
   (a) Vitamin B$_1$ (Thiamine), which is **non-fluorescent,** is converted to **fluorescent thiochrome** (blue fluorescence) by **oxidation** with oxidizing agents like potassium ferricyanide. The fluorescence is measured, which is directly proportional to concentration compounds.
   (b) Vitamin B$_2$ (Riboflavin) is determined based on the principle that **riboflavin on oxidation gives a non – fluorescent substance.**
5. **Organic analysis:** Qualitative and quantitative analysis of aromatic compounds present in cigarette smoke, air pollution, and automobile exhausts is done using fluorimetry.
   E.g., indoles, Naphthols, Proteins, plant pigments, and steroids.
6. **Pharmaceutical applications**
   (a) Direct Fluorescent analysis: In this method, Fluorescent drugs are determined directly. Eg: Aminacrine, P-amino salicylate, Griseofulvin, Quinine, Riboflavin.
   (b) Indirect method: The drugs are converted to fluorescent products by chemical reaction with other reagents.
   E.g., Chlordiazepoxide undergoes Photo-oxidation
   Hydrocortisone treated with 75%v/v sulphuric acid in ethanol
   Nicotinamide treated with cyanogen bromide.
   Diphenyl Hydantoin treated with alkaline Potassium permanganate.
   Thiamine is oxidized with potassium ferricyanide.
   (c) Analysis of Mixtures
      (i) Intensity and colour are chosen in such a way as to excite only one drug.
      (ii) Compounds can be separated and analyzed.
      (iii) Using chemical reaction: Both Codeine and Morphine give fluorescence at 355 nm. But in alkaline conditions, only codeine gives fluorescence.
      (iv) Derivatization: Atropine forms a complex with eosin which gives fluorescence when dissolved in chloroform.

7. Pharmaceutically important fluorescent compounds

Several pharmaceutically important compounds exhibit fluorescence properties, which make them valuable for various applications, including drug discovery, formulation, and analytical methods. Here are some examples:

Fluorescein: Fluorescein is a widely used fluorescent dye in pharmaceuticals and biotechnology. It's utilized in fluorescence microscopy, flow cytometry, and as a tracer in drug formulations.

Rhodamine 123: This compound is often used in cell biology and pharmacology as a mitochondrial stain. It's also employed in fluorescence microscopy and as a probe for membrane potential.

Fluorescent-labeled Antibodies: Pharmaceuticals often utilize fluorescent-labeled antibodies for various purposes, including immunofluorescence assays, flow cytometry, and in vivo imaging.

Fluorescent-labeled Nucleic Acids: Fluorescent-labeled nucleic acid probes are extensively used in molecular biology and diagnostics for detecting specific DNA or RNA sequences.

Green Fluorescent Protein (GFP): While not a pharmaceutical itself, GFP and its variants are crucial tools in drug discovery and development. They are used for visualizing protein localization, tracking cellular processes, and screening assays.

Fluorescent-labeled Ligands: Pharmaceutical compounds labeled with fluorescent tags are utilized in binding studies, receptor assays, and high-throughput screening to investigate drug-target interactions.

Fluorescent-labeled Lipids: Lipids labeled with fluorescent dyes are employed in drug delivery research to study cellular uptake, intracellular trafficking, and drug release kinetics.

Cyanine Dyes: Cyanine dyes are extensively used in fluorescence-based assays and imaging techniques in pharmaceutical research due to their stability, brightness, and tunable spectral properties.

Acridine Orange: Acridine Orange is used in pharmaceutical analysis for staining nucleic acids and as a marker for cell viability and apoptosis.

Fluorescent-labeled Peptides: Peptides labeled with fluorescent dyes are employed in studying peptide-protein interactions, peptide stability, and pharmacokinetics.

These compounds, among others, play vital roles in pharmaceutical research, drug development, and clinical diagnostics, owing to their unique fluorescence properties and diverse applications.

CHAPTER 26

Flame Photometry

INTRODUCTION

Flame photometry is a branch of spectroscopy where radiation emitted by the metallic atoms is measured. It is otherwise called **Flame atomic emission spectroscopy**. The flame photometry principle is based on the measurement of emitted light intensity when a metal is introduced into the flame. The colour of the emitted light is characteristic for each element and is used for qualitative analysis (identification). The intensity of the emitted radiation is directly proportional to the concentration of the metal and this forms the basis of quantitative estimation.

PRINCIPLE

When a sample solution containing metal salt is nebulised through a flame, a series of processes occur, which are given below

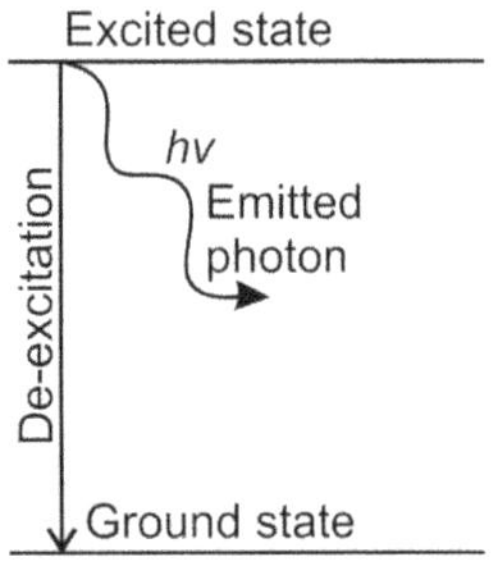

Fig. 26.1 Diagrammatic representation of flame photometry principle.

1. Spray leaves fine droplets of metal salt solution in flame – **nebulisation**
2. The solvent gets vaporised due to the thermal energy of the flame, leaving a fine residue of solid salt – **desolvation**
3. The salt is vaporized and gets converted to gaseous state – **vaporisation**
4. The gaseous molecules are dissociated to give neutral atoms, which are excited by the thermal energy of the flame – **atomization and excitation**
5. The excited atoms are unstable due to the high energy of the excited state, and they emit radiation while returning to the unexcited ground state - **Emission**.

The wavelength of emitted radiation is characteristic of the element emitting it. The wavelength of emitted radiation is used to identify the element (Qualitative analysis). As the intensity of the emitted radiation is directly proportional to the concentration of the element, the intensity is measured and used for quantitative analysis. The measurement of the emitted radiation forms the basis of flame photometry and the steps involved are given in the flow chart.

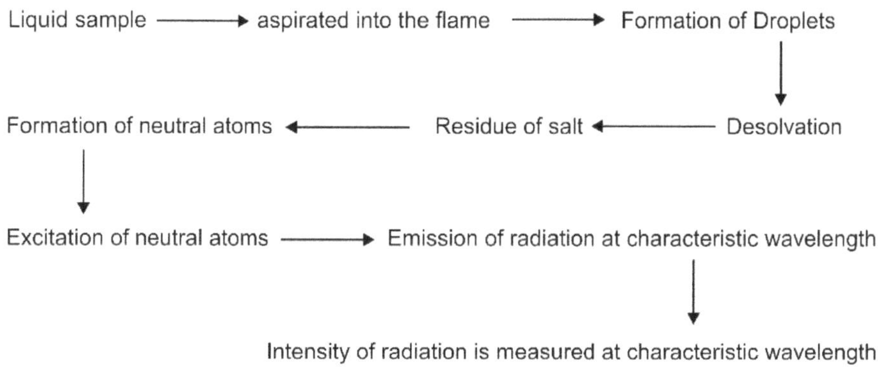

Boltzmann distribution governs the fraction of free atoms that are thermally excited and is given as

$$\frac{N^*}{N_0} = Ae^{-\Delta E/kT}$$

where

N^* – No. of excited atoms

N_0 – No. of remaining ground state atoms

A – Constant for the given element

ΔE – Difference in energy between the ground state and excited state.

k – Boltzmann constant

T – Flame temperature

Thus from Boltzmann distribution, it is understood that the energy of excitation is dependent on flame temperature. Thus, flame is useful only for the elements that require low excitation energy (like alkali metals and alkaline earth metals), i.e. Group I A (Li, Na, K) and Group II A (Ca,Mg etc.).

Since the emitted radiation is characteristic for each element, the wavelength of emitted radiation is different for different elements

For E.g., Sodium emits yellow colour radiation at 589 nm

Potassium emits lilac colour at 767 nm

Calcium emits brick red colour at 422, 554 and 626 nm

Lithium emits red colour radiation at 670 nm

The intensity of the emitted radiation is directly proportional to the concentration of the element present in the sample.

INSTRUMENTATION

The basic components of flame photometer are

1. Sample delivery systems
2. Source
3. Monochromators
4. Detector
5. Readout device

Table 26.1 Summary of Instrumentation.

Sample delivery systems	Source	Monochromators	Detector
(i) Nebulizer, (ii) Aerosol modifier, (iii) Flame or Atomiser	Burners 1. Mecker burner 2. Total consumption burner 3. Premix laminar flow burner 4. Lundergarph burner 5. Shielded burners	Filter wheel Quartz Prism Grating	Photovoltaic cells Phototubes Photomultiplier tube

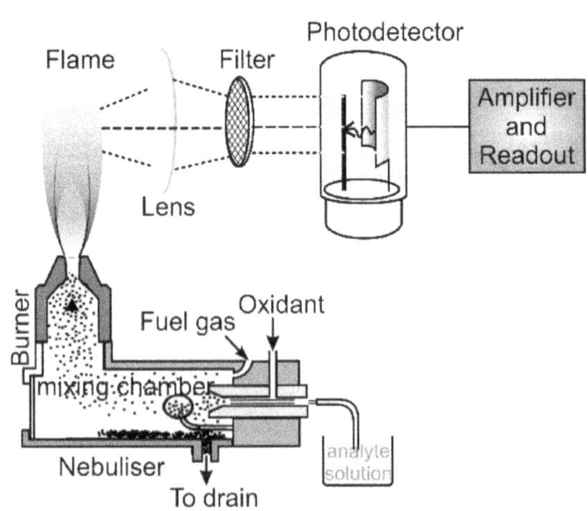

Fig. 26.2 Diagrammatic representation of Flame Photometer.

1. **Sample Delivery Systems**

   Three components are there in the sample delivery system.

   (i) **Nebulizer:** The conversion of sample solution into a mist of finely divided droplets (aerosol) is called nebulisation. The sample is carried to the atomizer from the nebuliser.

   There are three types of classification of nebulisers. The classification is based on

   1. The nebulisation process

      Pneumatic or ultrasonic nebulisers.

   2. Feeding of the sample

      Suction, gravity-fed, controlled flow reflux nebulizer

   3. Relative position of capillaries for the aspirated liquid and nebulising gas and the aspirated liquid

      Angular and concentric nebulisers

   (ii) **Aerosol modifier:** The large droplets are removed from the stream, and this modifier allows only the droplets smaller than the defined size to pass through.

   (iii) **Flame or Atomiser:** The atomizer performs the conversion of vaporized analyte into free atoms

   The different types are

   1. The type which introduces the sample directly into the flame.
   2. The type which introduces the sample in the chamber of an atomiser.

STRUCTURE OF FLAME

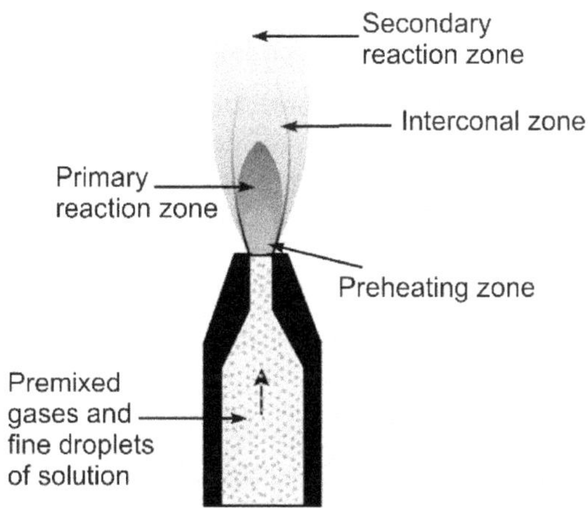

Fig. 26.3 Structure of Flame.

The flame is divided into

1. Preheating zone
2. Primary reaction zone/inner zone
3. Interconal zone
4. Secondary reaction zone

The maximum temperature is obtained above the tip of the primary reaction zone, and this zone is used for flame photometry.

Functions of flame

(i) To desolvate the liquid droplets from the sample forming residue.

(ii) To decompose the residue to form atoms

(iii) To excite the atoms so that they can emit radiation when returning to the ground state.

The temperature of the flame is responsible for all these events, and the factors controlling the temperature of the flame are

(i) Nature of fuel, oxidant and their ratio

(ii) Nature of the solvent used to dissolve the sample.

(iii) Amount of solvent entering the flame

(iv) Type of the burner

REQUIREMENTS FOR FLAME

1. Proper temperature should be maintained, so that the energy supplied is lesser than the ionization potential of the analyte atom
2. Temperature should be maintained constant throughout the procedure
3. No fluctuations in burning should be there.

Fuel and oxidant gases

The optimum temperature for the flame is important because the too low temperature may not be able to excite the atoms, and too high temperature may lead to ionization of the atoms causing the population of excited atoms to decrease (decreased intensity of emission). The different combinations of fuel and oxidant gases used are given in table 26.2.

Table 26.2 The different combination of fuel and oxidant gases.

Fuel	Temperature in oxygen	Temperature in air
Methane	2700	2000
Propane	2800	1925
Butane	2900	1010
Hydrogen	2780	2100
Acetylene	3050	2000
Cyanogen	4580	-----

Various hydrocarbon gases give satisfactory temperatures for metal analysis. Ordinary cooking gas can give a temperature of about 1700°C. Acetylene flame can give a temperature of about 2000-2300°C and is used to determine Li/Mg metals.

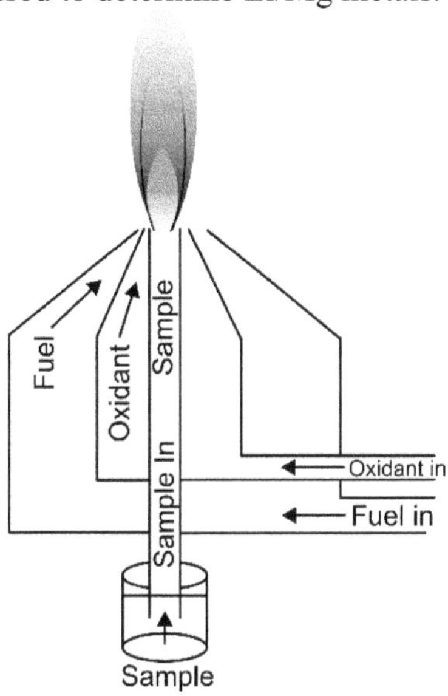

Fig. 26.4 Total consumption burner.

2. **Source-Burners:** The burners are used to spray the sample solution into the flame after mixing with fuel and oxidant. The different types of burners are
    1. Mecker burner
    2. Total consumption burner
    3. Premix laminar flow burner
    4. Lundergarph burner
    5. Shielded burners

    1. **Mecker burner:** This burner uses natural gas and oxygen and is not used nowadays. It produces low temperature and a non-homogenous flame.
    2. **Total consumption burner:** In these burners, hydrogen and oxygen gases are used as fuel and oxidant gases, respectively. The liquid sample is aspirated into the flame through a capillary tube. The oxygen and hydrogen enter through the side tubes and are burnt at the top of the burner to produce a flame. As soon as the sample enters the flame, it is vaporised, atomized and then excited.

       It is called a total consumption burner since the entire sample entering the capillary is consumed.

Advantages

1. Simple design and large sample size enhances sensitivity
2. Entire sample consumed
3. No explosive hazard.

Disadvantages

1. Large droplets not decomposed completely
2. Non- uniform and non-homogenous flame
3. Fluctuations in flame intensity
4. Viscosity of the sample affects the rate of sample introduction
5. Short path for the solute decreases sensitivity

3. **Premix laminar flow burners –most widely used burner:** In this burner, the sample, fuel and oxidant gas are mixed thoroughly and then introduced into the flame. The flow of the gases is laminar and not turbulent as in the total consumption burner. Only a small fraction of the sample droplets reach the flame. Easy decomposition of the sample takes place, leading to efficient atomisation. Large droplets are drained off the outlet.

Advantages

1. Noiseless, non-turbulent and stable flame.
2. Efficient atomisation
3. Clogging free
4. Long path provides sensitivity

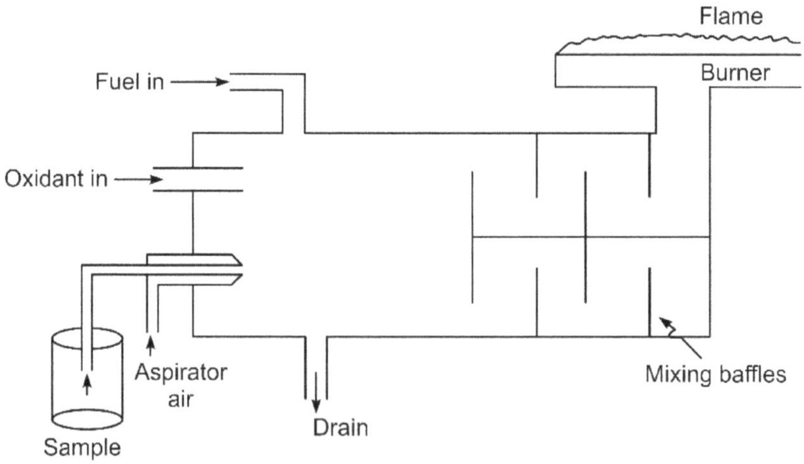

Fig. 26.5 Premix laminar flow burners.

Disadvantages

1. Only a small quantity of the sample reaches the flame
2. Rate of sample introduction is slow.
3. Explosive hazard during mixing

3. **Filters and monochromators**

   Prism: A quartz prism is used as quartz is transparent over the entire region.

   Grating: Grating monochromators can also be used

   A detailed description of filters and monochromators are given in UV Visible spectroscopy.

   A filter wheel present in a simple flame photometer contains several filters (Filters for each element) like Ca, Li, Na, or K. Specific filter will be selected based on the analyte to be determined.
4. **Detectors:** The emitted radiations are in the visible region. Hence detectors like **photovoltaic cells or phototubes** are used in the flame photometer. Flame spectrophotometer uses a photomultiplier tube as a detector. These detectors are explained in UV spectroscopy.
5. **Readout device:** The detector signal is displayed in a digital readout device. The emission at a specific wavelength will be displayed.

INSTRUMENTS

1. **Flame Photometer**

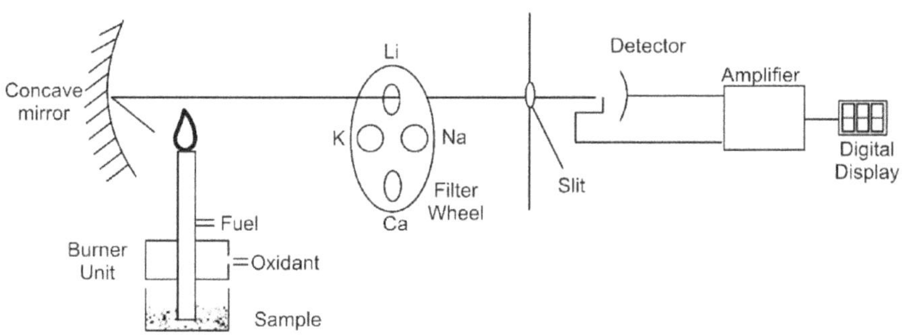

Fig. 26.6 Schematic diagram of a Flame photometer.

Working

The solution to be analysed is sprayed as fine droplets (aerosol) into the burner's flame after mixing with fuel and oxidant gases.

Air or oxygen and the fuel gas are compressed to a pressure of about 0.5kg/sq.cm using a compressor. This high pressure helps in the spraying of samples in fine droplets. This process is called nebulisation.

Next, the desolvation process occurs, followed by vaporization and atomisation.

The atoms formed are excited by the thermal energy of the flame.

These excited atoms are unstable, and they emit excess energy in the form of light to come back to the ground state.

A concave mirror focuses the light to the filter wheel containing Li,Na,K and Calcium filters. The specific filter for the analyte is selected, and the light is allowed to pass through it.

The emitted radiation is directly proportional to the concentration of the substance and is measured by the detector and displayed in the readout device.

2. **Flame Spectrophotometer:** The filter used in the flame photometer is replaced with a prism or grating monochromator in the flame spectrophotometer. A Photomultiplier tube is used as a detector.
3. **Double Beam Spectrophotometer:** This instrument is otherwise called as **internal standard flame photometer**. Lithium is used as an internal standard, and an equal concentration of lithium is added to both standard and sample. The emitted radiation is divided into two parts and measured by two different detectors. One part of the beam is due to lithium (internal standard), and the other is due to the sample. The ratio of the emission intensity of the analyte to the internal standard is recorded.

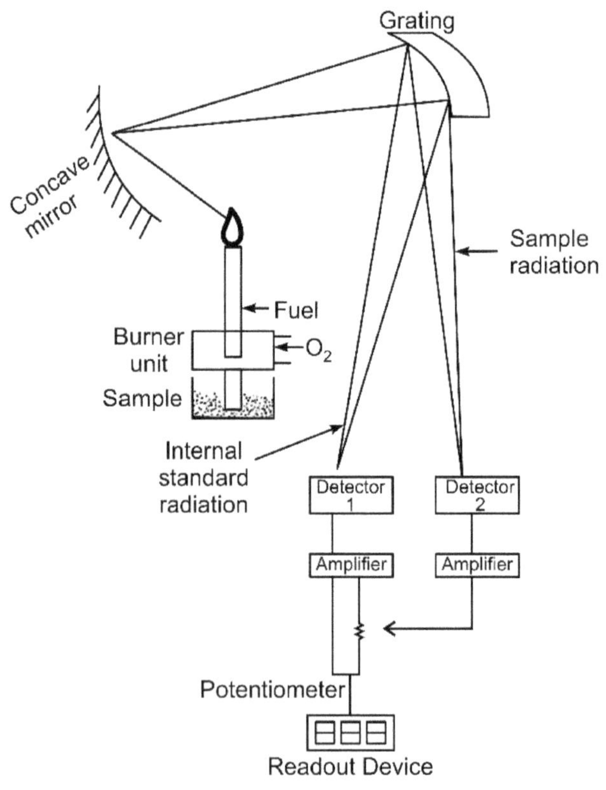

Fig. 26.7 Schematic diagram of a Double beam Flame spectrophotometer.

Advantages

1. Use of internal standards cancels out the error due to the fluctuations in flame.
2. Errors due to differences in viscosity and surface tension are also minimised.

APPLICATIONS

1. **Qualitative analysis:** Flame photometry is used to detect group I and group II elements of the periodic table. The sample is identified by the technique called peak matching. In this technique, a minimum of 3 peaks of emission spectrum should match the standard.

   E.g.: calcium emits radiation at 422,544, 626 nm. If the sample spectrum shows matching peaks in these wavelengths, then the sample is confirmed as calcium.
2. **Quantitative analysis:** Flame photometry is used for rapid quantitative estimation of Group I and II elements like lithium, calcium, sodium and potassium in samples.

   Some of the quantitative applications are determination of
   1. Concentration of calcium in serum
   2. Concentration of calcium, sodium, potassium in the urine
   3. Concentration of calcium, sodium, potassium and magnesium in IV fluids and oral rehydration salts.
   4. Estimation of potassium chloride in syrup.
   5. Serum lithium concentration in Therapeutic drug monitoring

   Experimental procedure

   There are four methods available for quantitative estimation
   1. Direct comparison method
   2. Calibration curve method
   3. Standard addition method
   4. Internal standard method

1. **Direct comparison method:** The emission of the sample solution is compared with standard solution emission.

   Advantages:
   1. Speed of analysis
   2. No need to prepare more standards.

   Disadvantages:
   1. Possibility of more errors.
2. **Calibration curve method:** A series of standard solutions are prepared from the stock solution. The appropriate filter is selected in

the instrument, and air pressure of about 0.4-0.5kg /sq.cm is set in the instrument. Distilled water is sprayed into the flame, and the instrument is set to 0% flame intensity. Using the highest concentration of standard, 100% flame intensity is set. Then the flame intensity of other standard solutions is determined. A calibration curve is constructed with a concentration of the standard on the X axis and flame intensity on the Y-axis. The % flame intensity of the sample is recorded, and the concentration of the sample is found out by the interpolation of the graph.

3. **Standard addition method:** An equal amount of the sample solution is taken in different standard flasks, and increasing concentrations of standard solutions of the same element are added to each standard flasks. The flame intensity of all the solutions is recorded, and the calibration graph is constructed with a negative x-axis (sample concentration). The extrapolated line meets the negative x-axis to give the concentration of the sample. A typical calibration curve is shown in figure 26.8.

Advantages:

1. Low concentrations of the elements can be determined.
2. Unexpected interfering substances will not affect the method.

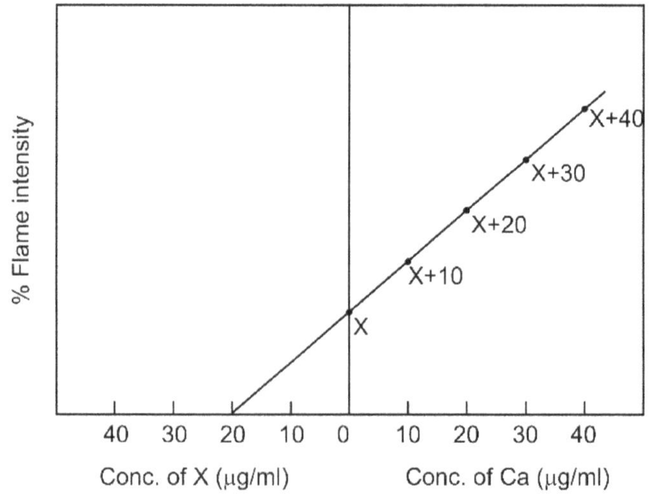

Fig. 26.8 Calibration curve in Standard addition Method.

4. **Internal standard method:** A known amount of the internal standard element is added to both the standard and sample solutions. The signal intensities of both sample and standard solutions are recorded. The ratio of the intensities is plotted against the concentration of the standard (calibration graph).The unknown concentration can be obtained from the graph by interpolation.

INTERFERENCES IN FLAME PHOTOMETRY

The presence of other materials in the sample causes some interferences in the recording of the spectrum. **Interference is a phenomenon that affects the measurement of the concentration of atoms in the ground state of an analyte.** The different types of interferences are

(i) **Physical interferences:** Background absorption, Spectral line interferences, matrix interference, viscosity and solvent interferences

(ii) **Chemical interferences:** Anionic interferences, vaporization interferences

(iii) **Scattering effects**

(iv) **Ionisation interferences**

(i) **Physical interferences**

1. **Background absorption:** The light absorption by the unvaporized solvent droplets in the flame causes background absorption. Absorption of unknown molecular species in flame and matrix interference (below 350nm) also causes background absorption.

   Correction: Using a deuterium lamp and grating monochromator minimizes these interferences.

2. **Spectral line interferences:** Occurs due to partial or complete overlap of the emission spectrum of two elements in the same wavelength. These interferences are more common in high flame temperatures.

   E.g., Iron 324.7 nm interferes with copper at 324.7 nm

   Iron 285.2 nm interferes with Magnesium 285.2 nm

   Aluminium interferes with emission lines of calcium and magnesium.

   Correction:

   1. Extraction of interfering material
   2. Using calibration curves of solutions with the interfering element
   3. Use of grating monochromators

3. **Matrix interference:** Sample matrix components other than the analyte react to form molecules to give this interference. Use of a blank to zero the instrument avoids this interference

   Changes in viscosity of the solution by a change in solvent or change in concentration causes matrix or bulk interference.

   Correction: Addition of an organic solvent decreases viscosity.

4. **Solvent interferences:** Metals in aqueous solutions give lower absorbance readings than the same metals in organic solutions.

(ii) Chemical interferences: When an analyte is not completely decomposed in flame to produce atoms, chemical interferences occur, leading to reduced absorbance of the analyte.

1. Vaporisation interferences

There are two types in this interference

(a) Chemical type

(b) Physical type

(a) Chemical type - occurs due to the incomplete dissociation and reaction with other ions in the sample.

These interferences are classified as

(i) Cation –Anion interferences

(ii) Cation – cation interferences

(iii) Oxide formation interferences

(i) Cation – Anion interferences: Thc intensity of emitted radiation is affected by the presence of certain anions like oxalate, phosphate, sulphate and aluminate.

E.g., calcium in the presence of phosphate – calcium signal is suppressed.

Correction:

1. Extraction of anions
2. Preparation of calibration graphs with a known concentration in the standard solutions (standard addition method).
3. Choice of flame, burners, atomizer and additives

   E.g., Acetylene nitrous oxide flame for phosphates, sulphates, silicates, and aluminates which are thermally stable.
4. Additives:

(a) Releasing agent: Use of Ionization suppressants like Lanthanum/ strontium to overcome interference due to Phosphates.

(b) Chelation or Masking Agents: Use of EDTA to mask calcium in the presence of phosphate

(ii) Cation – Cation interferences: These interferences are caused by the presence of other cations. These interferences are neither spectral nor ionic in nature.

E.g., Aluminium interferes with calcium and magnesium

Sodium and potassium have cation–cation interference

Correction:

1. Extraction of interfering cations
2. Construction of calibration graph

(iii) Oxide formation interferences: These interferences arise due to the formation of stable oxides of metal ions due to the oxygen present in the flame. Thus, the emission is decreased.

Metals like La, Al, and Ti give rise to oxides when aspirated into the flame.

Correction:

1. Use of high-temperature flames (Nitrous oxide-acetylene flames) to dissociate the oxides to give free atoms.
2. Oxygen free environment to produce atoms

(b) **Physical type** – High viscosity decreases intensity (interferes with atomisation.)

E.g., Dextrose, Sucrose.

This interference can be corrected by adding methanol to the sample, which enhances nebulisation and increases the sample concentration in flame leading to higher absorbance values.

(iii) **Scattering effects:** These effects also occur due to the higher concentration of the interfering element.

This effect can be eliminated by using a continuous light source (e.g., deuterium lamp) in addition to an HCL lamp.

Scattering occurs as a result of the particulate matter from the flame atomization scattering the incident radiation from the source. This can be corrected by using a blank during analysis.

(iv) **Ionisation interferences:** If the temperature of the flame is high, leading to ionization of the atoms, atomic emission intensity decreases. Ions have their own emission spectrum, which is different from atomic emission. This type of interference occurs only in I group elements (Na, K, Sr, etc.).

***Correction*:** By adding excess (100-1000 μg) of easily ionisable salts like potassium, caesium, and strontium to the sample and standard solutions. These ions act as suppressants for the ionization of the analyte and enhance the emission of analyte molecules. These ions have lower ionization potential, and they get ionized preferentially over the sample analyte.

LIMITATIONS OF FLAME PHOTOMETRY

1. No information is obtained about the molecular form of metal present in the sample.
2. Inert gases cannot be detected by this method
3. Only liquid samples can be analysed. (solubility of sample in solvent)
4. The number of elements that can be analysed by flame photometry are limited.

CHAPTER 27

Atomic Absorption Spectroscopy

Atomic absorption spectroscopy is a study of absorption of a specific wavelength of radiation by the atoms of metals in the ground state. It is a method of elemental analysis. It is a highly versatile technique so that 60-70 elements, including common rare earth metals can be determined by direct methods. Many non-metals can be detected by indirect methods. It is a very sensitive technique.

PRINCIPLE

The solution containing the metallic salt sample is nebulized into the flame, fine droplets are formed. The thermal energy of the flame causes desolvation leaving the salt residue, which decomposes to give the neutral atoms. These neutral atoms absorb the specific wavelength of light emitted by the source, Hollow Cathode Lamp (HCL). For each element determination, the same element is used as cathode in the HCL source.

The intensity of light absorbed by the atoms is directly proportional to the concentration of the element, which is measured by the detectors. In atomic absorption spectroscopy, beer's law is obeyed over a wide concentration range.

Total amount of light absorbed $\upsilon = \pi e^2 \times Nf/ mc$

Where,

e - charge on the electron of mass, m

c - speed of light

N - total no of atoms that are absorbed at a frequency υ in the light path

f - the ability of the atom to absorb at frequency υ

e,m,π and c are constants.

Thus, the total amount of light absorbed = constant × N × f

This means that the amount of light absorbed is dependent on the number of atoms absorbing the light and their ability to absorb at that particular wavelength. The equation also shows that the amount of light absorbed is independent of the wavelength of absorption and temperature. The flame is used for atomizing the sample only, and the excitation of the atoms are brought about by the HCL source radiation.

Table 27.1 Difference between atomic absorption spectroscopy and flame emission spectroscopy.

Atomic absorption Spectroscopy	Flame emission spectroscopy
1. Measures the intensity of radiation absorbed by unexcited atoms of the analyte at the ground state.	Measures the intensity of radiation emitted by the excited state atoms.
2. Atomic absorption depends on the no. of unexcited atoms.	Flame spectroscopy depends on the no. of excited atoms.
3. Independent of flame temperature.	Temperature-dependent.
4. Nearly a linear relationship between absorption and concentration. Beer's law obeyed over a wide concentration range.	Not true with flame emission
5. A wide range of elements can be analyzed.	Only group IA, IIA elements can be analyzed.

The flow chart representing the principle of AAS is given

Sample aspirated into flame → formation of droplets → solid residue → neutral atoms formation → absorption of specific wavelength by neutral atoms from HCL → measurement of the intensity of absorbed radiation by photometric detectors.

Advantages of Atomic absorption spectroscopy (AAS) over flame emission spectroscopy

1. AAS is specific for the element under analysis and spectral interferences are rare.
2. Independent of flame temperature.
3. More elements can be determined. Sensitivity is more.

Disadvantages

1. A separate lamp is required for each determination
2. Elements giving rise to oxides in the flame cannot be determined. E.g., Al, Ti, W, Si
3. Anionic interferences are present.

INSTRUMENTATION

Components of the AAS spectrophotometer are

1. Radiation source
2. Nebulizers
3. Atomizer - Burners
4. Monochromator
5. Detector
6. Readout device

Table 27.2 Summary of Instrumentation.

Radiation source	Nebulizers	Atomizer - Burners	Monochromator	Detector
(i) Hollow cathode lamp (HCL) (ii) Electrodeless discharge lamp (EDL)	Pneumatic or ultrasonic nebulisers Suction, gravity-fed, controlled flow reflux nebulizers Angular and concentric nebulisers	1. Flame atomizers: Total consum ption and premixed burners 2. Non-flame atomizers: Graphite tube atomizer carbon filament atom reservoirs	Filter Prism Grating	Phototubes Photomultiplier tube

1. **Radiation sources:** The two most commonly used radiation sources are
   (i) Hollow cathode lamp (HCL)
   (ii) Electrodeless discharge lamp (EDL)

   (i) Hollow cathode lamp: It is the most common AAS source.
   It contains a tungsten anode and a hollow cylindrical cathode.
   The cathode is made up of the element to be determined. Thus, a separate lamp is required for the determination of each element.
   The cathode may also be made up of alloy for the determination of the elements present in it. Then it is called a multi-element lamp.
   The anode and the cathode are sealed in a glass cylinder filled with argon or neon gas at low pressure. The opening of the glass cylinder has a silica/quartz window, transparent to the emitted radiation.

The potential applied between the electrodes causes a current in the mA range to flow through. The inert gas gets ionized at the anode, and these ions of gas are attracted to the cathode with high velocity. The impact with the cathode vaporizes the atoms of the cathode element. The vaporized atoms collide with the inert gas atoms or molecules and get excited. These excited atoms emit their characteristic radiation, and this emitted radiation is absorbed by the neutral atoms of the same element in the sprayed sample solution.

Advantages

1. It gives a bandwidth of 0.001 to 0.01 nm
2. The line width provided is less than the absorption line width of the element to be determined.

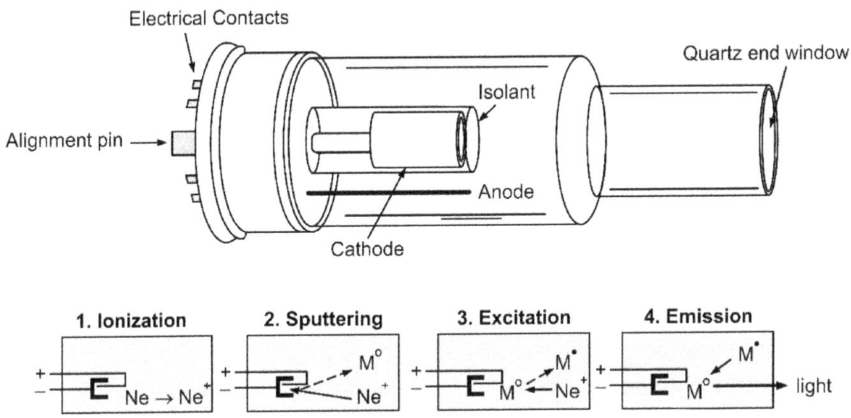

Fig. 27.1 Hollow cathode lamp.

Disadvantages

1. Finite lifetime due to the depletion of cathode
2. Adsorption of gas atoms on the inner surface of the glass cylinder.
3. For the determination of every element, a separate lamp should be used.

(ii) **Electrodeless discharge lamp:** This lamp consists of a small amount of the element or a salt of the element sealed in a quartz bulb with an inert gas atmosphere. The bulb is placed inside a small RF generator. When an RF field of sufficient power is applied, the inert gas is ionized. The coupled energy vaporizes the element and excites the atoms inside the bulb, resulting in the emission of the characteristic spectrum. EDC can be used to detect elements including Sb, As, Bi, Cd, Cs, Ge, Pb, Hg, P, K, Rb, etc.

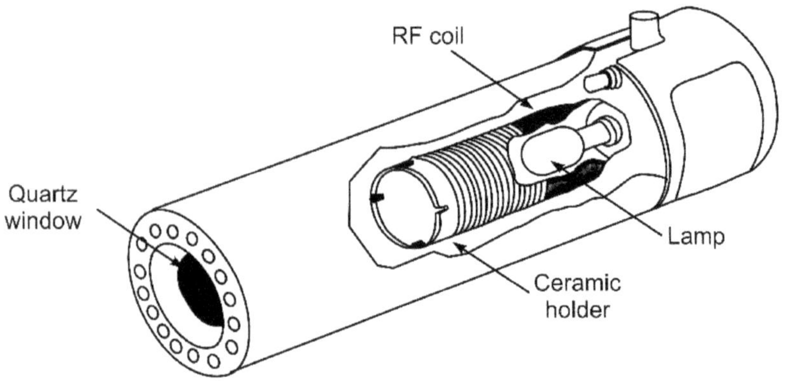

Fig. 27.2 Electrodeless discharge lamp.

Chopper: The function of the chopper is to create fluctuation in the output of the source. A chopper (rotating wheel) is placed between the hollow cathode lamp and the flame. This breaks the steady light from the lamp into pulsating light. This fluctuating light produces a pulsating current in photometric detectors. The light emitted by the flame produces a steady current. In the instrument, only the pulsating current is amplified and recorded. Thus, the interference due to light emitted by the flame is eliminated.

2. **Nebulizers:** The conversion of the liquid sample into small droplets is called nebulization. The liquid sample is drawn up the capillary by a high-velocity gas stream. A fine aerosol spray is mixed with fuel and oxidant gas thoroughly and then introduced into the flame.
3. **Atomizer burners:** In order to analyze the samples by AAS, the sample should be in an atomic state. This is achieved by the breaking down of the molecules into atoms. There are two types of atomizers.
   (i) Flame atomizers
   (ii) Non-flame atomizers.

   (i) Flame atomizers: Burners are used as flame atomizers

   The burners are used to spray the sample solution into the flame after mixing with fuel and oxidant. There are two types of burners, Total consumption and premixed burners.

   Total consumption burner: In these burners, hydrogen and oxygen gases are used as fuel and oxidant gases respectively. The liquid sample is aspirated into the flame through a capillary tube. The oxygen and hydrogen enter through the side tubes and are burnt at the top of the burner to produce a flame. As soon as the sample enters the flame, it is vaporized, atomized and then excited.

   It is called a total consumption burner since the entire sample entering the capillary is consumed.

Advantages

1. Simple design
2. Entire sample consumed
3. No explosive hazard.

Disadvantages

1. Large droplets not decomposed completely
2. Non- uniform and non-homogenous flame
3. Fluctuations in flame intensity
4. Viscosity of the sample affects the rate of sample introduction
5. Short path for the solute decreases sensitivity

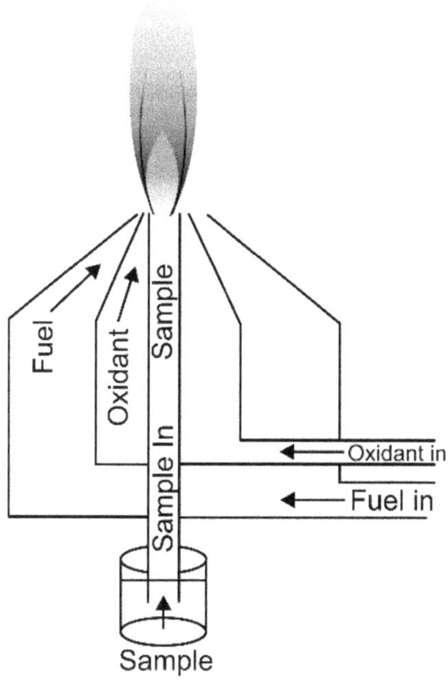

Fig. 27.3 Total consumption burner.

Premix laminar flow burners –most widely used burner: In this burner, the sample fuel and oxidant gas are mixed thoroughly and then introduced into the flame. The flow of the gases is laminar and not turbulent as in the total consumption burner. Only a small fraction of the sample droplets reach the flame. Easy decomposition of the sample takes place, leading to efficient atomization. Large droplets are drained off the outlet.

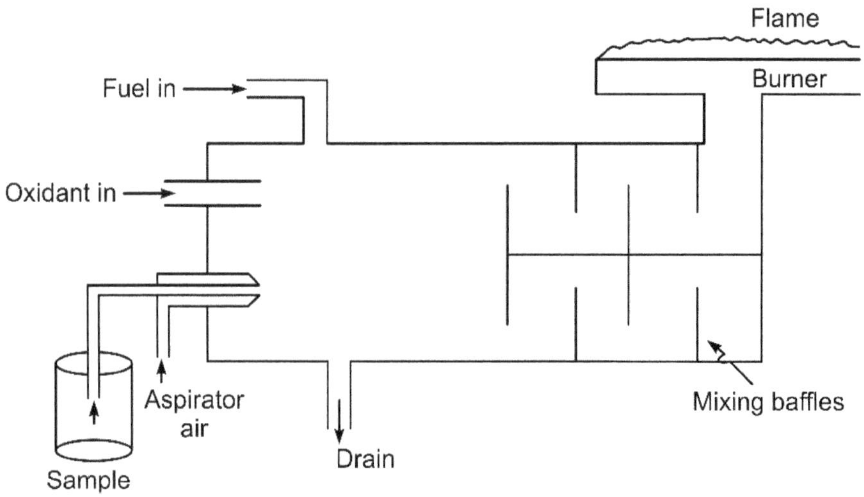

Fig. 27.4 Premix laminar flow burners.

Advantages

1. Noiseless, non-turbulent and stable flame.
2. Efficient atomization
3. Clogging free
4. Long path provides sensitivity

Disadvantages

1. Only a small quantity of the sample reaches the flame
2. Rate of sample introduction is slow.

(ii) **Non-flame atomizers:** E.g. of these types of atomizers are graphite tube atomizers and carbon filament atom reservoirs. A similar process is used in both the atomizers

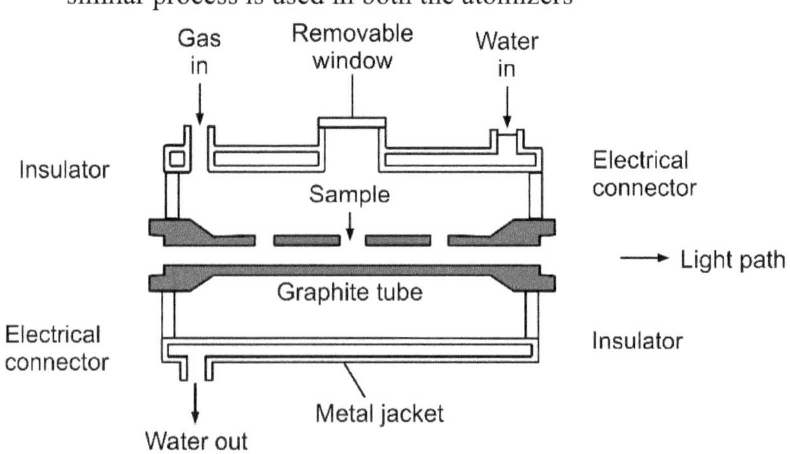

Fig. 27.5 Graphite tube atomizer.

Graphite tube atomizer: A small quantity of the sample (2-30μl) is loaded in the sample compartment. Here the sample undergoes desolvation, and it decomposes to form the atoms by electrical heating. Thus, the free atoms are vaporized and introduced into the optical light path, and the absorption of light is measured.

4. **Monochromators:** The most common monochromators are prism and gratings. These monochromators are explained in detail in the UV Visible spectroscopy chapter. It has to select the wavelength emitted by the element, excluding the emission by the gas in the HCL lamp or the background signal of flame.
5. **Detector:** The radiations absorbed by the elements are in the UV-visible range. The most suitable detector is a photomultiplier tube. In some instruments, phototubes are used.
6. **Readout device:** Readout devices display the absorption spectrum and the absorbance at a specified wavelength.

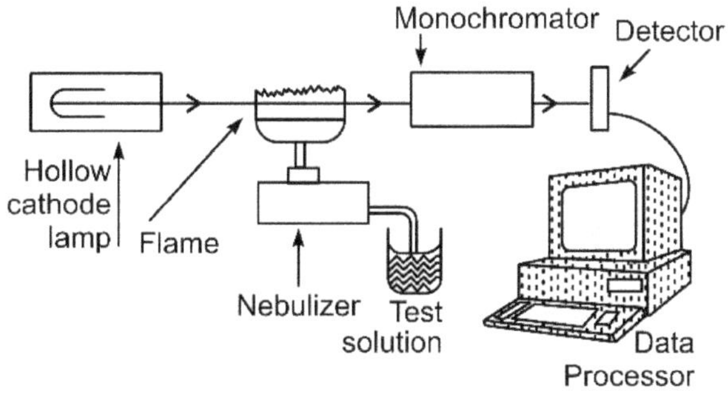

Fig. 27.6 Schematic diagram of atomic absorption spectrophotometer.

Two types of AA Spectrophotometers are available. They are

1. Single beam atomic absorption spectrometer
2. Double beam atomic absorption spectrometer

1. **Single beam atomic absorption spectrometer:** The light source is placed ahead of the flame with a chopper in between the light source and flame; when there is no sample in flame, the detector records the full intensity of the source emission. When the sample is introduced into the flame, there is a reduction in the emission due to absorption by the sample atoms. This output is recorded by the detector.

   Disadvantages

   Low stability.

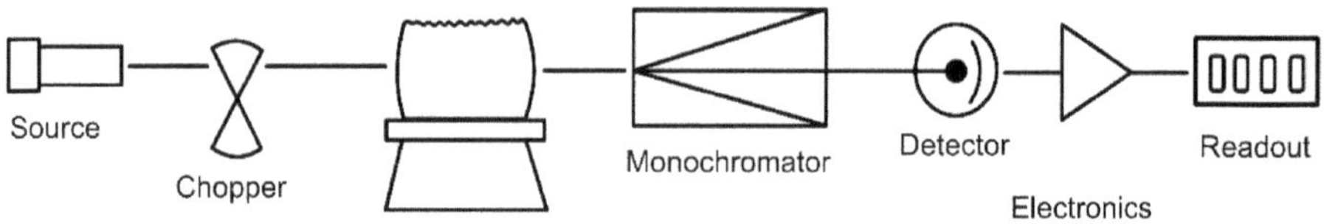

Fig. 27.7 Schematic diagram of Single beam atomic absorption spectrophotometer.

2. **Double beam atomic absorption spectrometer:** The chopped beam from the source (hollow cathode lamp) is divided into two parts. One part passes through the flame, and the other is the reference beam not passing through the flame. The two beams are recombined and reach the detector through a monochromator. The detector output is displayed in the readout system.

   Advantages

   1. Avoids fluctuations in the conditions of the flame
   2. Viscosity, temperature and spraying rate effects are eliminated.
   3. No change in detector sensitivity with time.

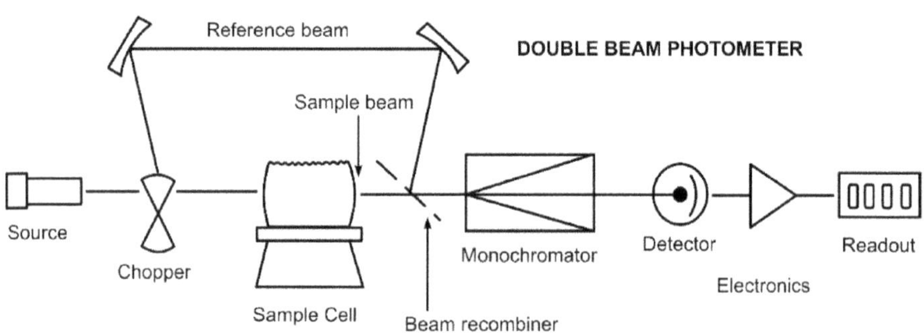

Fig. 27.8 Schematic diagram of Double beam atomic absorption spectrophotometer.

INTERFERENCES

Interference is a phenomenon that affects the measurement of the concentration of atoms in the ground state of an analyte.

The interference is less in AAS when compared to flame photometry. It is also free from cationic interferences due to the absorption of sharp resonance lines from HCL. The different types of interferences are

(i) **Physical interferences:** Background absorption, Spectral line interferences, matrix interference, viscosity and solvent interferences

(ii) **Chemical interferences:** Anionic interferences, vaporization interferences

(iii) **Scattering effects**

(iv) Ionization interferences

(i) Physical interferences

1. **Background absorption:** The light absorption by the unvaporized solvent droplets in the flame causes background absorption. Absorption of unknown molecular species in flame and matrix interference (below 350nm) also causes background absorption.

   Correction: The use of a deuterium lamp and grating monochromator minimizes these interferences.

2. **Spectral line interferences:** Occurs due to partial or complete overlap of the emission spectrum of two elements in the same wavelength. These interferences are more common in high flame temperatures.

   E.g., Iron 324.7 nm interferes with copper at 324.7 nm

   Iron 285.2 nm interferes with Magnesium 285.2 nm

   Aluminium interferes with emission lines of calcium and magnesium.

   Correction:

   1. Extraction of interfering material
   2. Using calibration curves of solutions with the interfering element
   3. Use of grating monochromators

3. **Matrix interference:** Sample matrix components other than the analyte react to form molecules to give this interference. Use of a blank to zero the instrument avoids this interference

   Changes in viscosity of the solution by a change in solvent or change in concentration cause matrix or bulk interference.

   Correction: addition of an organic solvent decreases viscosity.

4. **Solvent interferences:** Metals in aqueous solutions give lower absorbance readings than the same metals in organic solutions.

(ii) Chemical interferences: When an analyte is not completely decomposed in flame to produce atoms, chemical interferences occur, leading to reduced absorbance of the analyte.

1. Vaporization interferences: There are two types in this interference

   (a) Chemical type

   (b) Physical type

   (a) Chemical type - occurs due to the incomplete dissociation and reaction with other ions in the sample.

   These interferences are classified as

   (i) Cation –Anion interferences

   (ii) Cation – cation interferences

(iii) Oxide formation

(i) Cation – Anion interferences: The intensity of emitted radiation is affected by the presence of certain anions like oxalate, Phosphate, sulphate and aluminate.

E.g., calcium in the presence of Phosphate – calcium signal is suppressed.

Correction:

1. Extraction of anions
2. Preparation of calibration graphs with a known concentration in the standard solutions (standard addition method).
3. Choice of flame, burners, atomizer and additives

   E.g., Acetylene nitrous oxide flame for phosphates, sulphates, silicates, and aluminates which are thermally stable.
4. Additives:
   (i) Releasing agent: Ionisation suppressants like lanthanum/strontium to overcome interference due to Phosphates.
   (ii) Chelation or Masking Agents: Use of EDTA to mask calcium in the presence of Phosphate

(ii) Cation – cation interferences: These interferences are caused by the presence of other cations. These interferences are neither spectral nor ionic in nature.

E.g., Aluminium interferes with calcium and magnesium

Sodium and potassium have cation–cation interference

Correction:

1. Extraction of interfering cations
2. Construction of calibration graph

(iii) Oxide formation interferences: These interferences arise due to the formation of stable oxides of metal ions due to the oxygen present in the flame. Thus the emission is decreased. Metals like La, Al, and Ti give rise to oxides when aspirated into the flame.

Correction:

1. Use high-temperature flames (Nitrous oxide-acetylene flames) to dissociate the oxides and give free atoms.
2. Oxygen free environment to produce atoms

(b) Physical type – High viscosity decreases intensity (interferes with atomization.)

E.g., Dextrose, Sucrose.

This interference can be corrected by adding methanol to the sample, which enhances nebulization and increases the sample concentration in flame, leading to higher absorbance values.

(iii) **Scattering effect:** These effects also occur due to the higher concentration of the interfering element.

This effect can be eliminated by using a continuous light source (e.g., deuterium lamp) in addition to an HCL lamp.

Scattering occurs as a result of the particulate matter from the flame atomization scattering the incident radiation from the source. This can be corrected by using a blank during analysis.

(iv) **Ionization interferences:** If the temperature of the flame is high, leading to ionization of the atoms, atomic emission intensity decreases. Ions have their own emission spectrum, which is different from atomic emission. This type of interference occurs only in I group elements (Na, K, Sr, etc.).

Correction: By adding excess (100-1000 μg) of easily ionizable salts like potassium, caesium, and strontium to the sample and standard solutions. These ions act as suppressants for the ionization of the analyte and enhance the emission of analyte molecules. These ions have lower ionization potential, and they get ionized preferentially over the sample analyte.

APPLICATIONS OF AAS

1. **Qualitative analysis:** Since different HCL source has to be used for each element, AAS is not used in qualitative analysis.
2. **Quantitative analysis:** The calibration curve method is used. Serial dilutions of standard solutions are prepared, and their absorbances are measured.
3. A calibration curve is constructed with the concentration of elements and absorbance.
4. The concentration of the extrapolation of the graph. Beer's law is obeyed over a wide range of concentrations. Sample concentration upto 0.001 ppm can be analyzed quantitatively in AAS.
5. The other applications are

(i) Analysis of trace elements in biological fluids. (e.g., Blood, wine, etc.)

(ii) Estimation of elements like Ca, Ni, and Zn in food products.

(iii) In the pharmaceutical industry, it is used to estimate zinc in zinc insulin injection, Mercury in thiomersal injection.

(iv) Analysis of elements in soil samples, water, effluents, ceramics, etc.

(v) Determination of lead in $CaCO_3$, petrol etc.

CHAPTER 28

Atomic Emission Spectroscopy

Atomic Emission spectroscopy (AES) is based on the measurement of emitted radiation from the excited atoms to get the analyte concentration. After absorbing thermal or electrical energy, the sample gets excited and the emitted radiation is studied in both qualitative and quantitative analysis. This emission spectroscopy is called as AES because it is related to the emission of number of atoms present in the excited state. This technique is more useful in elemental metal analysis.

PRINCIPLE

When the atoms are excited by electric or thermal methods, the valence electrons move from lower energy orbitals to higher energy orbitals. The excited unstable electrons return to the ground state by emitting radiation in the form of discrete spectral lines. The emitted spectral line depends on the nature and type of the atom. This forms the basis of qualitative analysis. The intensity of emitted lines is directly proportional to the concentration of the atoms and this forms the basis of quantitative analysis in AES.

Quantitative estimation of metals as well as metalloids like arsenic, silicon and selenium can be carried out using AES. The high temperature provided by the atomization sources in AES, excite the atoms to the unstable higher energy level and the atoms emit radiations as they decay back to the stable ground states. In AES, all the atoms are detected simultaneously and this is the major advantage of AES when compared to AAS.

INSTRUMENTATION

The components of AES are

1. Source and sample holder
2. Monochromators
3. Detectors
4. Read out device.

Excitation Source	Sample holder	Monochromators	Detectors
1. Flame excitation source **High Temperature Plasmas** 2. Inductively coupled Plasma (ICP) 3. Direct current plasma (DCP) 4. Laser induced plasma 5. Laser induced breakdown (LIBS) 6. Microwave induced plasma (MIP) **Discharge sources-Arcs and sparks** **DC Arc, AC arc, AC spark** 7. Spark or Arc emission source	Solid sample holder Liquid sample holder a.porous cup container b.Rotating discs	Prism Grating Echelle monochromator	Photographic plates / films Photoelectric detectors.

I. Excitation Source

1. Flame excitation source

The higher temperature provided by the flame desolvates and vaporizes the sample to get free atoms. These free atoms are excited to higher energy level by the flame. There are many types of burners available and total consumption burner and premix burner are the commonly used burners. These burners along with the type of flames are discussed in flame photometry in detail. Air-acetylene flame is used for the determination of alkaline earth metals. It is inexpensive, stable and reproducible. Flame temperature fluctuation and lame composition causes interferences which affects the performance.

The temperature of the flame depends on

(i) Type of fuel and oxidant
(ii) Fuel oxidant ratio
(iii) Type of burner
(iv) Flame region.

Temperature of common flames

Fuel Gas	Oxidant	Temperature in K
Hydrogen	Air	2000-2100
Hydrogen	Oxygen	2600-2700
Acetylene	Air	2100-2400
Acetylene	Nitrous oxide	2600-2800

2. Inductively coupled plasma (ICP)

ICP-AES uses the argon plasma (6000-10000° C) for atomization and excitation of the sample atoms. ICP-AES is used to determine approximately all of the elements except gases and some non-metals (C, N, F, O, H). The components of ICP are Sample Introduction System to deliver the sample solution to the plasma which consists of pump, nebulizer and spray chamber and the Plasma to generate the signal. Plasma is formed in the torch from argon gas.

The high temperature offered by the ICP is efficient in desolvating, vaporizing, atomizing and exciting atoms. Molecular interferences are reduced to a greater extent in ICP source.

Plasma is defined as a homogenous mixture of gaseous atoms, ions and electrons at very high temperature. Usually neutral gas like argon is used. Plasma is generated in a device called torch. Plasma is initiated by a spark from a tesla coil. Argon ions, once formed in a plasma, are capable of absorbing sufficient power from an external source to maintain the temperature at a level at which further ionization sustains the plasma indefinitely. The plasma temperature is about 10 000 K

The inductively coupled plasma torch consists of 3 concentric silica quartz tubes. The Inner tube contains sample aerosol and Argon stream passes through the middle tube. The outermost tube contains flow of gas as a coolant.

An oscillating current is produced in an induction coil that wraps around the tubes by the radiofrequency (RF) generator (typically 1-5 kW @ 27 MHz or 41 MHz). The induction coil creates an oscillating magnetic field which in turn sets up an oscillating current in the ions and electrons of the argon gas. These ions and electrons collide with other atoms in the support gas to create high temperature plasma.

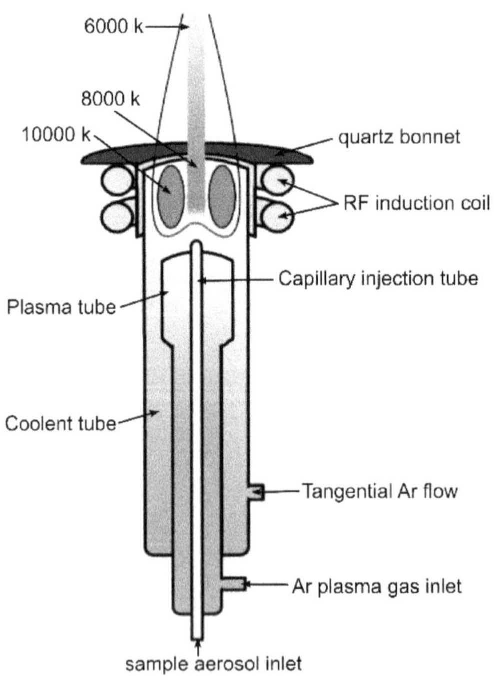

ICP excitation source

Different regions of ICP torch

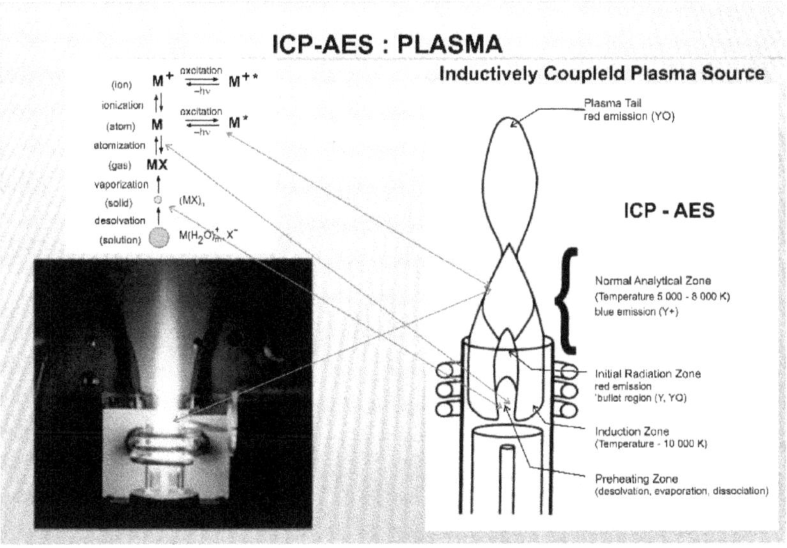

Based on the view, **ICP-AES is classified into**

(a) Radial (SOP) - **SOP: Side-on-Plasma**

In this type, optical system and plasma are indirect to each other-indirect view. Radial plasma looks through the side of the plasma and is best suited for high matrix tolerance and concentration.

It is Robust and has less interference.

Radial torch is more suitable for hard matrices (concentrated samples);

In alkali metals (Na, K, Li) calibration is more linear;

It has less spectral interferences and robust. Its sensitivity is low (Limit-of-Detection is
higher);

Used in the fields of Petrochemical and Metallurgy.

(b) Axial (EOP) - **EOP: End-on-Plasma**

In Axial type, Optical system and plasma are direct to each other - direct view. Axial view plasma looks down the central channel of the plasma, this provides the best sensitivity and lowest detection limits.

Axial torch is more suitable for light matrices

In alkali metals (Na, K, Li) calibration is less linear;

It shows more spectral interferences;

It has got higher sensitivity (Limit-of-Detection is lower);

Used in the areas of Environmental and Chemical.

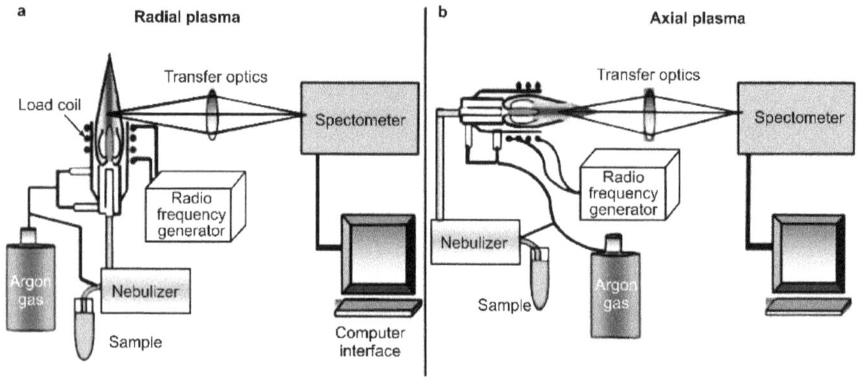

3. Direct Current Plasma (DCP)

It is one of the versatile excitation device for both qualitative and quantitative analysis.

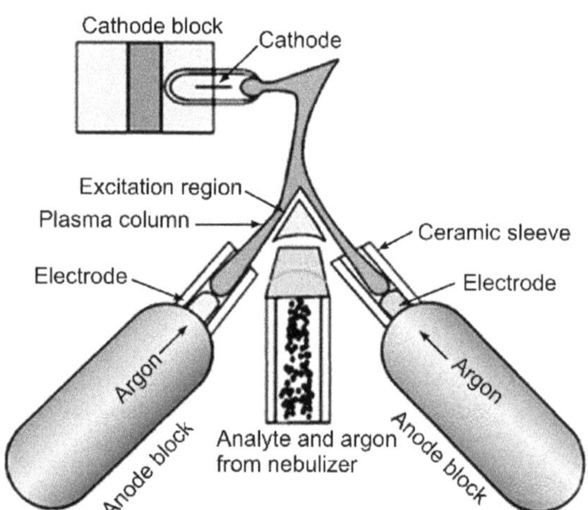

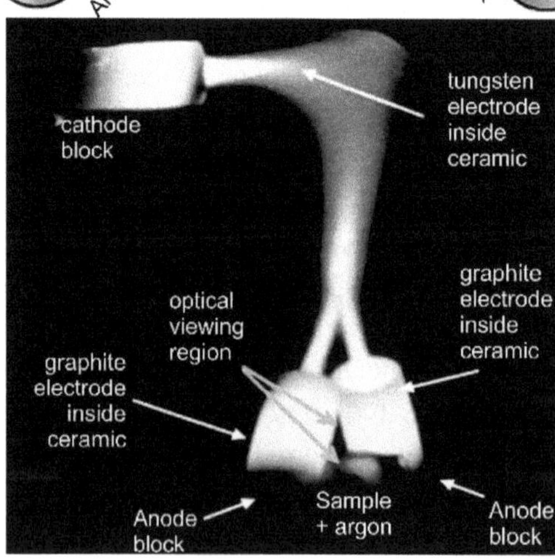

In direct current plasma (DCP) the dc source is an external power supply. The recent DCP is the three electrodes DCP or inverted -Y shaped plasma. It has two anodes set at an angle of about 60° and a cathode. Anode is made up of graphite and is placed inside ceramic sleeves. A cathode block consists of a little tungsten electrode also placed inside ceramic sleeve. The argon gas is introduced through the sleeves around the anodes and it transfers the discharge to the cathode block and plasma is obtained by momentarily bringing the cathode in contact with the anodes. Argon gas ionizes and a high current passes through the cathode and anodes. The temperature obtained is about 5000°C.

The electronic release of the two electrodes creates the DCP. The sample is placed on an electrode. In this technique the emission of the sample by the converted gas atoms is encouraged by placing the solid samples near the discharge.

The electrical discharge between two electrodes creates direct current plasma. Argon gas is used as plasma support gas. The ionized gas atoms excite the analyte atoms in the gaseous phase. The process is also called as glow discharge excitation.

Advantages of DCP

- Consumption of argon gas is less.
- Simpler instrumental requirements
- Less spectral line interference

Disadvantages of DCP

- DCP sources usually have fewer lines than ICP sources
- Lower sensitivities than ICP sources
- The graphite electrodes need frequent replacement because they tend to decay with continuous use.

4. Laser induced Plasma

In this source highly energetic CO_2 laser pulse is used to generate optical sample excitation. Laser is focused on to the support gas like argon to maintain the plasma, which atomizes and excites the sample present in the support gas until it ionizes and analyzed by a spectrometer.

5. Laser induced breakdown (LIBS) excitation source

In this type of AES a highly energetic laser pulse is used as the excitation source. When laser beam is focused on a small spot of a sample (liquid, solid and gases) the temperature of heated region increases inducing the formation of hot plasma. The laser pulse rapidly vaporizes the sample material and converts it into the gaseous phase. The plasma formed atomizes and excites the analyte molecules. These atoms are then detected by the detector in AES. The obtained spectra consist of lines corresponding to the elements evaporated from the sample surface.

6. Microwave Induced Plasma excitation source

This source consists of a quartz tube surrounded by microwave guide. The carrier gas and aerosol enter the inner tube while the outer tube serves as the microwave cavity. The plasma is formed at top of the torch and extends out like a flame. It allows the introduction of wet aerosols at lower power.

MIP operates with a low helium flow rate. Microwaves generated by the magnetron fill the microwave cavity and oscillates the electrons in the plasma support gas. These oscillating electrons, collide with the flowing gas atoms creating and maintaining the high temperature plasma. The excited atoms emit radiation as they leave the microwave cavity and this emitted radiation is measured.

This plasma is suitable for the determination of halides and other nonmetals.

Discharge sources- Arcs and sparks

The spark sources use a current pulse and the arc sources use a continuous electrical discharge between two electrodes. They vaporize the sample and excite the atoms of the sample.

Arc source: These sources consist of two electrodes made of metal or graphite. If the sample is a metal, that itself can be used as a electrode. For the samples which are non conducting, the sample is ground with graphite powder and kept on the cup tipped lower electrode. The first discharge sources produce a direct current (DC) arc by electrically heating the sample in the electrode cup and vaporizing the analytes into a low-voltage, high-current discharge. The temperature of the arc plasma varies from 4000 to 5000K. There are two types of Arc sources

(i) Direct current arc
(ii) Alternating current arc.

Spark source: Spark sources produce lower average temperature than arcs, but the local temperature can be as high as 40000 K. An AC potential in the order of 10-50 kV is discharged through a capacitor which is charged and discharged through the graphite electrodes about 120 times resulting in a discharge current of about 1000 A.

Arc and spark sources are widely used in metal industries.

Electrodes

Two types of electrodes are used in atomic emission spectroscopy

1. Self electrode
2. Graphite electrodes

1. Self electrodes

If the sample is a good conductor and if it can withstand high temperature, the sample material itself is used as electrode. This type of electrodes is called as self electrodes. For example, alloys and metal powders can be made into solid cylinders or discs to be used as electrodes.

2. Graphite electrodes

These electrodes are used when the analyte is thermo labile at high temperature and not a good conductor. The sample is placed in a small cavity of the lower graphite electrode. Both upper and lower electrodes are made of graphite with narrow neck. The upper electrode has sharpened end to reduce wandering of the arc. This improves the reproducibility and the narrow neck increases the sensitivity.

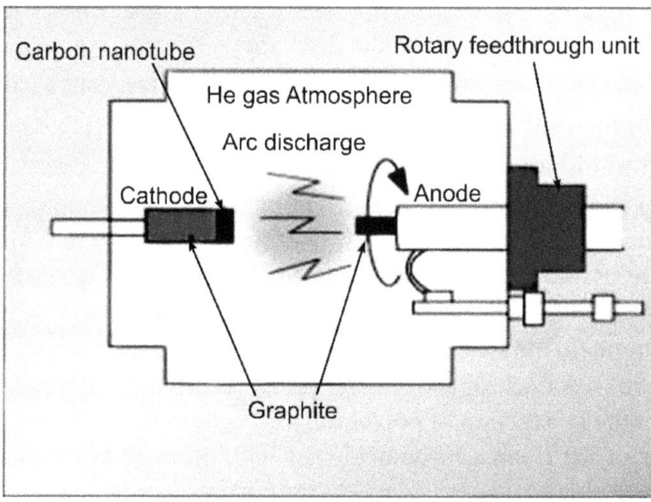

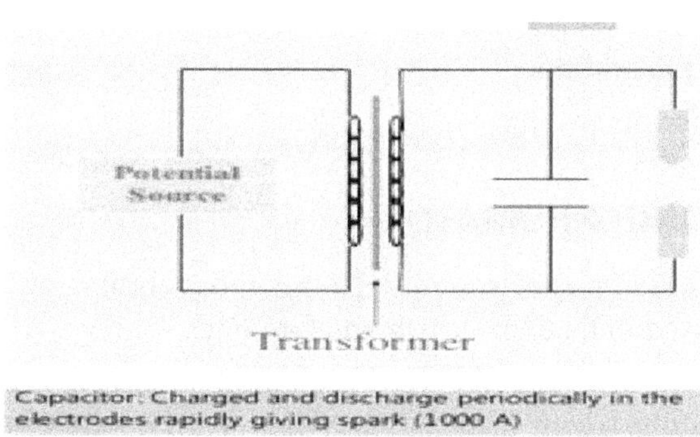

II. Sample Holders

Solid sample Holders

The different kind of samples analyzed by AES is metals, alloys wood, plastic paints, polymers, soil and seawater. The sample is dissolved in suitable solvent like Al_2O_3, SiO_2 or C and dried to form powder. This sample is loaded in to the sample holder. Sample is vaporized when the electrical discharge takes place and it starts spectroscopic emissions.

Organic compounds in biological are reduced to ash by burning in furnace or chemical decomposition. The ash is mixed with carbon, alumina or silica powders and this forms the matrix when the mixture is fed in to the discharge.

Metallic samples can be used directly as one of the electrodes by converting into suitable shape.

Liquid sample holders

There are two types of liquid sample holders. One is porous cup container in which the sample enters the discharge through the porous base. The second type is the rotating disc sample holders, where the disc rotates through the sample and carries the sample to the discharge.

In ICP and DCP determinations, pneumatic nebulizers are used.

III. Monochromators

Prism Monochromators

Two half prisms are used to avoid the splitting of emission light. The light is split into two beams by the first half and the two beams are combined to a single beam by the second half prism. This type of prism is known as cornu type of prism.

Grating monochromator

These grating monochromators give better resolution. Gratings are **more efficient** in the conversion of polychromatic light to monochromatic light. A **resolution of ±0.1 nm** can be achieved with gratings and hence they are used in spectrophotometers.

There are two types of Gratings

(i) Diffraction grating

(ii) Transmission grating

ECHELLE MONOCHROMATOR

It is used in emission spectroscopy. In this monochromator, two dispersive elements are used in tandem (Prism and Grating).

The prism disperses the light in one plane. The dispersed light is made to fall on the grating which disperses the light at right angles to the plane of dispersion of prism. The final dispersion of wavelengths happens over a two dimensional plane. Multiple numbers of photomultipliers are used to measure the radiation intensity.

Data obtained from echelle monochromator is very useful but it is not versatile and it is expensive.

Slits

Two types of slits are present. They are entrance slit and the exit slit.

Entrance slit is placed at the entrance of light from source and eliminates stray light by permitting only the light from the sample to enter the optical path length.

Exit slit placed after the monochromator and allows only the required wavelength to reach detector.

IV. Detectors

Two types of detectors are used in AES. They are

1. Photographic detectors - plates or films.
2. Photoelectric detectors.

Photographic detectors

These detectors are used in most of the spectrographs other than direct reading spectrographs. Photographic emulsion is used to register the intensity of spectral lines in this type of detectors. Suitable developers are used to develop the emulsion at the given temperature in recommended time. These are used for qualitative analysis.

Photographic emulsion consists of light-sensitive crystals of silver halides suspended in gelatin. These are useful for shorter wavelengths like blue and violet. The emulsion is modified by adding suitable dyes, so that it can be used for other wavelengths like green, red and IR regions.

The density of the developed photographic film is measured by a densitometer. The log ratio of intensity of light passing through clear film to the light passing through blackened film is calculated. The log exposure is plotted against calculated density.

Advantages:

1. All spectral features are recorded simultaneously over wide range of wavelengths.
2. Impinging radiations are integrated over the entire time of exposure.
3. It is a permanent record and can be used over a period of time
4. It offers high sensitivity in UV, Visible region
5. Less cost

Disadvantages:

1. Long exposure times
2. Processing and analyzing is difficult
3. Non linear response
4. Precision and sensitivity is less in quantitative measurements.
5. Limited range

Photoelectric detectors

Photomultiplier tubes and solid state photodiodes are this type of detectors. These detectors are used in quantitative analysis.

Advantages

1. Linear response
2. Precision and sensitivity is high.

Limitations

1. High cost
2. Only one spectral line can be measured at a given time. So more no of PMT are required for detecting different emission lines.

Atomic emission spectrometers

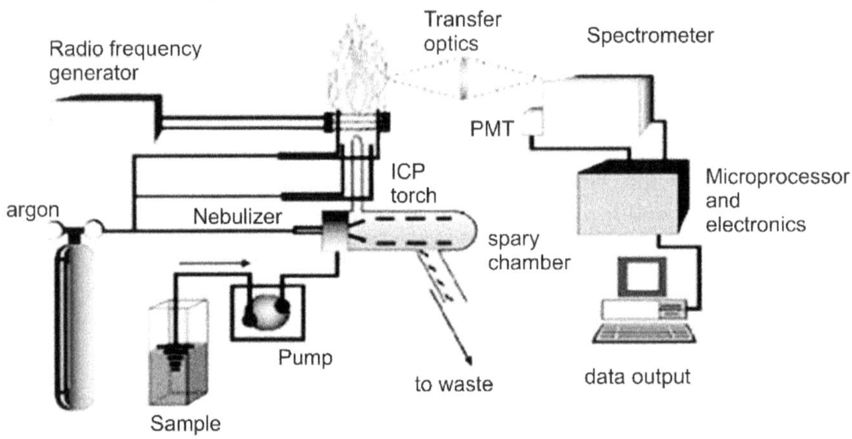

Schematic diagram of ICP-AES is shown above.

Based on the monochromators used, the instruments can be classified as Prism instruments and Grating instruments.

PRISM INSTRUMENTS

The components of prism instruments are excitation source, an entrance slit, a collimator lens, dispersing prism, and camera lens and detector photographic plate.

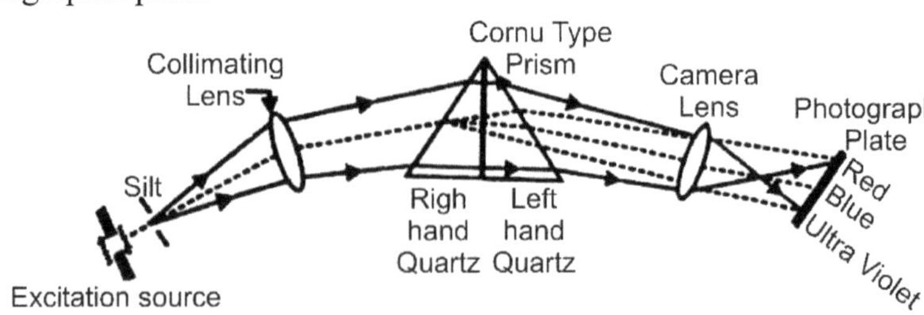

Working: The light from excitation source passes through the slit and collimated by the lens. The parallel beam of light passes through the prism.

The refracted light from the prism is detected on the photographic plate with the help of camera lens.

To avoid polarization splitting in prism, cornu type prisms and littrow type prism are used.

Grating instruments

In these instruments, Grating monochromator is used in the place of prisms. Gratings give linear dispersion and the resolution is constant and independent of wavelength. There are two types of instruments

1. Concave grating instruments
2. Plane grating instruments

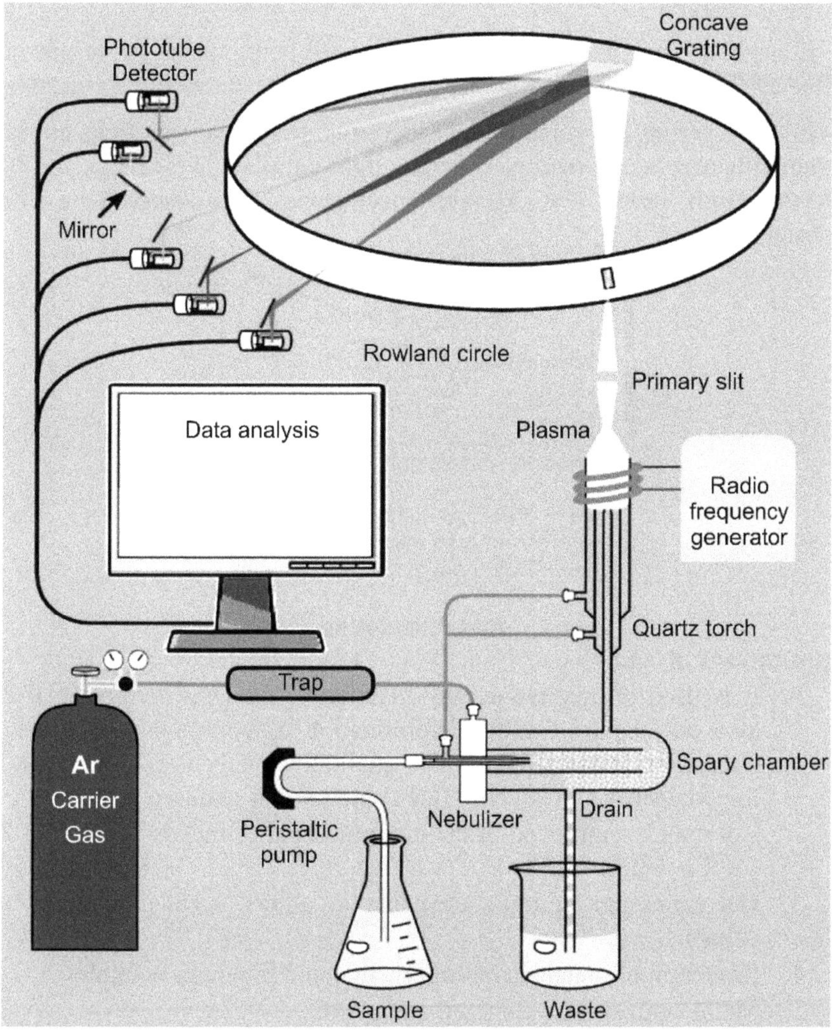

Rowland circle

The different mountings of concave grating instruments are

1. Rowland circle
2. Wadsworth mounting
3. Eagle arrangement of Rowland circle

In Rowland mounting, the film and the grating are present at right angles to the slit. Thus all these three parts come in a circle called as Rowland circle. The diameter of the circle is equal to the radius of curvature of the surface of concave grating. The images are detected by PMT detectors on the Rowland circle. To get the maximum signal, the detector can be moved along the circle.

In Wadsworth mounting, along with the concave grating, a concave mirror is used.

In eagle arrangement of Rowland circle, all components lie on one side of the circle, resembling littrow prism arrangement.

In plane grating Instrument like Elbert mounting, plane gratings are used along with concave mirror to make the light parallel. Their range is 1800-3000Å. High order UV Visible spectra can be observed in these instruments.

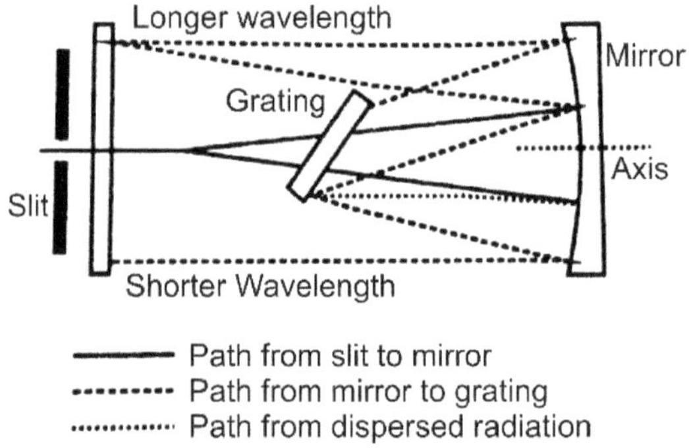

Elbert mounting

Applications of AES

1. It is used in qualitative and quantitative analysis of metals. It can also be adapted for the determination of non-metals like carbon, phosphorous and sulphur. The qualitative analysis is carried out by the comparison of spectral lines with known standard samples.
2. Commonly employed in the determination of metals like K, Na Zn, Cu ,Ca and Li
3. Determination of trace elements in alloys, metals, reagents and solvents.
4. Detection of metals in environmental and biological samples
5. Metal analysis in water, soil and plants

Advantages of AES

1. Excellent for elemental trace analysis
2. All metals and metalloids can be detected using AES.
3. No chemical separations are required.
4. Small sample size is sufficient (1-10mg)
5. Analysis time is less with suitable standards.
6. Can be used for routine qualitative analysis
7. Variety of samples like geological, metals, plants, alloys, forensic samples, soil, environmental and biological samples can be analyzed.

Disadvantages

1. High cost
2. Destructive technique. Sample recovery is not possible
3. Only dilute solutions only can be analyzed
4. Limited to the analysis of elements.

CHAPTER 29

NMR Spectroscopy and ESR Spectroscopy

It is a branch of spectroscopy that deals with the interaction between the nuclei and Radiofrequency waves. The transitions between the magnetic energy levels of the nuclei of the molecules induced by the radio frequency waves are studied in this spectroscopy. The magnetic energy levels are created when the nucleus is placed in the magnetic field.

In the absence of the magnetic field, the spin states of the nuclei degenerate. i.e. They possess same energy (both +1/2 and -1/2). When a magnetic field is applied, the energies of the spin states separate from each other and the absorption of radiofrequency waves cause transition between these energy levels.

Radio waves are the lowest energy EMR in the range of 10^7 to 10^8 cps. The energy of radio waves is so less, that it is insufficient to cause changes in the rotational or excitational energies of an atom or a molecule. But this energy is powerful enough to alter the nuclear spin of the atoms of the molecule. NMR spectroscopy gives information about the number and types of atoms in the molecule.

The important criteria for the compound to be NMR active

All the nuclei are not NMR active. The Nuclei with spin Quantum number $I = \frac{1}{2}$ are only active in NMR. For example ^1H and ^{13}C nuclei.

If I = 0, the nuclei is not NMR active.

All nuclei with an odd number of protons (^1H, ^2H, ^{14}N, ^{19}F, ^{31}P...) or nuclei with odd number of neutrons like ^{13}C are NMR active. These nuclei have asymmetrical charge distribution. Nuclei with even number of protons and neutrons (^{12}C and ^{16}O) are not NMR active.

QUANTUM NUMBERS AND NMR

According to Quantum Theory, the spin angular momentum of a spinning nucleus is

Spin angular momentum = $[I\,(I+1)]^{1/2}\,\dfrac{h}{2\pi}$ ......(29.1)

Where I is the spin quantum number of the nucleus

h- Planck's constant

But $\mu = \gamma \times$ spin angular momentum

$$\mu = \gamma \times [I\,(I+1)]^{1/2}\frac{h}{2\pi} \qquad \text{......(29.2)}$$

where μ = magnetic moment of the nucleus, γ = gyro magnetic ratio

The nucleus with the magnetic moment, when introduced in to the magnetic field (H_0), the energy levels are separated as

$m_I = -\frac{1}{2}$ (against the direction of applied magnetic field)

$m_I = +\frac{1}{2}$ (along the direction of applied magnetic field)

For a nucleus with I=1/2, energy levels of the two spin states are given as

$$E_1 = -\frac{1}{2}\left(\frac{\gamma h}{2\pi}\right)H_0 \qquad \text{......(29.3)}$$

$$E_2 = +\frac{1}{2}\left(\frac{\gamma h}{2\pi}\right)H_0 \qquad \text{......(29.4)}$$

Energy levels for a nucleus with spin quantum number 1/2

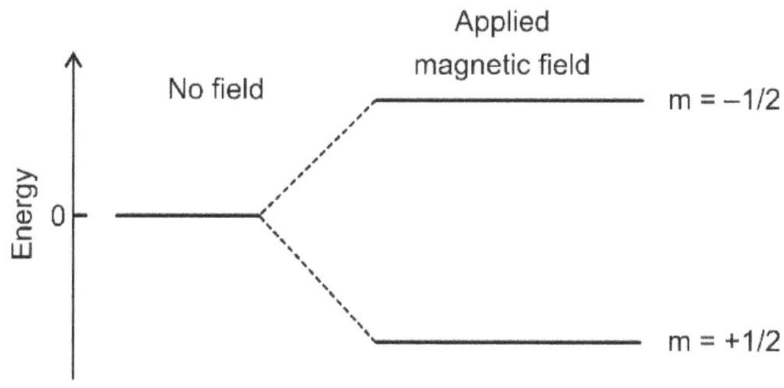

The nucleus absorbs EMR (energy) and it is excited from lower energy level E_1 to higher energy level E_2. The difference in energy is

$$\Delta E = E_2 - E_1$$

It means that the amount of energy required to change the magnetic moment of the nucleus from parallel (+1/2) to anti parallel (-1/2) state is equal to ΔE.

The nucleus which is in the upper energy state E_2 after the absorption of energy ΔE, comes back to energy level E_1 by emitting energy equivalent to ΔE.

The frequency of the absorbed or the emitted radiation is given by the Bohr's relationship

$$\nu = \frac{E_2 - E_1}{h} \qquad \text{......(29.5)}$$

On substituting for E1 And E2 in this equation

$$\nu = \frac{\frac{1}{2}\left(\frac{\gamma h}{2\pi}\right)H_0 + \frac{1}{2}\left(\frac{\gamma h}{2\pi}\right)H_0}{h}$$

$$\nu = \left(\frac{\gamma}{2\pi}\right)H_0 \qquad \text{......(29.6)}$$

Equation (29.6) is the Larmor equation and it is the mathematical basis of NMR.

This equation shows that the frequency/energy absorbed or emitted by a nucleus in moving from one energy level to another is directly proportional to the applied magnetic field. Absorption of the energy is determined in NMR.

RESONANCE

When a nucleus is placed in the magnetic field, it aligns itself against or along the magnetic field. The nucleus spins in a particular frequency which is called as the precessional frequency. This precessing nucleus is irradiated with RF radiation. When the applied RF radiation matches with the precessional frequency of the nucleus, the nucleus starts absorbing the energy, become excited and goes to the higher energy level. It returns to the ground state by losing the excess energy. This process of excitation and relaxation repeated again and again as long as the sample is irradiated with IR radiation. The nucleus is said to be in resonance during this process.

To determine the resonance frequency, the energy absorbed by the nucleus is measured at different magnetic field strengths (H_0). The energy is absorbed by the nucleus when the precessional frequency of the nucleus is equal to the applied RF radiation. The absorbed energy produces a signal at the detector which is recorded as a peak in spectrum.

An NMR spectrum is a plot of absorption signal against the frequency.

PRINCIPLE

Any nucleus with an odd mass number has asymmetrical charge distribution and it spins on its own axis. When this nucleus is placed in a magnetic field, a magnetic moment is created and the nucleus is spinning on its axis with precessional frequency in the precessional orbit. This happens in the ground state or parallel orientation where the magnetic field created by the spin of the nucleus is aligned with the direction of applied magnetic field.

When the precessional frequency is equal to the applied frequency, the absorption of radio frequency waves occur and a signal is obtained in NMR spectrum. This absorption of energy causes the excitation of the nucleus from ground state to excited state, causing reversal of the spin orientation of the nucleus to anti parallel orientation (excited state). In this state, magnetic field created by the spin of the nucleus opposes the direction of applied magnetic field. The nucleus is now in the state of resonance and it returns to the ground state when the RF frequency is stopped. Increase in the strength of magnetic field, increases the precessional frequency.

Excitation process in NMR spectroscopy

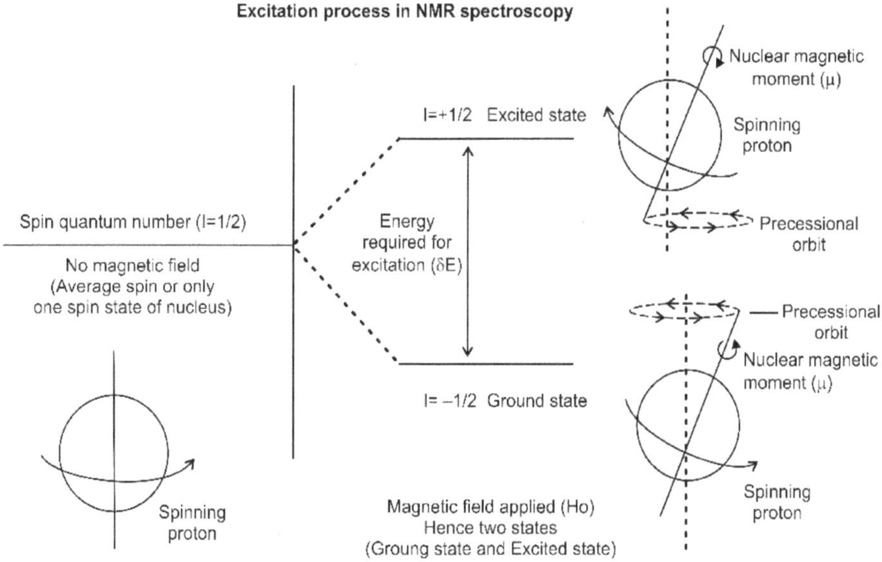

$$\delta E = \frac{\gamma h H_o}{2\pi}$$

$$\delta E = h\nu_o$$

where H_o = Strengh of applied magnetic field

γ = magnetogyric ratio

h = Plank's constant

ν_o = Larmour frequency or precessional frequency

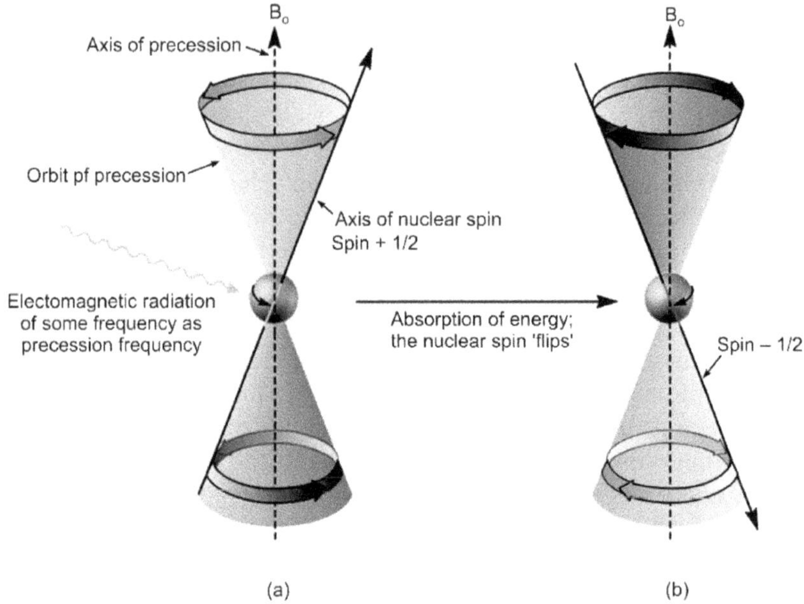

A typical NMR spectrum is shown in the picture. Intensity of the signal obtained is plotted against the applied magneti field.

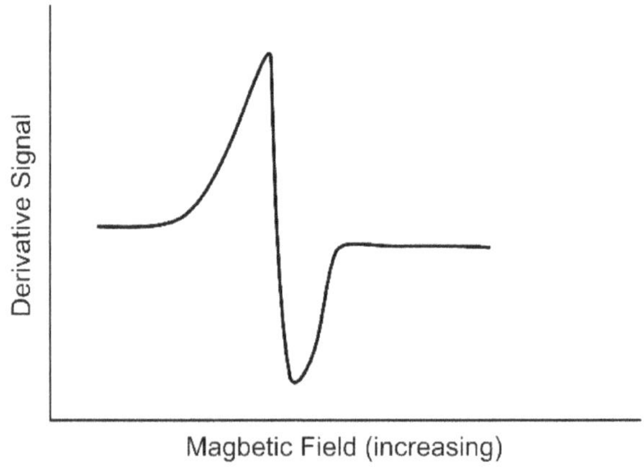

NUMBER OF SIGNALS

Equivalent and Non-Equivalent protons

Equivalent protons are the set of protons in the similar environments. These protons absorb at the same field strengths. These protons are completely interchangeable by an axis or plane of symmetry (enantiomeric protons).E.g. Hydrogen atoms in Methane molecule.

Non- equivalent protons are the protons with different environments. These protons absorb at different applied field strengths.

E.g.: CH_3OH ---- Hydrogens in the CH_3 group are equivalent but the hydrogen in OH is non equivalent.

The different kinds of protons present in the given molecule can be identified by the number of signals in PMR spectrum. (^1H NMR). Each type of proton give rise to one signal.

The number of NMR signals equals the number of different types of protons in a compound

Some examples are given below

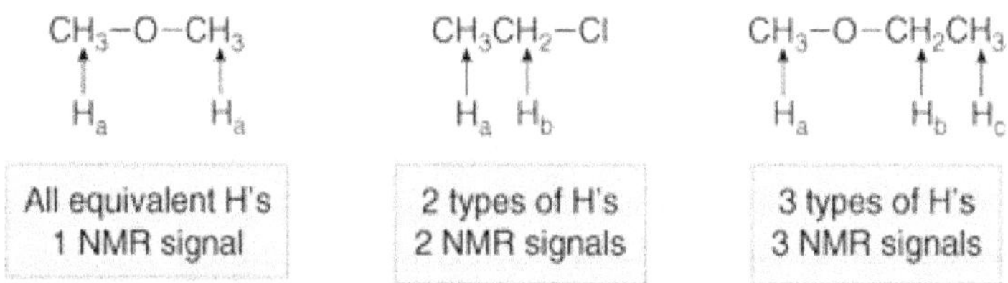

Protons on the same carbon atom can also be non-equivalent. Methyl protons are equivalent (H_a) and they are non-equivalent to other protons (H_b, H_c).

SHIELDING AND DESHIELDING

The nucleus in any atom is surrounded by electrons. When the molecule is placed in a magnetic field, the surrounding electrons (double bond, triple bond, aromatic or any other ring system) circulate and generate counter field which either opposes or reinforces the applied magnetic field.

The actual magnetic field experienced by the proton decreases in conditions like

(i) The proton is present inside the magnetic field produced by the surrounding circulating electrons (secondary field produced by the circulating electrons oppose the direction of applied magnetic field)

(ii) When the proton is closer to an electropositive atom

In these conditions more applied magnetic field is required to cause excitation in the nucleus. These protons are called as shielded protons and the effect is called as shielding effect.

There are two types of shielding

(i) Local Shielding

The shielding effect caused by the magnetic field of the electron density in the immediate vicinity of the protons is called as local shielding.

E.g. Effect of electro negative and electropositive atoms in the vicinity.

(ii) Low range Shielding

The secondary fields produced by the induced circulation of π electrons in aromatic compounds can affect the fields experienced by the nuclei which are not directly associated with the π electrons. This kind of shielding is called Low range shielding.

The actual magnetic field experienced by the proton increases in conditions likes

(i) The proton is present outside the magnetic field produced by the surrounding circulating electrons (secondary field produced by the circulating electrons aligned along the direction of applied magnetic field)

(ii) When the proton is closer to an electronegative atom

In these conditions, lesser applied magnetic field is sufficient to cause excitation in the nucleus. These protons are called as deshielded protons and the effect is called as deshielding effect.

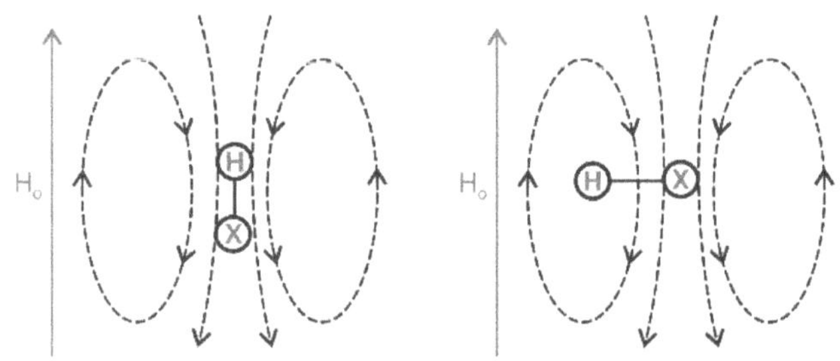

Shielding effect Deshielding effect

Chemical Shift (Position of Signals)

Theoretically, All the protons present in the organic compound should give only one signal in NMR spectrum. But the hydrogen atoms in the molecule are not in the same environment and the applied magnetic field is not felt equally by all the hydrogen atoms uniformly. This is because of the presence of π electrons, aromatic electrons, hetero atoms and electronegative atoms. The different magnetic fields felt by different types of hydrogen atoms make the precessional frequency different for different protons and consequently their excitational frequency also becomes different for each type of proton. Thus each kind of proton gives signal in different positions.

The shift in the position of NMR signal in comparison with a standard reference due to the shielding or deshielding of protons by surrounding electrons is called as Chemical shift.

For measuring chemical shifts of various protons in a molecule, the signal of TMS is taken as reference. TMS is Tetra Methyl Silane $(CH_3)_4$ Si and it is used as internal reference in NMR. The low electro negativity of the Si atom and the shielding of the equivalent protons give one NMR signal which is greater than most of the organic compounds and the signal appears at 0 ppm. A small quantity of TMS is added to the sample while recording PMR spectrum.

The difference in the absorption position of the proton with respect to the TMS signal is called chemical shift and it is denoted by the symbol δ

In organic compounds, protons resonate at lower field than the protons of TMS. The signal of the TMS protons appears at zero δ value at the extreme right side of the spectrum.

The δ values for the protons which absorb at lower field than TMS is given a positive value for δ

$$\text{Chemical shift ppm } \delta = \frac{\text{Shift downfield from TMS (HZ)}}{\text{Spectrophotometer frequency (MHz)}}$$

In terms of frequency

$$\delta_{sample} = \left(\frac{v_{sample} - v_{reference}}{v_{reference}} \right) \times 10^6$$

The value of δ is expressed in ppm units and the values lie between 0 to 10 in δ scale.

An alternative scale used for the measurement of chemical shift is τ scale. In τ scale, signal for reference standard TMS is taken as 10 ppm.

These two scales are related by the expression

$$\tau = 10\text{-}\delta$$

TMS – Tetra Methyl Silane – Internal standard $(CH_3)_4$ Si

Tetra methyl silane is used as the internal reference standard to measure the chemical shifts of different types of protons. TMS gives only one signal. It is called as internal standard because a small quantity is added to the sample during the recording of the spectrum.

The reasons for using TMS as a reference standard are

1. TMS is chemically inert in nature
2. TMS has got 12 equivalent protons and hence give a single intense signal.
3. TMS peak is not interfering with the other compounds.
4. TMS can be easily removed by evaporation (boiling point 300K)
5. Sample recovery is easy
6. It does not take part in intermolecular associations with sample.
7. Its resonance position is far away from absorptions due to protons in most organic molecules, thus signal of TMS = 0 ppm.

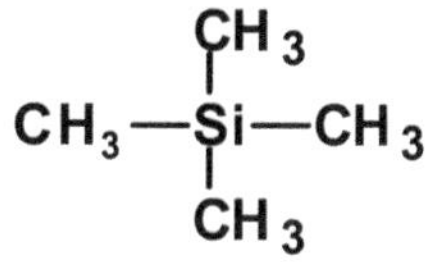

Tetramethylsilane (TMS)

As the electro negativity of silicon is low when compared with carbon (Si- 1, C- 2.5), the equivalent protons are shielded more than most of all the organic compounds. Thus the signal of other organic compounds appears downfield of TMS signal.

TMS is not soluble in aqueous solutions. Hence for water soluble substances, DSS (2,2-methyl)-2-silapentane-5-sulphonate can be used as reference. The protons of DSS give a single signal and the methylene protons of DSS give a series of small peaks which can be ignored.

SOLVENTS USED IN NMR

The NMR spectroscopy is used to study the nature, type, number and environment of protons (Hydrogens) in the sample and hence the solvent used should be **free from Hydrogen atoms.** Therefore solvents like **Carbon tetra chloride (CCl_4), Deutrated chloroform ($CDCl_3$), Deutrated water (D_2O), Deutrated Methanol (CD_3OD), Deutrated Dimethyl Sulphoxide (CD_3) SO, Deutrated acetic acid (CD_3COOD), Deutrated trifluoro acetic acid (CF_3COOD) etc are used.**

Substitution of D for hydrogen in the solvents eliminates the proton signal from the solvent in the spectrum. Deuterium does not give the signal in the same region as the hydrogen nucleus.

Requirements of solvents used in NMR

1. The solvent should be inert
2. It should be magnetically neutral
3. It should be volatile in nature, so that the sample recovery is possible
4. It should not contain hydrogen atoms
5. It should be easily available and inexpensive

Factors affecting Chemical Shift

The factors that influence chemical shift are

A. Intra molecular factors

(i) Inductive effect
(ii) Vanderwaal's shielding
(iii) Anisotropic effect

B. Intermolecular factors

(i) Hydrogen bonding
(ii) Temperature
(iii) Solvents

A. Intra molecular factors

(i) Inductive effect

In shielding, when the molecule is placed in the magnetic field, the induced magnetic field produced by the circulating electrons opposes the applied magnetic field. Thus the shielded protons require more applied field to resonate and this causes the up field shift of the absorption.

The presence of electronegative atoms like **halogens, oxygen and nitrogen, reduce the electron density around the proton due to inductive effect. This makes the protons deshielded and the absorption shifts downfield.**

E.g.: Protons in Dimethyl ether (CH_3OCH_3) give a down field signal than the protons of ethane (CH_3CH_3)

The electro negativity and the proximity of the electronegative atom to the proton dictate the extent of deshielding.

Higher the electro negativity, greater will be the deshielding and thus the **δ** value will also be more.

i.e., F > Cl > Br > I

Eg: The protons of CH_3-F are deshielded more than the protons of CH_3-Cl

In CH_3CH_2Cl, the methylene (CH_2) protons are more deshielded than methyl (CH_3) protons

CH_3-F	CH_3-Cl	CH_3-Br	CH_3-I
δ = 4.26	δ = 3.0	δ = 2.82	δ = 2.16

The electron withdrawing groups reduce the electron density around the proton leading to **deshielding. E.g.: NO_2, COOH.**

The electron releasing group increases the electron density around the proton leading to **shielding. E.g.: alkyl group.**

Hybridization of adjacent atoms

The deshieldingeffect in different types of the protons are given in decreasing order

Aldehyde (SP_2) > Vinylic (SP_2) > Acetylenic (SP) > Allylic (SP_3) > Alkyl (SP_3)

	RCHO >	R2C=CHR $R_2C=CH_2$ >	RC≡CH	> $R_2C=C(R)\ CHR_2$ >	RCH_3, R_2CH_2, R_3CH
δ Values	9.5-10.1	4.6-5.7	2.0-3.0	1.6 -2.6	0.8-1.7

Deshielding → Shielding

The triple bond shields the acetylenic hydrogen and shifts its signal to lower frequency (to the right) to a smaller δ value that is up field shift.

The C-C double bond deshields the vinylic hydrogens and shifts their signal to higher frequency (to the left) to a larger δ value that is downfield shift.

(ii) Vanderwaal's shielding

The presence of bulky groups in a molecule can cause deshielding due to the week Vander Waal's forces and give slightly higher value of **δ** than predicted.

(iii) Anisotropic effect (Space effect)

Anisotropic effect arises due to the orientation of nuclei with respect to the applied magnetic field. Electrons around the nucleus can set up the magnetic field, and the effect of this field on the chemical shift depends upon the spatial arrangements.

Alkene

When an alkene is placed in a magnetic field, the loosely held circulating π electrons of the double bond create a magnetic field in perpendicular direction of circulating electrons. This magnetic field reinforces the applied field in the vicinity of the protons.

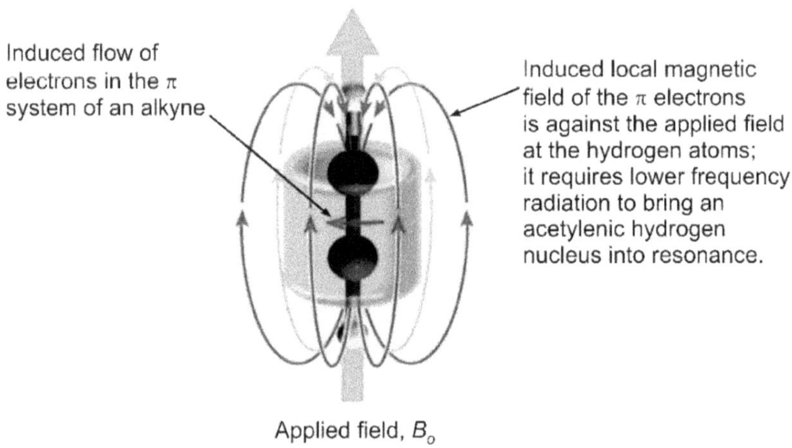

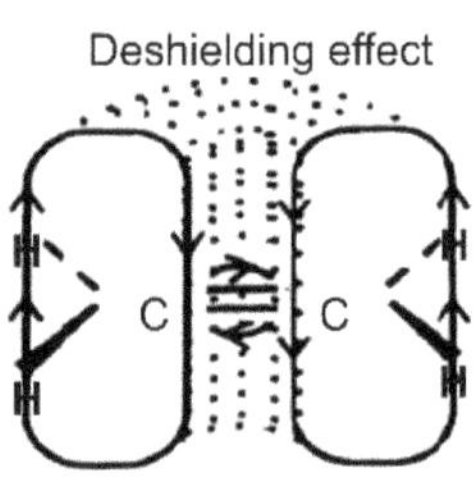

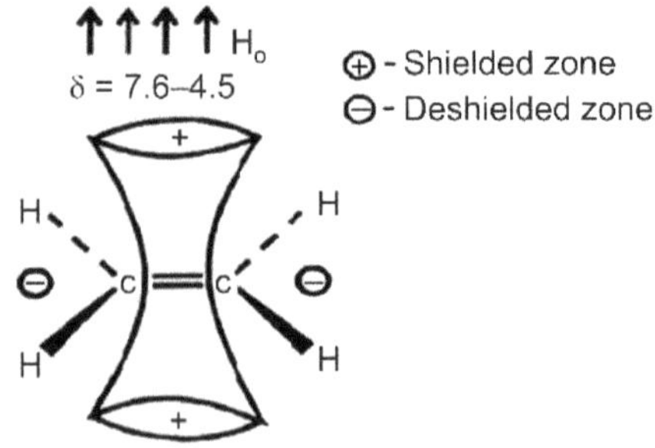

The reinforcement of the magnetic field makes the protons to feel a strong magnetic field and hence the protons require a higher frequency to resonate.

Thus the protons are deshielded and the absorption occurs downfield.

The ethylenic protons are in the deshielded region (4.6-5.7) and the absorption occurs at downfield. Ethyl carbons are in the shielded region

ALKYNE- ACETYLENE

When acetylene molecule is placed in magnetic field, the π electrons of the C≡C triple bond are induced to circulate and the induced magnetic field opposes the applied magnetic field. Hence the proton feels less magnetic field and it requires lower frequency to resonate. Thus the protons are shielded and the absorption occurs up field.

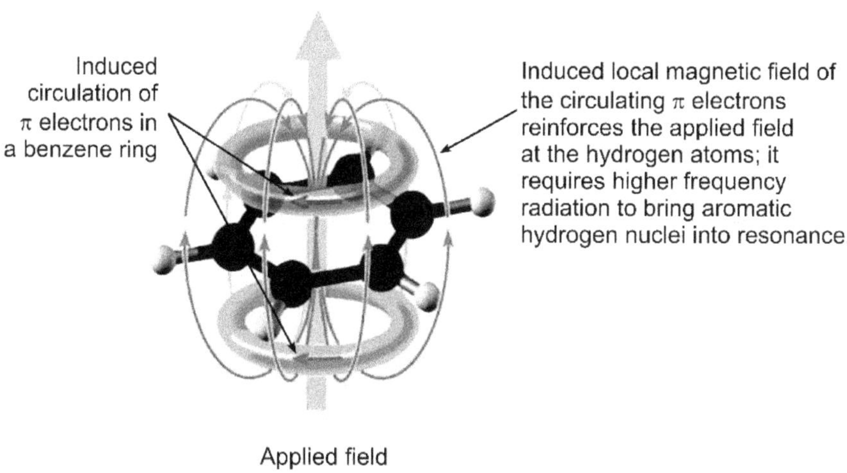

Shielding effect

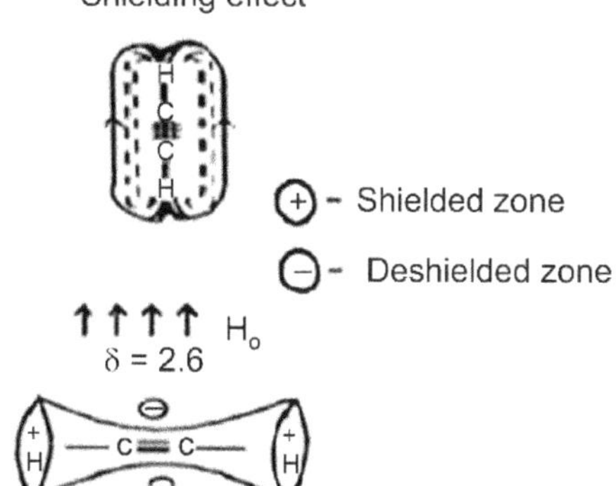

The acetylenic protons are in the shielded region and the protons are resonating at relatively high field (2-3) as compared with ethylenic protons.

BENZENE

The six π electrons in the benzene circulate around the ring creating a ring current when the molecule is placed in magnetic field. The magnetic field induced by these moving electrons reinforces the applied magnetic field in the vicinity of protons. Thus, the protons feel a stronger magnetic field and a higher frequency is needed for resonance. The protons are highly deshielded and absorb downfield when compared to alkenyl protons and acetylenic protons. (6-8.5 δ)

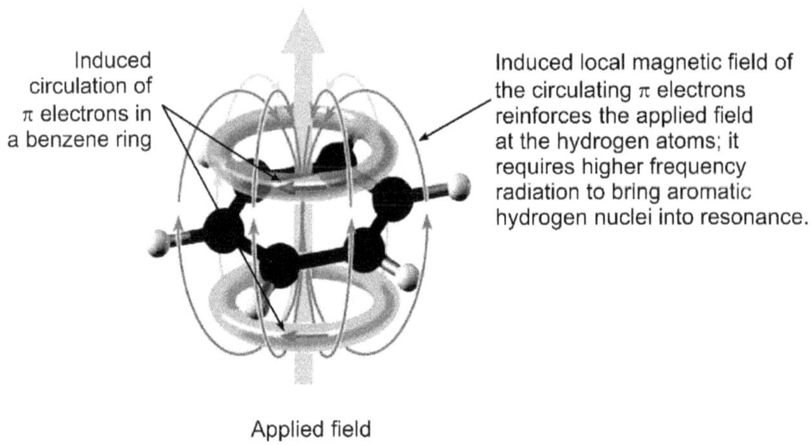

A. Intermolecular factors

(i) Hydrogen Bonding

Intra-molecular hydrogen bonding does not show any change in absorption due to change in concentration. But the hydrogen atom involved in the intermolecular H-bonding shares its electrons with two electronegative elements and as a result it is deshielded and get higher **δ** value that is downfield absorption.

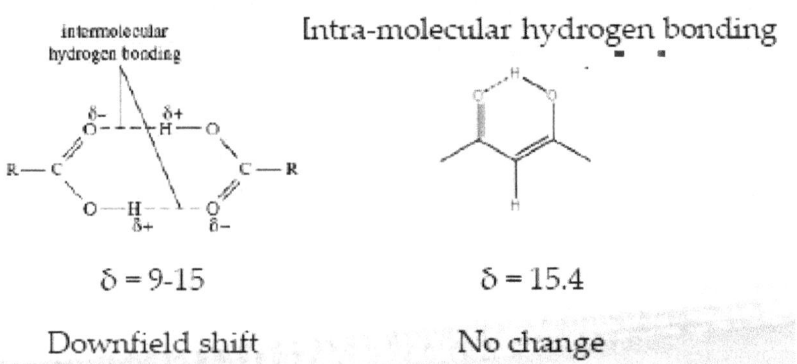

(ii) Temperature

The change in temperature has little effect on Chemical shift.— OH, —NH—, and —SH protons show up field shift at higher temperature.

(iii) Solvents

The solvents used in NMR spectroscopy should be chemically inert, magnetically isotropic, devoid of hydrogen atom and should dissolve the sample to a reasonable extent.
E.g. CCl_4, CS_2, $CDCl_3$ etc.

CHEMICAL SHIFT REAGENTS

These are the reagents that are used to cause shift in the NMR spectra. The amount of shift depends on,

- Distance between the shift reagent and proton
- Concentration of shift reagent.

ADVANTAGES OF SHIFT REAGENTS

- Shift reagents give spectra which are much easier to interpret
- No chemical manipulation of sample is required
- More easily obtained.

Paramagnetic materials can cause chemical shift, e.g., Lanthanides. Complexes of Europium, Erbium, Thallium and Ytterbium shift resonance to lower field. Complexes of Cerium, Neodymium and Terbium shift resonance to higher field.

Europium is the most commonly used metal to cause shift in the NMR spectra. Two of its widely used complexes are, 1. Eu (dpm)3. 2. Eu (fod)3

Regardless of the molecule in which it is present, the proton with a particular environment will have the same chemical shift. Thus the position of signals in the PMR spectrum of compound gives information about the electronic environment of the molecule.

SPIN COUPLING- SPLITTING OF SIGNALS

The number of signals in a NMR spectrum indicates the number of types of protons present in the given sample. Each type of proton gives separate signal. For example; methyl protons (CH_3), methylene protons (CH_2) and methine protons (CH) give different signals in their respective chemical shift values. In certain molecules, instead of a single peak a group of peaks are observed. This phenomenon of splitting of proton signals into two or more sub-peaks are referred as splitting.

Characteristic Chemical Shifts of Common Types of Protons

Type of proton	Chemical shift (ppm)	Type of proton	Chemical shift (ppm)
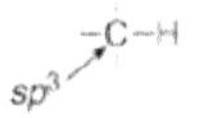	0.9–2	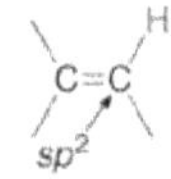	4.5–6
• RCH_3 • R_2CH_2 • R_3CH	~0.9 ~1.3 ~1.7	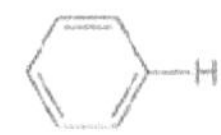	6.5–8
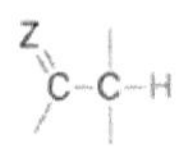 Z = C, O, N	1.5–2.5	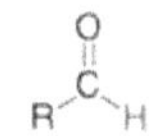	9–10
—C≡C–H	~2.5	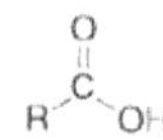	10–12
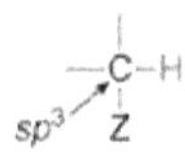 Z = N, O, X	2.5–4	RO–H or R–N–H	1–5

The spins of the neighboring nuclei in a molecule interact with each other causing splitting of signals (peaks) in NMR spectrum. This is called as spin-spin coupling. Coupling occurs through bonds. Coupling is not effective more than three bonds.

Chemically equivalent protons do not show spin-spin coupling due to interaction among themselves. i.e., only the nonequivalent protons show the property of coupling. Spin-spin splitting occurs only between nonequivalent protons on the same carbon or adjacent carbons.

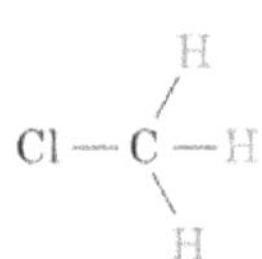

Three C–H protons are chemically equivalent; no splitting occurs.

Nonequivalent protons

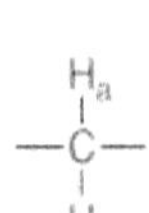

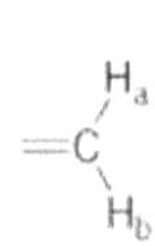

H_a and H_b are on the **same** carbon.

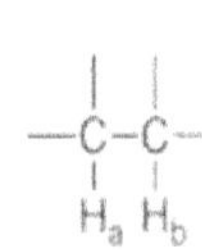

H_a and H_b are on **adjacent** carbons.

To understand the spin spin splitting take the example of 1, 1, 2 tribromo ethane.

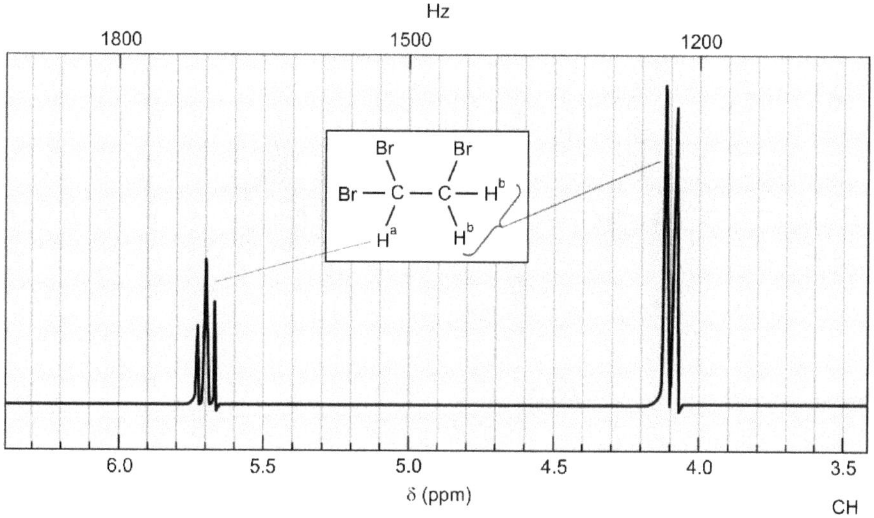

CH Br_2CHCH_2BR

In this molecule two types of protons are present (CH2, CH). So the NMR spectrum is expected to have two peaks one for each type of protons. But practically when the NMR spectrum is recorded, it shows five peaks. Thus it is shown that the signal for each proton is split according to a pattern. This is called as ***splitting of signals***.

The splitting pattern of a given proton can be predicted by the ***n+1* rule**, where ***n*** is the number of equivalent protons on the neighboring carbon.

As per the (n + 1) rule in **1, 1, 2- tribromo ethane**, the methine proton (H_a) has two equivalent protons of Methylene (H_b) on the carbon next to it. Therefore, n = 2 and hence it will split the signal of the methine proton (H_a) into (2+1) = 3 peaks (Triplet).

The Methylene protons are having n = 1 and therefore it will be split into (1+1) = 2 peaks (Doublet).

Thus the methylene protons appear as doublet and the methine proton appears as a triplet. The peak intensities in the doublet are 1:1 and in triple it is 1:2:1.

The simplest multiplicities are **singlet** ($n = 0$), **doublets** ($n = 1$ or coupling to just one proton), **triplets** ($n = 2$), **quartets** ($n = 3$), **quintets** ($n = 4$), **sextets** ($n = 5$) and **septets** ($n = 6$).

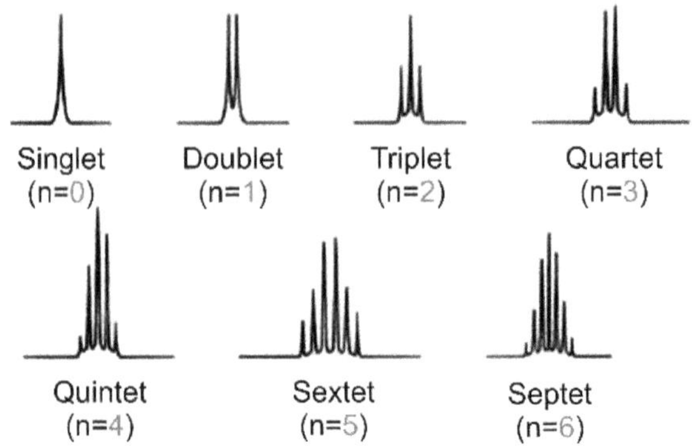

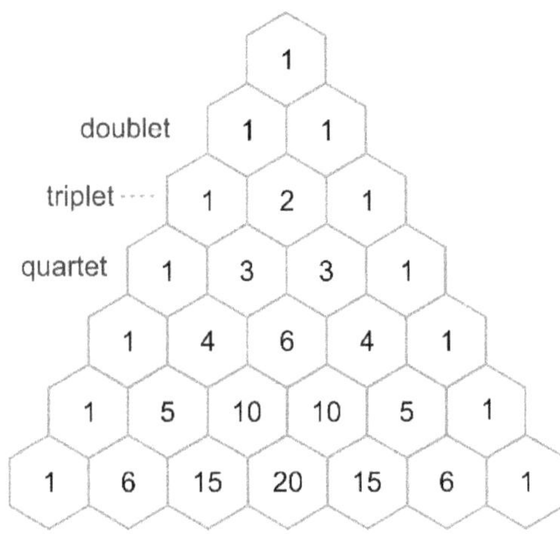

Pascal's Triangle

The intensity of individual peaks can be predicted theoretically using Pascal's triangle.

REASONS FOR SPLITTING

Signal splitting is dependent on the environment of the absorbing proton with respect to the neighboring proton. The actual magnetic field experienced by the given proton is affected by the different spin states of the neighboring protons. This spin spin coupling between the absorbing proton and the neighboring proton is responsible for the splitting of signals in NMR.

In the example

(a) (b)
CH-CH_2

The magnetic field experienced by the secondary protons (b) is influenced by the spin of the neighboring tertiary proton (a). If the spin of the a proton is aligned along the applied magnetic field, the net field experienced by b protons increases and vice versa. At any given moment, half of the tertiary protons (a) will be aligned along the magnetic field and the other half will be aligned against the magnetic field. Thus in half molecules, the (b) protons feel increased field and the other half will feel decreased field, leading to splitting of the signal to peaks called doublet with equal intensities (1:1)

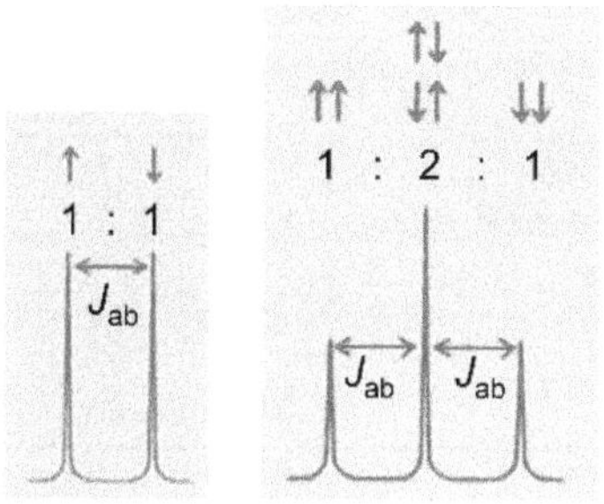

Spin states of (a) proton as felt by b protons
Spin states of (b) protons as felt by (a) proton
(b) Protons –doublet
(a) proton - triplet

The spin states of 2 secondary protons (b) give rise to four possible combinations as show in figure. Two spin alignments are equal. Thus, the three effective combinations, split the signal of tertiary proton (a) and the tertiary protons signal appear as triplet with peak intensities as 1:2:1

COUPLING CONSTANTS

The extent of the splitting effect is given by the distance between the peaks in a multiplet which is called as coupling constant. It is the distance between two adjacent sub-peaks in a split signal. It is denoted by the letter J shown in figure above. The unit of J is Hertz (Hz) or cycles per second (cps). The J values are dependent on the molecular structure and they are independent of applied field strength.

INSTRUMENTATION

The components of NMR spectrophotometer are

(i) Sample holder
(ii) Magnet
(iii) Sweep generator
(iv) Radiofrequency generator
(v) Radiofrequency receiver (RF detector)
(vi) Recorder

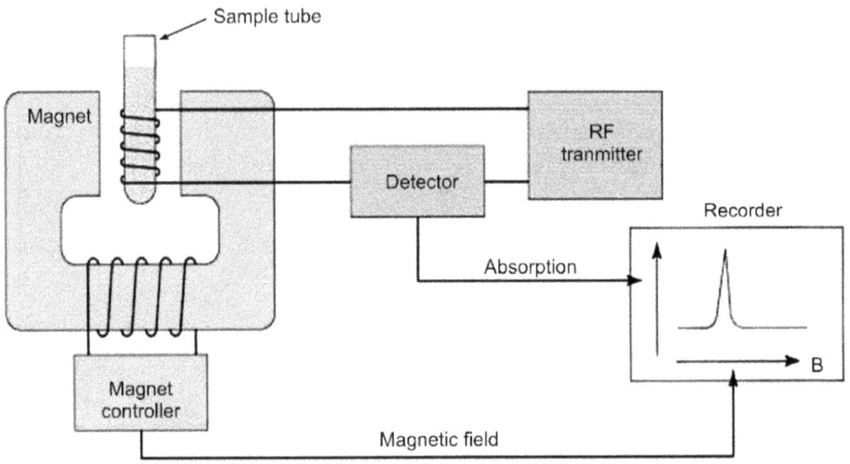

Schematic Diagram of NMR Spectrophotometer

(i) Sample holder

The sample holder should be chemically inert and transparent to RF radiation. Mostly it is a glass tube of about 15 cm long and 5 mm in diameter. The solvent used should not contain hydrogen. A sample size of 1-30 mg in the form of dilute solution (2-10%) is used.

(ii) Magnet

A strong magnet is used which provides a stable and homogenous magnetic field. The magnet is of about 15 inches in diameter and it is capable of producing strong magnetic fields up to 23,500 gauss (G) for a 100 MHz instrument.

Magnetic coils or Helmholtz coils are present in the poles of the magnet to produce secondary magnetic fields reinforcing with the main field in the same direction. These coils are used to vary the magnetic field in Field sweeping.

(iii) Sweep generator

It is used to supply dc current to secondary magnets. Resonance occurs when the precessional frequency of the nucleus matches with the applied RF frequency. This can be achieved by two methods

1. **Frequency sweep method**

   Applied magnetic field H_0 is kept constant, and hence the precessional frequency of the nucleus is fixed. The R_f frequency is varied to match the precessional frequency, so that resonance is achieved.

2. **Field Sweep method**

   In this method the RF frequency is kept constant and the magnetic field H_0 is varied using helmhaltz coils. This is the easier and most commonly used method.

(iv) Radiofrequency generator

The radiofrequency oscillator used is installed perpendicular to the magnetic field by wounding around the sample holder. It transmits radio waves of frequencies in the range of 60,100,200 and 300MHz.

(v) Radiofrequency receiver (RF detector)

The RF detector is installed perpendicular to the magnetic field and oscillator coil. It is tuned to same frequency as transmitter coil. When the precessional frequency matches with the RF frequency, the nuclei resonate and it induces an emf in detector. This signal is amplified and recorded.

(vi) Recorder

It records the signal after amplification and gives the spectrum as a plot of signal strength in y-axis and magnetic field strength in x-axis. The intensity of the signal produced is directly proportional to the number of nuclei resonating at that particular field strength.

Applications of NMR

1. NMR is used in structural diagnosis. It gives information about number, nature of protons and possible arrangement of groups in a molecule.
2. Identification of Organic compounds
3. It is used to determine the molar ratio of the components of a mixture
4. NMR is useful in study of hydrogen bonding in organic compounds.
5. It is used in structure determination of complexes
6. Used in the study of Keto-enol tautomerism
7. It is helpful to study intra molecular conversion
8. Used to evaluate exchange effect
9. Determination of activation energy
10. NMR is also used in elemental analysis, to study rate of reactions, to differentiate cis-trans isomerism and detection of aromaticity.

ESR SPECTROSCOPY

Electron spin resonance (ESR) spectroscopy is a type of absorption spectroscopy in which the paramagnetic substances absorb microwave frequency radiation to undergo electronic transitions (spin changes) between magnetic energy levels.

ESR is also called electron paramagnetic resonance (EPR) and Electron magnetic resonance (EMR).

Comparison between ESR and NMR

S.No	NMR	ESR
1.	Magnetic resonance Phenomenon is observed in Nucleus.	Magnetic resonance Phenomenon is observed in electrons
2	Radiofrequency (300-1000 MHz) is used to cause spin changes in the nucleus	Radiofrequency (3-400 GHz) is used to cause spin changes in electrons
3	Applicable to both paramagnetic and diamagnetic substances	Applicable only to molecules with unpaired electrons (paramagnetic).
4	Used for the study of nature and the number of protons/carbon in molecules	Used for organic/inorganic substances, free radicals, ions of transition metals, rare earth elements, and molecules like NO, O_2, and NO_2
5.	The magnetic field is held constant and the radio frequency is varied. (Frequency sweep)	Frequency is held constant and the magnetic field is varied. (Field sweep)

Substances that can be studied using ESR

1. The molecules with unpaired electrons such as paramagnetic substances – (stable) molecules like NO, O_2, and NO_2 ions of transition and rare earth metals.
2. Free radicals or radical ions:-These are unstable entities produced as intermediates in chemical reactions. If the lifetime of these free radicals is greater than 10^{-6} sec, they can be studied by ESR or their lifetime can be prolonged using the matrix technique (low temperature in solid-state) and then studied.

Theory

ESR spectra can be applied only to molecules having unpaired electrons. For an electron having a spin of s=1/2, in the absence of the magnetic field, the spin quantum numbers +1/2 and -1/2 will have doubly degenerate (equal) spin energy states. On application of a magnetic field,

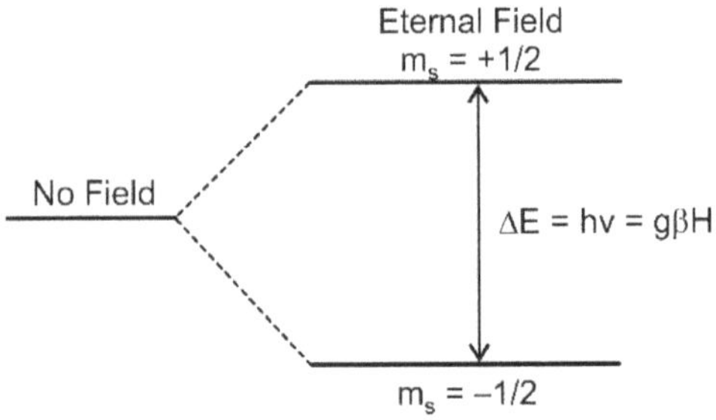

the degeneracy is removed and two non-degenerate (unequal) spin energy states are created, similar to NMR (Nuclear spin energy states).

In a lower energy state, the spin energy state (magnetic moment is aligned along the field and the quantum number is m_s=-1/2. The high energy state corresponds to the quantum number m_s=+1/2 and the magnetic moment opposes the applied magnetic field. The two energy levels will have energy that is split up from the original energy state (absence of magnetic field).

The transition from the ground state (-1/2) to the excited state (+1/2) occurs by the absorption in the microwave frequency region. The microwave frequency range used in ESR is 9500MHz to 35,000MHz. The magnetic field strength is 500- 3400 gauss. The energy of transition

$$\Delta E = h\nu = g\beta H$$

where

H-applied magnetic field

ν -frequency of absorbed radiation in cycles/sec

g- Proportionality factor called Lande's splitting factor or spectroscopic splitting factor. This g value gives an idea about electron's environment.

$g = g_{std}(1-\Delta H/H)$, where H – resonance frequency used, ΔH-Field separation between the standard and sample, g_{std} –g value of the internal standard.

β- Bohr's magneton factor,

$$\beta = eh/4\pi mc$$

where e - electronic charge
m - Mass of electron
c - Velocity of light
h - Planck's constant

INSTRUMENTATION

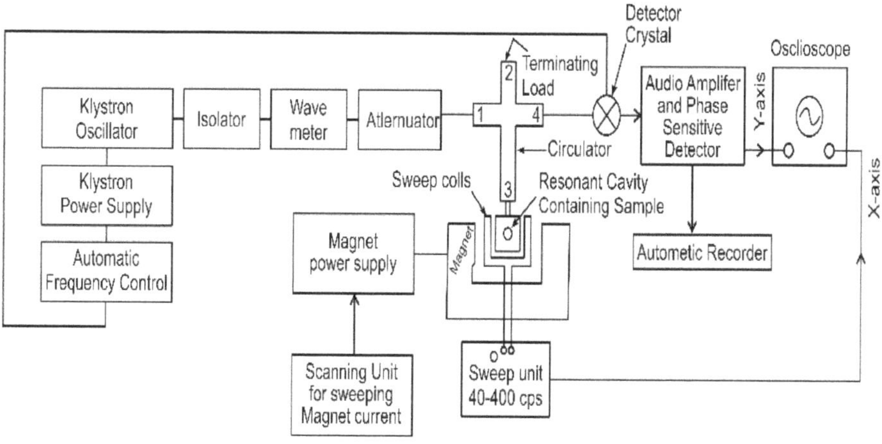

Block diagram of a typical ESR spectrometer

The various components of ESR Spectrometer are

1. **Source**
2. **Circulator or Magic T**
3. **Sample cavity**

4. **Magnet system**
5. **Crystal detector**
6. **Amplifier and Phase sensitive detector**
7. **Oscilloscope and recorder.**

1. **Source**

   The different components of source in ESR are

   (i) **Klystron**

   A klystron oscillator is a vacuum tube that produces microwave oscillation in the frequency region determined by the applied voltage. Generally, it operates at a frequency of 9500 MHz.

   (ii) **Isolator**

   It is a strip of ferrite material and a non-reciprocal device. It minimizes the vibrations in the microwave frequency produced by klystron. It isolates the narrow range of microwave frequency.

   (iii) **Wave meter**

   It is placed between Isolator and attenuator. The wavemeter identifies the frequency of microwaves produced by the klystron oscillator. It is calibrated in frequency units (MHz) instead of wavelength.

   (iv) **Attenuator**

   It controls the amount of incident radiation incident upon the sample. It is similar to a filter in spectrophotometers. The attenuator is placed between and circulator.

2. **Circulator or Magic T**

   After passing through the isolator, wave meter, and attenuator the microwave radiations from the klystron enter into the circulator through a waveguide. This waveguide is coupled with the magnetic field by a loop of wire and this sets up a corresponding field in the waveguide.

   The waveguide is a hollow rectangular copper or brass tube with silver or gold plating inside.

   In the four-arm circulator, the microwave radiations enter through arm 1 to arm 3 which is connected to the resonant cavity, and sample Arm 2 has a terminating load to absorb the radiation reflected from arm 4 connected to the detector.

3. **Sample cavity**

   It is the resonant cavity containing the sample and it forms the heart of the ESR spectrometer. The sample cells are flat with a thickness of 0.25 mm and a sample volume of 0.05 ml- 0.5 ml is generally used. Dual sample cavities are also used for both sample and reference. The sample can be gas, liquid, or solid. The solvents used should have a low dielectric constant. Frequency sweep coils are mounted inside the sample cavity. The concentration of the sample should be 10^{-9}M. Water, alcohol, and solvents with high dielectric constant cannot be used as they absorb microwaves strongly. Examples of solvents that can be used in ESR are Glycerol, toluene, Triethanolamine, Nujol, etc.

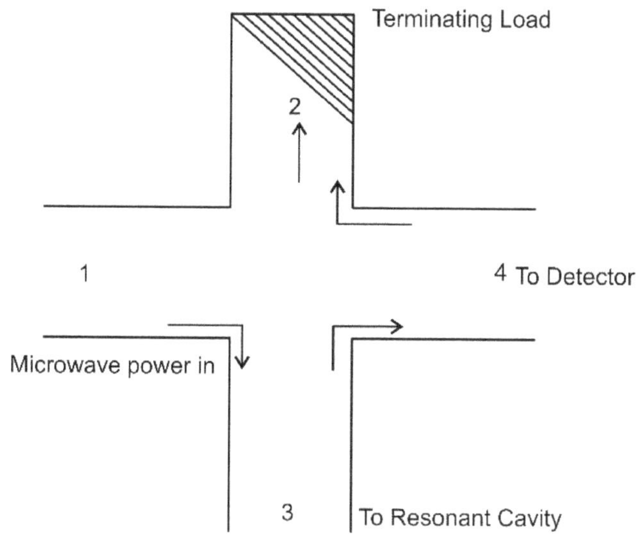

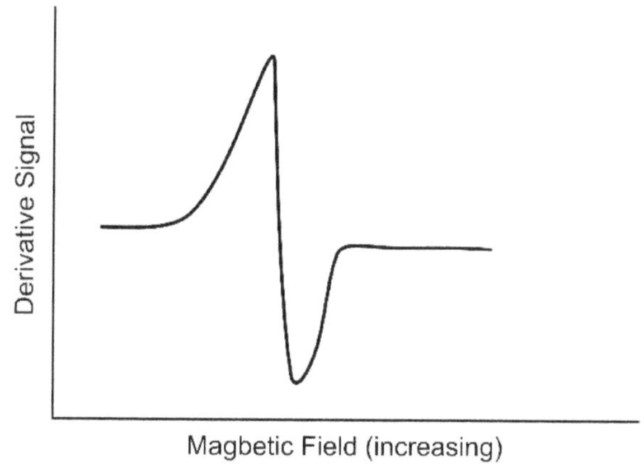

A typical ESR spectrum

4. **Magnet system**

   The magnetic field can be varied from 0-500 gauss/0-3400 gauss. For sweeping magnetic fields, sweep coils are used.

5. **Crystal detectors**

   Silicon crystal is the most commonly used detector and this crystal acts as a microwave rectifier. The microwave frequency is converted to DC output by this crystal.

6. **Amplifier and Phase sensitive detector**
   The signal detected by the crystal detector is amplified by the amplifier. The noise components of the amplified signal are rejected and the narrow band of the signal is separated by the phase-sensitive detector.
7. **Oscilloscope and Recorder**
   The signal from the phase-sensitive detector is recorded by an oscilloscope or pen recorder.

Working of ESR

1. The sample is placed in the resonant cavity which is a long path-length cell and the waves are reflected to and fro more than a thousand times in the cavity.
2. The klystron oscillator produces microwaves.
3. These waves after passing through the isolator, wavemeter, and attenuator reach the arms of the circulator.
4. The microwaves entering through arm 1 divide themselves between arm 2 and arm 3.
5. Arm 2 contains the balancing load.
6. If there is no sample in the resonant cavity, the impedance of arm 2 and arm 3 will be the same, the microwaves are absorbed completely and no power is received by the detector in arm 4.
7. If there is a sample in the resonant cavity, it will absorb some microwave radiation, which causes a change in the impedance of arm 3 and some quantity of microwave energy reaches the detector arm 4.
8. The detector is the rectifier which converts the microwave energy falling on it to direct current
9. When the magnetic current is equal to the resonance frequency, the signal will appear as an absorption peak.
10. By making the magnetic field sweep slowly over a period of several minutes, the derivative spectrum against the magnetic field can be recorded.

Due to the interferences of the noise from the instrument, the ESR spectrum is generally recorded as the first derivative spectrum.

Hyperfine splitting

It is the interaction between the spinning electrons and the adjacent spinning magnetic nuclei. The number of splittings is given as (2nI+1) where n- is the number of equivalent nuclei interacting magnetically with the electron, and I –spin quantum number of the nuclei.

For example, consider one hydrogen atom having one electron and one proton and the I value is equal to ½ for the proton. Using the formula 2nI+1 =(2x1x1/2)+1 =1+1 =2.

Thus the ESR spectrum of hydrogen consists of two peaks.

Reference standard

To determine the g –value of an unknown substance, a reference substance of known g-value is used in ESR. In most cases, DPPH is used as the standard and its g value is 2.0036. The reference is placed along with the unknown substance in the dual cavity cell. Two signals appear in the ESR spectrum with a field separation of ΔH. The g value is calculated using the formula

$G = g_s\left(1-\frac{\Delta H}{H}\right)$ where H is the resonance frequency

ESR spectrum

The information obtained from the ESR spectrum is

1. It gives information on the location of unpaired electrons
2. The type and number of neighborhood nuclei of the odd electron are given by the number of line components.
3. The total number of free electrons in the sample can be evaluated by the addition of intensities of spectral lines. Relative intensities give the type of nuclei splitting the spectrum.

Applications of ESR spectroscopy

1. **Study of free radicals** – Free radicals can be detected even in low concentrations. The structure of organic and inorganic free radicals can be determined.
2. Structural elucidation of organic and inorganic molecules including the shape of radicals.
3. Determination of reaction velocities and mechanism.
4. Study of biological systems such as leaves, seeds, and tissue preparations.
5. Miscellaneous application
   (i) Action of semiconductor
   (ii) To study conduction electrons in solutions of alkali metals
   (iii) To study complexes of copper, Nickel, cobalt, and sodium with malenonitriledithiolate.
   (iv) To study the oxidation state of metal ions in complexes.
6. Quantitative analysis

   It is carried out using a dual sample cavity. Reference standard like DPPH and Peroxylamine disulphonate are used.

CHAPTER 30

Mass Spectroscopy

It is a spectroscopic technique that can provide information on the molecular structure of organic and inorganic compounds. Mass spectroscopy can be used to determine molecular weight directly. In this technique, the analyte is bombarded with a beam of electrons to produce molecular ions and ionic fragments. The resulting ions are then separated based on their masses. It is one of the important qualitative analytical tools for the study of organic substances.

THEORY

There are two steps involved in mass spectroscopy. In the first step, the neutral molecule is converted to positively charged ions. In the second step, the ions are separated based on their masses using an electrical field or magnetic field or both.

A molecule M is bombarded with electron e

$$M + e^- \rightarrow M^+ + 2e^-$$

M^+ - ionised molecule, e- electron

The ions are accelerated in an electric field at voltage V.

The energy of each particle is eV and this is equal to the kinetic energy $\frac{1}{2}mv^2$

$$\frac{1}{2}mv^2 = eV \quad .....(30.1)$$

$$V^2 = \frac{2eV}{m} \quad .....(30.2)$$

$$v = \sqrt{2eV}/m \quad .....(30.3)$$

Where v is the velocity of the particle, m is the mass of the particle, e is the charge on the electron and V is the accelerating voltage.

The energy eV and kinetic energy of all particles are the same.

It can be written as

$$\frac{1}{2}m_1v_1^2 = \frac{1}{2}m_2v_2^2 = \frac{1}{2}m_3v_3^2 = \qquad .....(30.4)$$

Where m_1, m_2, and m_3 are the mass of different particles and v_1, v_2, and v_3 are the velocities of respective particles.

From the equation (30.4), it is understood that the velocity of particles varies with the mass of the particles.

After acceleration by the applied voltage, the particles pass through a magnetic field H for size separation. In this field, the particles move in a circle due to the attractive force of the magnetic field. This attraction is Hev, and the balancing centrifugal force is mv^2/r. When the particle moves uniformly around the circular path, both forces are equal.

$$\frac{Mv2}{r} = Hev \qquad .....(30.5)$$

$$\frac{1}{r} = Hev/mv^2$$

$$r = \frac{mv}{eH} \qquad .....(30.6)$$

Where r- radius of the circular path.

Substituting equation (30.6) in equation (30.3)

$$r = \frac{m}{eH}(2eV/m)^{½} \qquad .....(30.7)$$

Squaring on both sides

$$r^2 = m^2/e^2H^2\ (2eV/m) = m/e\ (2V/H^2) \qquad .....(30.8)$$

$$r = [(2V/H^2)\ (m/e)]^{1/2} \qquad .....(30.9)$$

From the equation (30.9), it follows that the radius of the circular path of particles depends on Voltage V, Magnetic field H and m/e. As e, V and H are constants, it shows that r is dependent on mass m. This equation forms the mathematical basis of Mass spectrometry.

COMPONENTS OF MASS SPECTROMETER

1. The inlet system
2. Ion source (ionisation chamber)
3. Electrostatic accelerating system
4. The magnetic field
5. The ion separator (mass analyzer)
6. The ion collector (detector)
7. The vacuum system

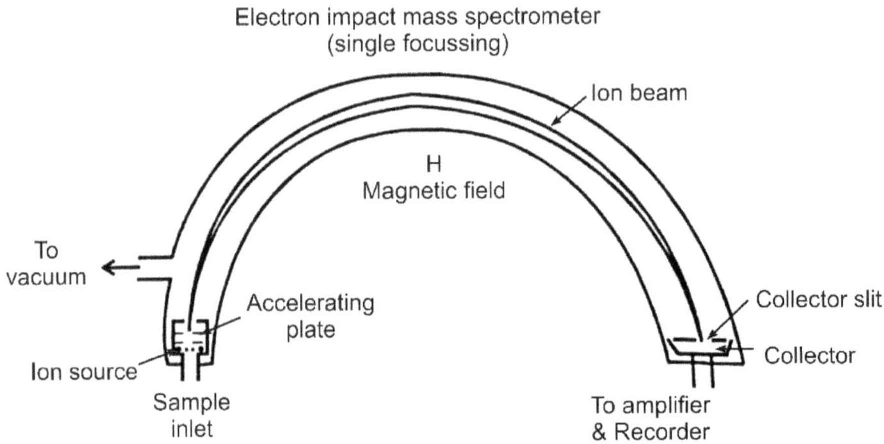

180°mass spectrophotometer (single focussing EI mass spectrometer)

Single focusing EI mass spectrometer is a horseshoe-shaped glass tube. A vacuum is applied to the tube. The instrument contains the sample inlet, electron gun and accelerating plates on one side and the collector slit is situated on the other end. The electric and magnetic fields are applied at the curvature of the tube.

The sample is introduced into the sample inlet where it is converted to a vapour state and is bombarded with an electron beam of 70 eV. Positively charged ions are formed by the knocking out of one electron due to this bombardment of the sample molecules by fast-moving electrons. The ions are accelerated by the accelerating plates and travel in a straight path. The application of a magnetic field deflects the path of the ions and they are separated based on their masses. The separated ions are collected by an ion collector and detected by the detectors.

1. **The Sample Inlet system**

   The sample is converted to a gaseous state in the inlet system. The sample inlet system is heated. The sample size is usually 1 micromole. The sample may be a gaseous sample or a liquid sample. Gases are simply allowed to leak into the reservoir and the liquids are introduced using hypodermic needle injection.

2. **Ion source (ionisation chamber)**

   The sample in the vapour form is introduced into the ionisation chamber. As the sample vapours enter the chamber, it is bombarded by fast-moving electrons of 70eV emitted by an electron gun. It is an electrically heated filament which emits electrons and they are attracted by the anode. The electron gun is situated perpendicular to the sample vapour flow path. The collision of the sample molecules by electrons results in the formation of positive ions. Different mass spectrophotometers make use of different ionisation techniques. There are various ionisation techniques used are

$$M + e^- \longrightarrow M^+ + 2e^-$$

Based on the nature of the substance and the method by which ions are generated the ion sources are classified as

- Gas Phase Sources.
  Electron Impact Ionization (EI).
  Chemical Ionization (CI).
  Field Ionizations (FI).
- Desorption Sources.
  Field Desorption (FD).
  Electrospray Ionization (ESI).
  Matrix-assisted Laser desorption Ionisation (MALDI).
  Plasma desorption (PD).
  Fast Atom Bombardment (FAB).
  Thermo spray Ionization (TS).
  Secondary Ion Mass Spectrometry (SIMS).

3. **Electrostatic accelerating systems**

   The positive ions are repelled away from the positive ionization chamber and pass through three slits with voltage in decreasing order which are called accelerating plates. The middle plate carries some intermediate voltage and the final at '0' volts. All the ions are accelerated into a finely focused beam. The ions come out of the accelerating system as an accelerated collimated ribbon of ions

4. **The Magnetic field**

   The accelerated collimated ribbon of ions from the electrical field enters the magnetic field. The magnetic field deflects the straight path of the ions into a curved path. The radius of the curved path is dependent on the mass m, accelerating voltage V and the change in the ion (e) and the strength of the magnetic field H.

5. **The ion separator (Mass Analyzer)**

   The mass analyzer separates the ions according to their masses. The different mass analyzers are
   Magnetic Sector Analyzer (MSA)
   Quadrupole Analyzer (Q)
   Time-of-Flight Analyzer (TOF)
   Ion Trap Mass Analyzer (QSTAR)
   Ion Cyclotron Resonance (FT-ICR)
   Orbitrap Mass Analyser (OTA)

6. **The ion collectors (detector)**

   These are the detectors used in mass spectrophotometers. The different detectors used in mass spectrophotometers are photographic plates, Faraday cylinders and PMT detectors.

RECORDING OF A MASS SPECTRUM

The sample is introduced into the ionization chamber. The positive ions are formed and they are accelerated into the magnetic field by applying accelerating voltage V to the accelerating plates. The particles with the lowest mass no will be deflected by the magnetic field. The ions formed are separated based on their m/e values by the analysers and the separated ions are collected by the detector

The mass spectrum is a graph in which the relative abundance is plotted in the ordinate and the m/e ratio in the abscissa.

Fig mass spectrum of ethanol

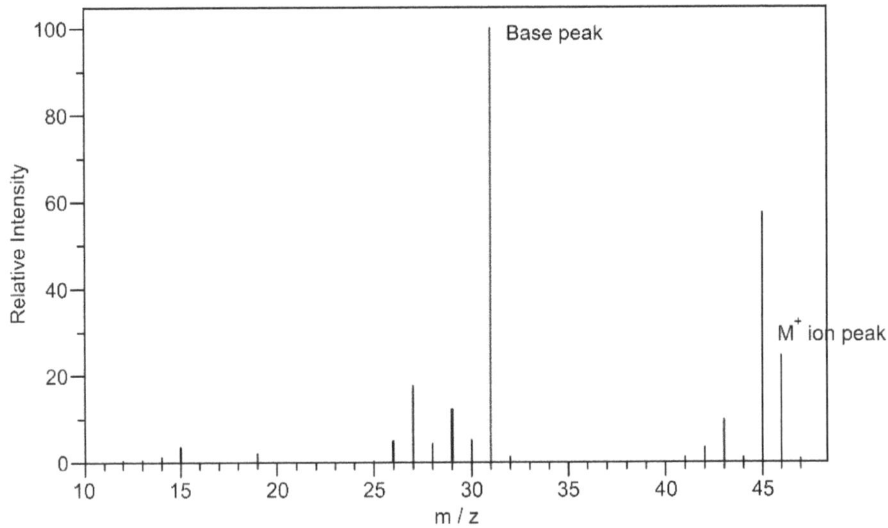

Types of ions produced in Mass spectrometer.

1. **Molecular ion or parent peak**

   These ions are called M^+ ion peaks. The loss of a single electron from the molecule produces a molecular ion. The peak with the highest m/e value is called the molecular ion peak. The m/e value of this peak corresponds to the molecular weight of the compound.

2. **Base peak**

   The peak with the highest relative abundance (100%) is called as base peak.

3. **M+1 Peak**

   These peaks appear at one value of m/e above the molecular ion peak in the mass spectrum. M+1 peaks are due to isotopes like ^{13}C, ^{2}H, ^{15}N & ^{33}S

4. **M+2 Peak**

   These peaks appear two values above the molecular ion peak. M+2 peaks appear in the spectrum if the sample contains isotopes like ^{18}O, ^{34}S, ^{37}Cl and ^{81}Br.

5. **Fragment ions**

   These ions are formed by the further fragmentation of the M^+ ions. The excess energy left in the molecular ion results in fragmentation leading to the formation of fragment ions.

6. **Rearrangement of ions**

   These ions are formed by the rearrangement of atoms in the fragments. These ions are not a fragment of the original molecules.

7. **Multiply charged ions**

   The usual ions formed in a mass spectrometer are singly charged ions. Sometimes doubly or triply charged ions are formed and these are the multiply charged ions. This type of ion is more common in hetero aromatics.

8. **Negative ions**

   These ions are formed rarely in the mass spectrophotometer

9. **Meta-stable ions**

   Meta-stable ions are formed due to the decomposition of an ion during the passage between the source and detector in the spectrometer. Meta-stable ions appear as a weak-intensity broad peak at non–integral mass numbers.

APPLICATION OF MASS SPECTROMETRY

1. **Molecular weight determination**

   The M^+ ion peak in the mass spectrum gives the molecular weight of the sample. The highest m/e value corresponds to the molecular weight of the sample.

2. **Isotopic abundance**

   A mass spectrophotometer is used to determine the isotopic abundance of easily vaporizable elements.

3. **Isotopic dilution method**

   This method is used to determine the amount of a component of a complicated mixture.

4. **Qualitative analysis**

   The intensity of peaks corresponds to the proportion of fragments. Quantitative estimation can be carried out by comparison with a standard.

5. **Detection of cis-trans isomerism**
6. **Evaluation of heat of sublimation**
7. **To determine the ionization potential**
8. **Impurity detection**
9. **Identification of unknown compound**
10. **Reaction kinetics studies**
11. **Reaction mechanism studies**
12. **Latent heat of vaporization of liquids**
13. **Determination of bond dissociation energies**
14. **To get information on bonding**
15. **Characterization of polymers.**

CHAPTER 31

Polarimetry

Polarimetry is a non-destructive sensitive technique used for the measurement of optical activity exhibited by organic and inorganic compounds. Optical activity is the ability of certain substances to rotate the plane of polarized light. For example, sugar and quartz crystals. Substances that rotate the plane of polarized light towards the right side (clockwise) are called dextrorotatory (+) while substances that rotate the plane of polarized light towards the left side are called Levorotatory. A mixture of the sample containing both forms in equal proportions is called racemic modification and it is optically inactive.

The magnitude of rotation depends upon the following factors

(i) Nature of the substance

(ii) The path length of light (l)

(iii) Concentration

(iv) Temperature

(v) Nature of solvent

(vi) The wavelength of light used.

The rotation of the substance is expressed as specific rotation $(\alpha)^{+}{}_{D}$. Specific rotation is defined as the number of degrees of rotation of plane-polarized light produced by 1 decimeter length of the solution with one gram of substance/ml.

$$(\alpha)^{+}{}_{\lambda} = \frac{100x\theta}{lxc}$$

where,

λ- wavelength- length in decimeters,

θ - the angle of rotation observed,

c- concentration in gms /100ml of the solution.

Optical rotation is usually measured with sodium D light. Specific rotation varies with concentration and temperature.

The sample should possess the following characteristics to be analyzed by polarimetry

1. Sample should be optically active
2. Sample must have asymmetric carbon (chiral center).
3. The structure should be non-superimposable on its mirror image.

To be optically active, the molecule **should not possess** any of the following symmetry elements.

(i) Centre of symmetry
(ii) Plane of symmetry
(iii) Axis of symmetry

INSTRUMENTATION

The compounds with the ability to rotate the plane of polarized light are called optically active compounds. This property is called optical activity. The optical activity of the compound is measured by a polarimeter.

COMPONENTS OF POLARIMETER

The following components are present in Polarimeter

(i) Light source – sodium vapor lamp
(ii) Polarizer – Quartz or Nicol prism
(iii) Polarimeter sample tube – Glass tube
(iv) Analyzer – Nicol prism
(v) Circular scale – to measure the rotation angle.

The polarimeter is made of two Nicol prisms, a polarizer, and an analyzer. The polarizer is fixed and the analyzer is rotatable.

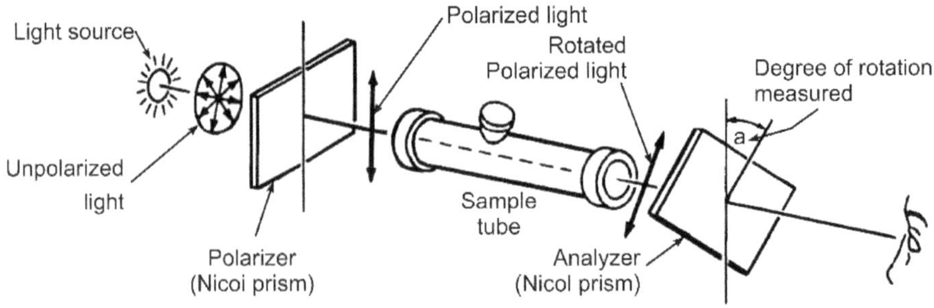

WORKING

The light from the source passes through the polarizer which allows only the light vibrating in one plane to pass through it. Thus, the light becomes plane-polarized. When the position of the analyzer is the same as the polarizer, the light from the polarizer passes through it. The field in the eyepiece looks illuminated. When the analyzer is rotated through the right angle, no light is passing through it and the field in the view becomes dark. Now, the sample tube containing the optically active sample solution is placed between the polarizer and the analyzer. The sample rotates the plane of polarization of light and the field of view is illuminated again. The analyzer is rotated again to get a dark view. The angle through which the analyzer is rotated to get a dark view is noted in a circular scale. This gives the angle of rotation (θ).

OPTICAL ROTATORY DISPERSION

Natural light is made of two components (electrical and magnetic). Both are perpendicular to each other and these two components are perpendicular to the direction of propagation of the wave. The electrical component is made up of two component vectors called left (E_L) and right (E_R) circularly polarized light.

In an ordinary medium, the electrical vector E is confined to the single plane because the E_L and E_R both have the same speed. But in an optically active medium, E_L and E_R rotate at different speeds, making an angle α with the original plane of E, though the light is plane polarized.

The refractive index n of the medium is different for the left and right circularly polarized light, $n_L \neq n_R$, leading to different speeds of rotation. The difference in the refractive indices of RCPL (Right circularly polarized light) and (Left circularly polarized light) LCPL is known as circular birefringence. The medium is said to be birefringent and the angle of rotation α is

$$\alpha = \frac{1800}{\lambda}(n_L - n_R)$$

where λ is the wavelength of incident light.

It is known that [α]= (αx100)/l x C, where α is specific rotation in degrees, l is path length in decimeters, and C is concentration in gms/100ml

$$\textbf{Molar rotation } [\phi] = \frac{(\alpha)M}{100}$$

where M is the molecular weight of the optically active compound.

The change in optical rotation with the wavelength is called as optical rotatory dispersion (ORD). It is defined as the rate of change of specific rotation with a change in wavelength. ORD is used in the structural determination of compounds.

When plane-polarized light is passed through an optically active compound, due to the circular birefringence of the medium, the RCPL and LCPL travel with an unequal rate of propagation. This results in deviation of plane-polarized light leading to optical rotation.

ORD CURVES

It is a plot of specific rotation x10^{-2} against wavelength λ. ORD is dependent on the refractive index.

A plain ORD curve has no maxima or minima. It is an ORD curve of a chiral compound without chromophore. Chiral compounds with chromophores give anomalous or cotton effect curves.

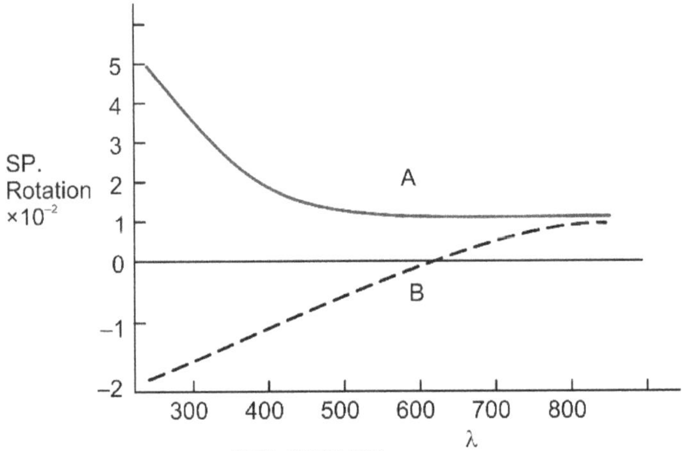

ORD CURVES

Curve A – Specific rotation increases with a decrease in wavelength (plain positive curve)
Curve B- Specific rotation decreases with an increase in wavelength (plain negative curve)

INSTRUMENTS

The instruments used for Optical rotatory dispersion are Polarimeter and a spectropolarimeter. In spectropolarimeters, monochromators are placed before Polarizer. The detector used is PMT detector.

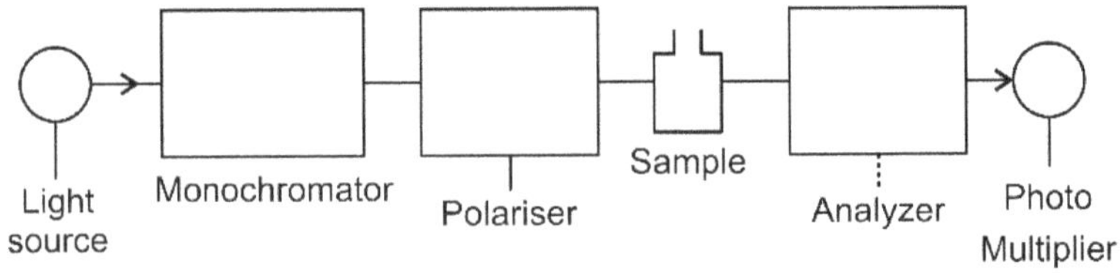

Diagram of the optical components of a spectropolrimeter

CIRCULAR DICHROISM

Apart from the unequal rate of propagation in a birefringent medium, E_L and E_R also exhibit **different absorption coefficients.** Due to this differential absorption of light, the magnitude of E_L is not equal to the magnitude of E_R and it changes the circularly polarized light to elliptically polarized light.

The difference between the absorption of left and right circularly polarized light is measured as a function of wavelength. If the sample contains a chiral chromophore, then one CPL will be absorbed greater than the other CPL.

Circular dichroism (CD) is the difference in the absorption of left-handed circularly polarized light (L-CPL) and right-handed circularly polarized light (R-CPL) and occurs when a molecule contains one or more chiral chromophore (light-absorbing groups).

Circular dichroism = ΔA (λ) = A(λ)LCPL - A(λ)RCPL

where λ is the wavelength

The difference between the absorption of left and right-handed circularly polarized light is measured as a function of wavelength. CD is measured as a quantity called mean residue ellipticity and its unit is degrees-cm^2/dmol.

A CD signal can be positive or negative depending on which CPL is absorbed more. If LCPL is absorbed more than RCPL then the CD signal is positive and if LCPL is absorbed less than RCPL then the CD signal is negative

The technique in which circular dichroism is measured as a function of wavelength is termed circular dichroism spectroscopy (CD spectroscopy).

COTTON EFFECT

The medium exhibiting circular birefringence exhibits Circular Dichroism. The combination of circular birefringence and CD in the absorption region of the sample gives the phenomenon called the cotton effect. The absorption bands are observed in this region.

Chiral compounds with chromophores give anomalous cotton effect curves. These curves are divided into two types

1. Single cotton effect curves
2. Multiple cotton effect curves

Molar rotation increases with a decrease in wavelength for one isomer of an optically active medium. This is called the positive cotton effect. The optical molar rotation peak is at a higher wavelength than its trough.

In the negative cotton effect, the optical molar rotation is higher at a lower wavelength than its trough. The absorptive CD is restricted to a narrow zone of wavelength whereas ORD covers more range in wavelength.

SINGLE COTTON EFFECT

In these curves maxima and minima, both occur in the region of maximum absorption. On moving from a longer wavelength, maxima (peak) come first than the minima (trough). It is a positive cotton effect. The peak is at a higher wavelength than the trough.

If the peak is at a shorter wavelength than the trough, then the curve is negative cotton effect curve.

Zero cross over points corresponds to normal UV λ_{max}.

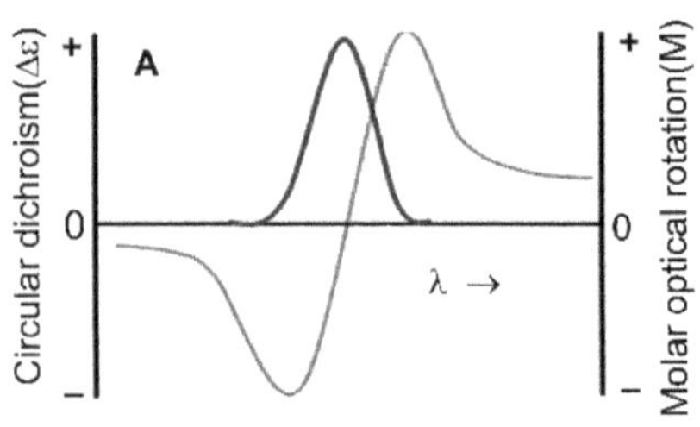

Figure A ---- positive cotton effect.

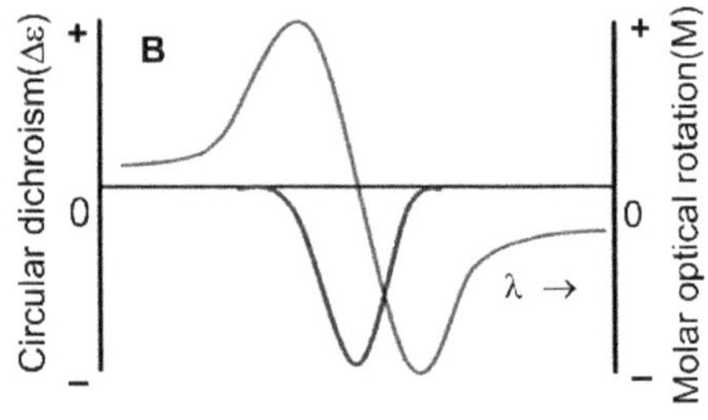

Figure B -----negative cotton effect.

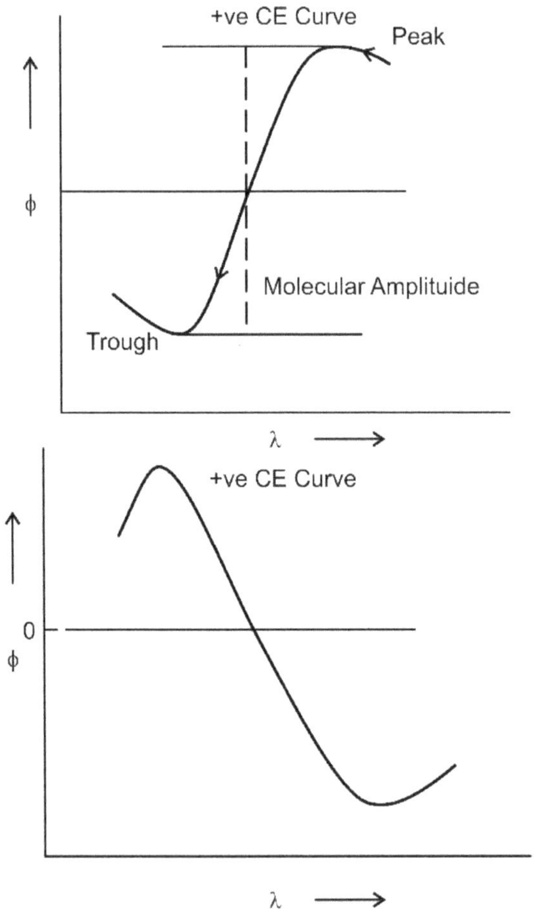

Single cotton effect curves

MULTIPLE COTTON EFFECT

Two or more peaks and troughs are obtained in these types of curves. For example, the curves of keto steroids, camphor, etc.

CD INSTRUMENTATION

To measure circular dichroism, the ordinary spectrophotometer can be adapted with some changes. Production of right and left circularly polarized light is done using a quarter wave plate. A plane polarized beam can be passed through the quarter-wave plate which is rotated from -45° to +45° to produce right and left circularly polarized light of one wavelength. To cover a wave length region, several quarter wavelength plates are used.

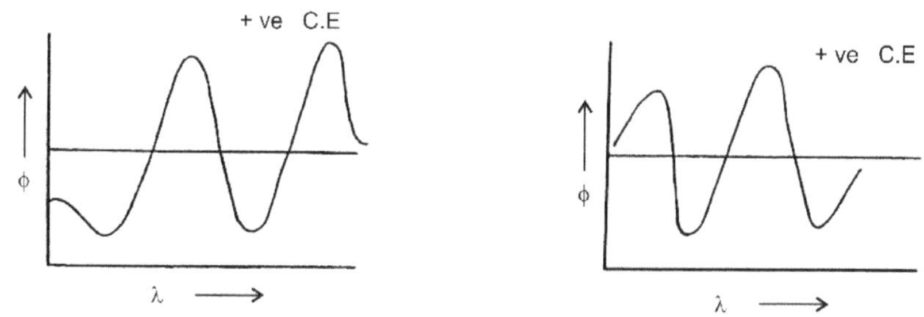

Multiple cotton effect curves

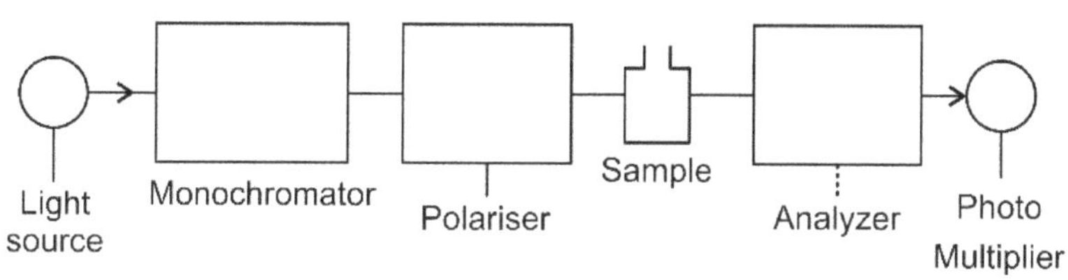

Diagram of the optical components of a spectropolrimeter

Difference between ORD and CD

Optical Rotatory Dispersion	Circular Dichroism
The plane-polarized light is rotated through an angle θ due to the difference in the refractive indices of the sample for RCPL and LCPL.	Differential absorption of RCPL and the LCPL by the sample gives rise to CD
These are dispersive spectra	These are absorptive spectra
Circularly polarized light is not converted to elliptically polarized light	Circularly polarized light is converted to elliptically polarized light
Specific rotation is plotted against wavelength to get graphs	Molar ellipticity is plotted against wavelength to obtain graphs

Applications

1. Determination of the structure of amino acids, polypeptides proteins
2. ORD is used in quantitative analysis
3. ORD is used in the determination of absolute configuration and conformational studies
4. Equilibrium studies also make use of ORD
5. CD is used in the determination of Protein conformation
6. Conformation of nucleic acids determined using CD.

CHAPTER 32

X-Ray Diffraction

X-ray diffraction (XRD) is the technique which is based on the diffraction (scattering) of x-rays by crystals. The diffraction pattern of x-rays gives an idea about the arrangement of atoms within the crystal structures. This technique is used in qualitative analysis including structural elucidation of organic and inorganic compounds.

THEORY

The x-ray region in EMR spectrum is ranging from 0.1 to 100 Å. The range used for analytical purpose varies from 0.7 to 2.0 Å.

PRODUCTION OF X-RAYS

When high velocity electrons collide with a metal target x-rays are generated. The x-rays are generated using Roentgen tube. When a high voltage (15-60 kv) is applied, the hot tungsten filament (cathode) produces high speed electrons. These electrons are made to hit the metal target (anode) like copper aluminium molybdenum or magnesium. Water circulation is used to cool the copper block containing the target material.

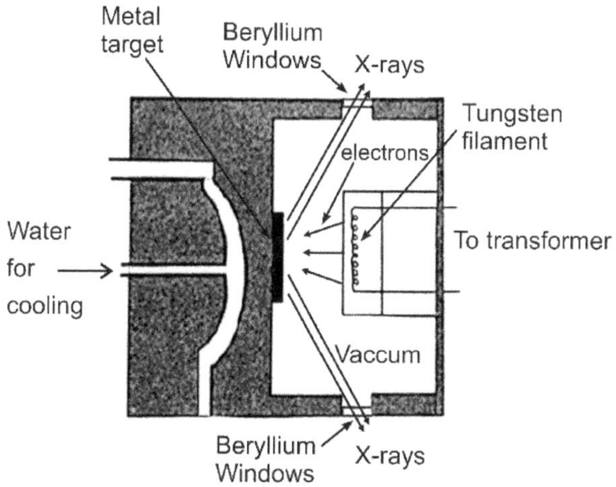

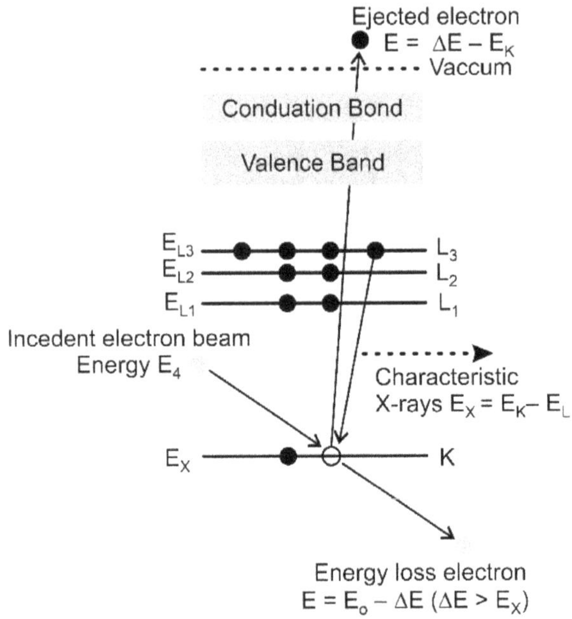

When the fast-moving electrons collide with the atom in the metal target, it knocks out an electron completely from the inner shell of the atom. Loss of inner shell electron causes one of the outer shell electron to fall into the vacated orbital with the emission of x-ray. The energy of emitted x-ray is equal to the difference in energy between the two electronic energy levels.

For e.g. $E_k = E_L - E_k$ where k shell loses electron and the electron from the L-shell replaces it. E_k is the energy of emitted x-ray radiation.

SCATTERING AND DIFFRACTION

The phenomenon of scattering forms the basis of diffraction. When an X- ray beam is incident on a sample, the electrons which are oscillating at the same frequency of incident x-ray emit EMR in all directions at the frequency of the incident radiation. Some of these scattered waves coming from atoms which are arranged in regular manner in a crystal lattice undergo constructive interference and they are said to be diffracted by the crystal plane. The diffraction pattern of x-rays is unique for every crystalline substance and hence it is the finger print of the atomic and molecular structure of the crystals. Bragg's law governs the diffraction conditions. If the path lengths of two rays are equal to the whole number of wave length, then constructive interference takes place.

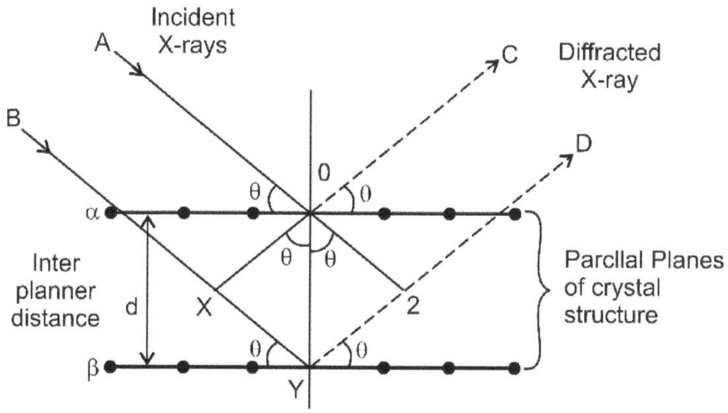

A beam of x-rays falls on the crystal at an angle of θ, then some of these rays will be reflected from the upper layer at the same angle θ. The angle∠XOY =θ and ∠ZOY= θ.

Here AO=BX, CO = DZ

From the figure it can be seen, that the path difference between the two rays reflected from the planes is equal to XY+YZ.

Path difference = XY+YZ .....(32.1)

Path difference is defined as the integral multiple of wavelength = nλ .....(32.2)

Thus, nλ= XY+YZ .....(32.3)

Sinθ=L/H

In ΔXOY, sin θ = XY/OY

That is XY=OY × sinθ

XY = d sinθ .....(32.4)

In ΔZOY sin θ = ZY/OY

ZY=OY × sinθ

ZY = d sinθ .....(32.5)

∴ nλ = d sinθ+ d sinθ .....(32.6)

nλ = 2d sinθ .....(32.7)

this is the Bragg's equation where

n- Order of diffraction, λ = wavelength, d = inter planar distance, θ = glancing angle.

Thus, Bragg's equation gives the relationship between

(i) Wavelength of x rays (λ)

(ii) Inter planar distances in crystals (d) and

(iii) Angle of reflection (θ)

CRYSTAL LATTICE

A series of points that are arranged in a distinct pattern is called as a lattice. A crystal lattice structure is similar to a lattice, but instead of points, it is composed of a series of atoms. A crystal lattice is typically arranged in a sort of symmetrical geometric shape, with each vertex representing an atom. Many solids possess a lattice structure because the total intermolecular energy is lowest when the atoms are arranged in these types of geometrical shapes.

A **lattice point** is a point in a Cartesian coordinate system such that both its x and y coordinates are integers. A lattice point is a point at the intersection of two or more grid lines in a regularly spaced array of points, which is a **point lattice**.

In a plane, point lattices can be constructed having unit cells in the shape of a square, rectangle, hexagon, and other shapes.

Lattice parameter refers to the physical dimension of unit cells in a crystal lattice. Lattices in three dimensions generally have three lattice constants, referred to as *a*, b, and c.

Unit cell is the smallest repetitive unit that contains the complete lattice pattern of a crystal. There are seven crystal systems (cubic, tetragonal, orthorhombic, hexagonal, monoclinic, triclinic, trigonal) and 14 crystal lattices.

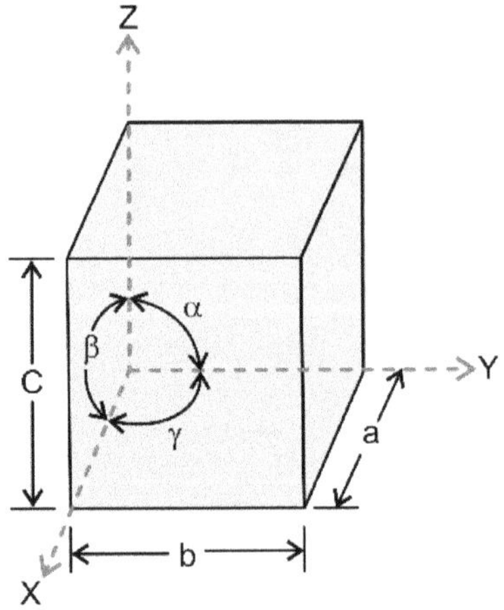

a,b,c are the lattice constants. Crystalline materials fit into one of fourteen recognized lattice arrangements. These are known as **Bravais lattices**.

The names of the crystal lattice systems are as follows:

1. Primitive cubic
2. Body centered cubic
3. Face centered cubic
4. Primitive tetragonal
5. Body centered tetragonal

6. Primitive orthorhombic
7. Base centered orthorhombic
8. Body centered Orthorhombic
9. Face centered Orthorhombic
10. Primitive monoclinic
11. Base centered monoclinic
12. Triclinic
13. Rhombohedral
14. Hexagonal

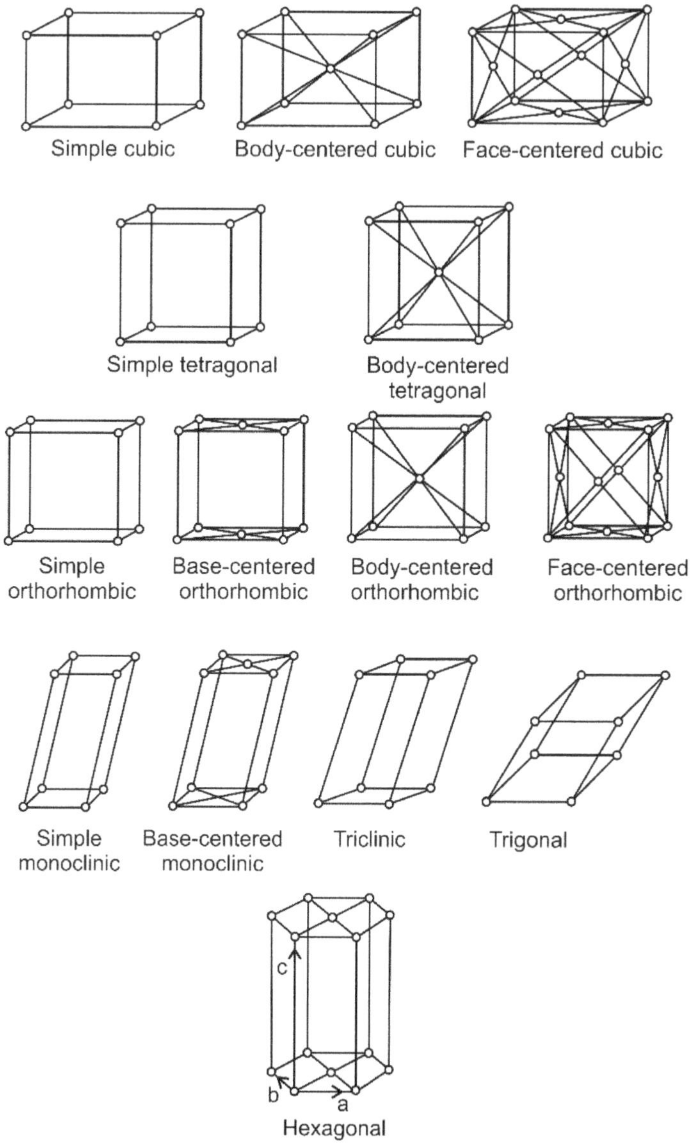

Miller indices

The application of set of rules led to the allotment of miller indices (hkl) in a crystal lattice. These miller indices (hkl) in crystallography help to define the orientation of a crystal plane with respect to main crystallographic axis. These are a set of numbers which can quantify the intercepts and are useful in identifying the planes in a lattice structure. They specify both orientation and the spacing of parallel planes. The orientation of a crystal plane can be defined by how the plane intersects the main crystallographic axis of the crystal.

For cubic crystal

$$d = a/\sqrt{h^2+k^2+l^2}$$

where

a = lattice constant that is the constant difference between unit cells in a lattice, hkl are the miller indices and d is the inter planar spacing

Reciprocal lattice

A crystal resides in a real space. The diffraction pattern of the crystal is in the reciprocal space. Reciprocal lattice is always one of the 14 bravis lattices.

As the miller index of the plane increases, the interplanar distance decreases and there is a crowding of planes around the origin in real lattice. Hence reciprocal lattice is used when dealing with planes in crystal lattices.

The reciprocal space lattice is a set of imaginary points which are constructed in the manner that the vector direction from one point to another corresponds with the direction of normal of real space planes. The distance between these points is the reciprocal of real interplanar distance

The reciprocal lattice is geometrically constructed from real lattice. The properties of the reciprocal lattice are inverse of the real lattice. E.g.: Far away planes in real crystal are closer to the origin in reciprocal lattice. Planes in real lattice become points in reciprocal lattice and vice versa.

Reciprocal crystal = Reciprocal lattice (diffraction spots) + Motif (intensities).

Including Miller indices, the Bragg's equation becomes as

$$n\lambda = 2d_{hkl} \sin \theta ,$$

where

θ- angle of incidence

d_{hkl} – Space between crystal planes of miller indices hkl

n- integer

When n= 1,2,3, a series of angles (θ) is obtained for the given set of plane spacing d_{hkl}. They belong to first order, second order, third order etc.

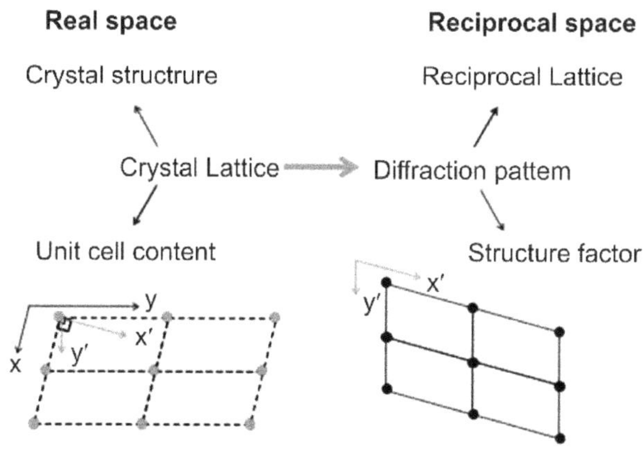

Instrumentation

1. Production of X-rays

X-ray tubes are used for the production of x-rays. Coolidge tube is the typical x-ray tube used. It consists of a cathode (c) made of tungsten filament which is heated by battery (b) to emit thermionic electrons. The emitted electrons are attracted towards the anode having target a. The electrons on striking target a, they transfer their energy to the metallic surface giving off X-ray radiation.

The target material should have atomic number greater than the sample elements and the x-rays emitted by the target material should be energetic enough to excite the elements under study.

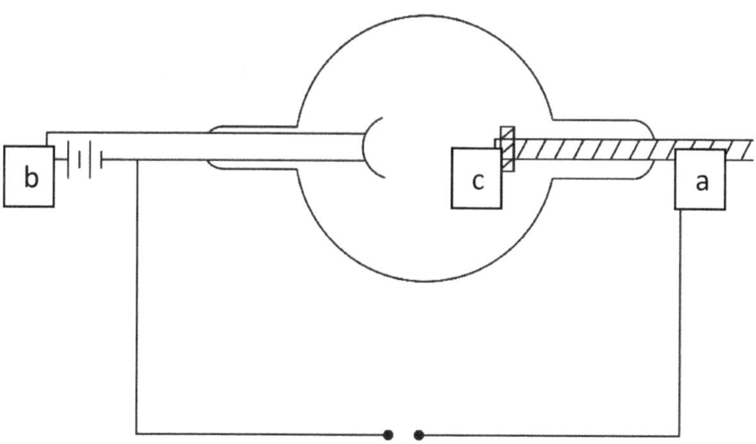

Coolidge tube.

2. Collimator

A narrow beam of x-rays are produced by passing the x-rays emitted by the target material through a collimator. It is made up of two sets of closely packed metal plates with a small gap in between. Only a narrow beam of x-rays passing through are allowed to pass through the gap and all the other x-rays are absorbed.

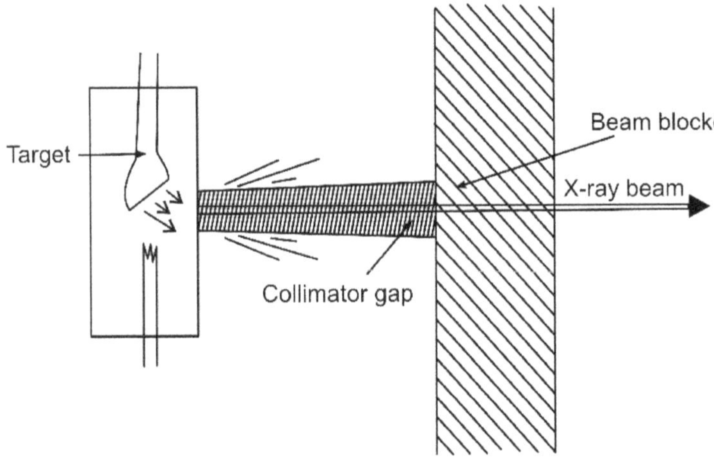

3. Monochromator

Two types of monochromators are used in X-ray Diffractometer.

(i) Filter

(ii) Crystal monochromator

(i) Filter: It allows only the required wavelength to pass through and absorbs the other unwanted radiations. E.g.: Zirconium filter is used for molybdenum radiation

Iron filter for cobalt radiation

Nickel filter for copper radiation

(ii) Crystal Monochromator

These monochromators are crystals made of sodium chloride, lithium fluoride and quartz etc. To get the required wavelength, the crystal monochromator is placed in the x-ray beam in such a way that the angle of reflecting planes satisfies the Bragg's law.

There are two types of crystal monochromators.

(a) Flat crystal monochromators (b) Curved crystal monochromators.

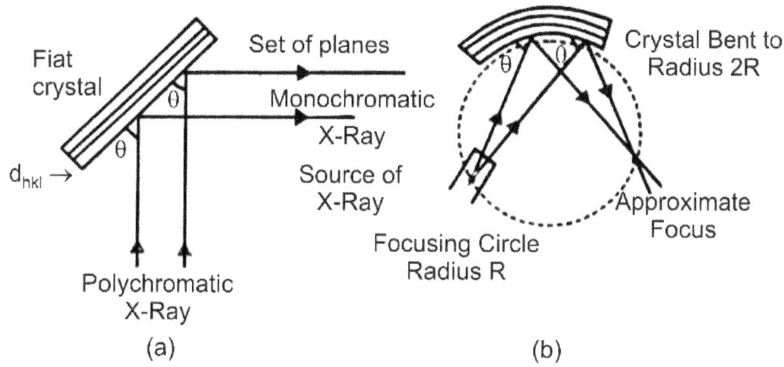

4. Sample Preparation and Sample holder

Sample should be in the form of crystal of about 0.3 mm in cross section. Powders or polycrystalline substances are ground to particle size of 0.002 to 0.005 mm compressed in to a thin film and placed in sample film holder.

In the instruments, the sample holder is fixed at a place and the x-ray source and detector are rotated at certain angle.

5. Detectors

X-ray diffraction patterns are obtained as the x-rays diffracted from the sample strike the detectors. There are two methods to detect the diffracted x-ray intensities. They are

1. Photographic Methods
2. Counter methods

Different detectors used in Counter methods are

(a) Geiger-Muller counter
(b) Proportional counter
(c) Scintillation detector
(d) Solid state semiconductor detector
(e) Semiconductor detectors

1. Photographic Methods

The position and intensity of x-ray beam is recorded using a plane or cylindrical film. The photographic film after exposure to diffracted x-ray from sample is developed. The amount of darkening in developed film is given as

$$D = \log I_0/I$$

where

D-Density, I_0- incident intensity, I- transmitted intensity. A densitometer is used to measure D.

Advantage: Entire diffraction pattern is obtained on a single film.

Disadvantage: Time consuming

Not useful for quantitative measurements

There is a possibility of encountering errors.

2. Counter methods

(a) Geiger-Muller counter

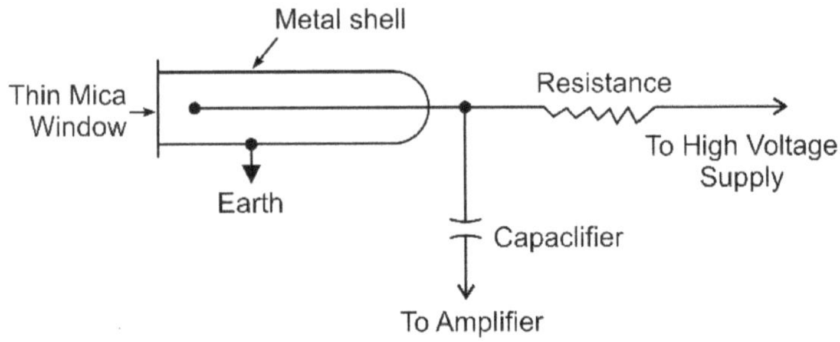

Schematic diagram of a geiger tube

Inert gas like argon is filled in the metal Geiger tube. The anode is a tungsten wire in the centre of the tube and it is maintained at a positive potential of 800-2500 v. The x-rays as they enter the tube, collide with gas molecules and produce electrons. The electrons are attracted by the anode. The avalanche of electrons travelling towards the anode produces a current which is measured.

Disadvantages:

1. Used only for counting low rates
2. Geiger tube efficiency fails below 1 Å wavelength.
3. It cannot be used to measure the energy of the ionizing radiation.

Advantages:

1. Inexpensive and trouble free
2. Gives maximum signal for the applied x-ray intensity.

(b) Proportional Counter

It is constructed in the same way as Geiger counter. A heavier gas like Xenon or Krypton is filled in the counter and the gas is getting ionized when a voltage is applied. The output pulse is proportional to the intensity of incident x-ray radiation and the energy can be measured directly. The dead time of proportional counter is very short and it can be used to count high rates.

The sensitivity and efficiency o this counter is comparable to Geiger tube.

Advantages:

Electronic circuit is complex and expensive.

(c) Scintillation detector

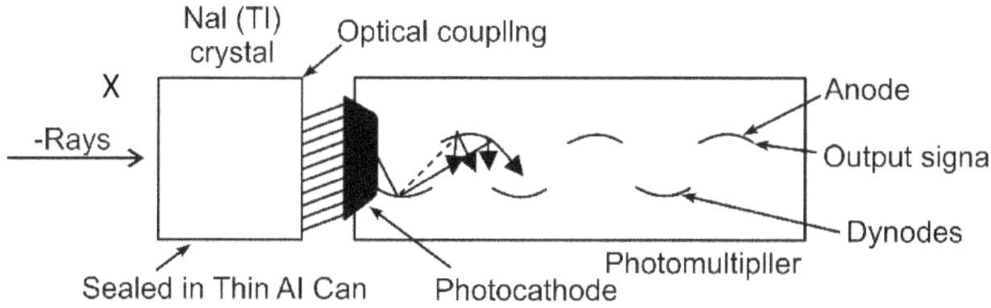

A large sodium iodide crystal activated with a small amount of thallium is present in scintillation counters. When the diffracted x-rays from the sample falls on the crystal, pulses of visible light are emitted and these are detected by a PMT detector. The other crystals that can be used are anthracene, naphthalene and p-terpenol in xylene.

High rates can be counted using scintillation detector, since it's dead time is short. X-rays of shorter wavelength can be measured using this detector.

(d) Solid state semiconductor detector

The current flowing through the conductor is caused by the electrons produced by x-ray beam and is proportional to the x-ray beam incident on the detector. The conductor should be maintained at low temperature to minimize noise and to reduce the decrease in detector performance.

(e) Semiconductor detectors –Si (Li) and Ge (Li)

A thin film of lithium metal coated to one end of silicon block. X-rays falling on this lithium drifted silicon displaces an electron and a hole is generated. Now, voltage is applied and the electrons move towards the positively charged electrode and the holes move towards the negative electrode.

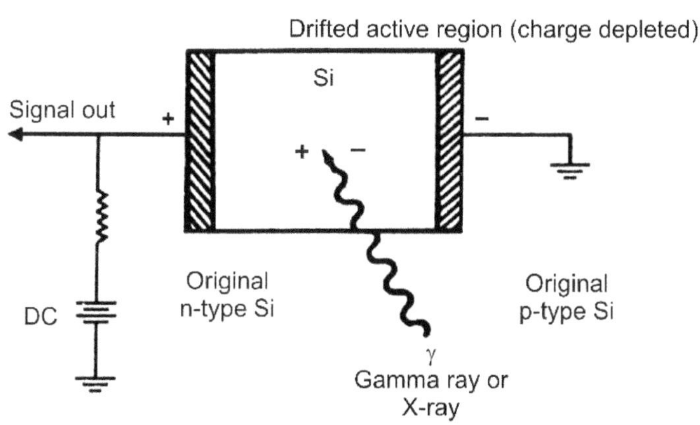

When the electrons arrive at the lithium coating, the generated pulse is equal to Q/C, where q- total charge collected and c-detector capacity. The number of pulses is a direct measurement of photons of x-rays falling on the detector.

X-RAY DIFFRACTION METHODS

The crystal structures of various types of solids are studied using these diffraction methods. The different diffraction methods are

1. Laue photographic method.
2. Bragg x-ray spectrometer method
3. Rotating crystal method
4. Powder method

1. Laue Photographic method

There are two methods available in Laue's method of crystal diffraction.

(a) Transmission method
(b) Back reflection method.

(a) Transmission method

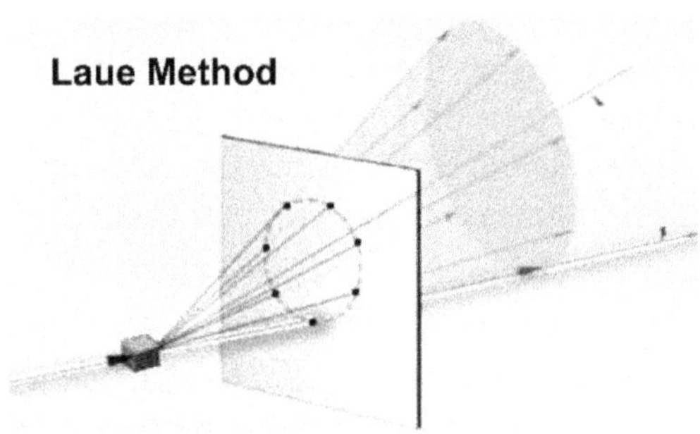

The x-rays from the tungsten source maintained at 60,000 volts are allowed to pass through a pinhole collimator. This thin beam of x-rays falls on the crystal under investigation. The x-ray after passing through the crystal gets diffracted and recorded on a photographic plate.

In the transmission Laue method, the film is placed **behind the crystal to record** beams which are transmitted through the crystal. The incoming radiation and the film are perpendicular to each other. One side of the cone of Laue reflections is defined by the transmitted beam. The film intersects the cone, with the diffraction spots generally lying on an ellipse.

This method can be used to orient crystals for solid state experiments. It is the most suitable method for the investigation of preferred orientation of the sheet particularly confined to lower diffraction angles. This method is also used in determination of symmetry of single crystals.

(b) Back reflection method.

Large and thick crystals can be investigated by this method. In the back-reflection method, the film is placed **between the x-ray source and the crystal**. The beams which are diffracted in a backward direction are recorded. One side of the cone of Laue reflections is defined by the transmitted beam. The film intersects the cone, with the diffraction spots generally lying on an hyperbola.

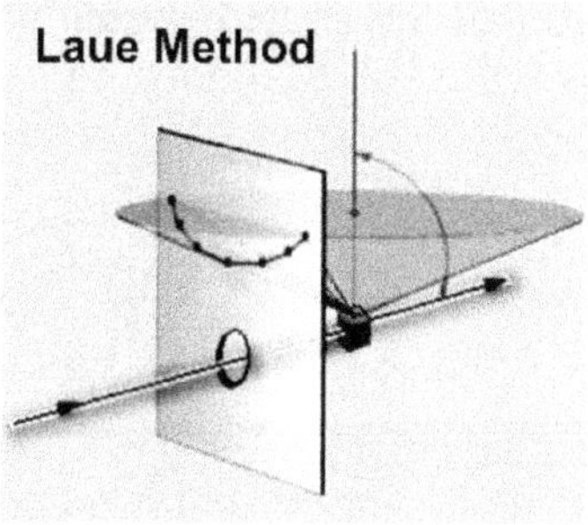

Crystal orientation is determined from the position of the spots. Each spot can be indexed, i.e. attributed to a particular plane, using special charts. The Greninger chart is used for back-reflection patterns and the Leonhardt chart for transmission patterns. The Laue technique can also be used to assess crystal perfection apart from the size and shape

The disadvantage of this method is that it requires large crystals.

2. Bragg x-ray spectrometer method

The principle behind this method is the Bragg's equation.

$$n\lambda = 2d\sin\theta$$

where

λ- Wavelength of x-rays, n- Integer, d- Inter planar spacing,θ - Angle of reflection.

COMPONENTS AND WORKING

The x-rays from the anode A passes through the slits to fall on the crystal C. The crystal is mounted in such a way that it can be moved along the circular scale S. The reflected x-rays from the crystal enter the ionization chamber E through window w after passing through slit F. The ionization chamber is connected to a battery. The ionization current produced is measured by the electrometer Q connected to the ionization chamber. The ionization current produced is directly proportional to the intensity of the incident diffracted x-rays.

Initially, the crystal is mounted in such a way that $\theta = 0$ and the ionization chamber is adjusted to receive the x-rays. The crystal and the ionization chamber are moved in small increments. The chamber is moved twice the angle than the crystal. X-ray spectrum is obtained by plotting a graph between ionization current and the glancing angle. The obtained peaks correspond to Bragg's reflection. Different order glancing angles are obtained with known values of d and n and from the observed value of θ, λ can be measured.

Single plane generates several diffraction lines and the sum total of diffraction lines gives diffraction patterns. From the pattern different distances between planes and the angle between planes can be deduced in each of three dimensions.

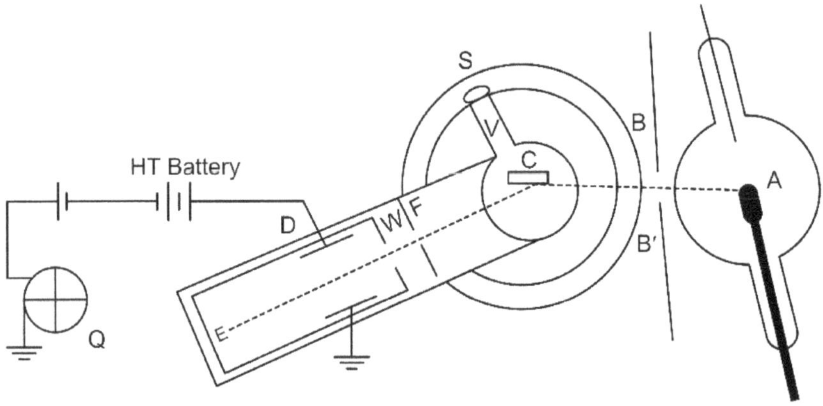

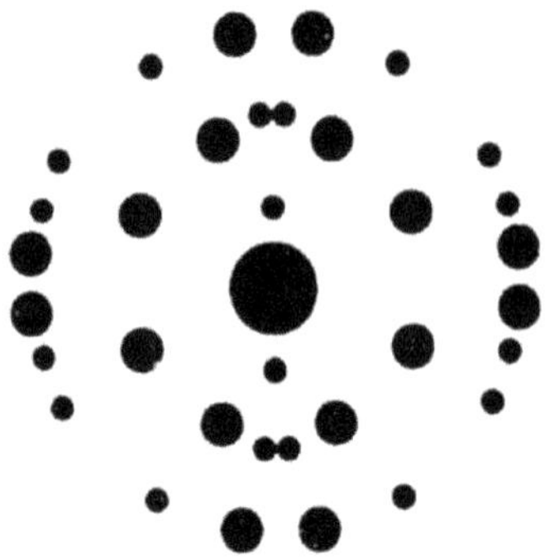

Diffraction pattern of a single crystal of an inorganic salt.

The wavelength of x-rays determined by,

$$2d \sin \theta = n\lambda$$

From the θ values of various order spectra produced by reflection from a crystal, the mean value of λ/d is determined. The value of λ/d is known as lattice constant.

Lattice constant = λ/d

With known d, wavelength λ can be determined.

3. Rotating crystal method

The generated x-rays pass through monochromator, collimator and then made to fall on the crystal mounted on a rotatable shaft. When the crystal is rotated, the sets of adjacent planes come to their reflecting positions. Each plane produces a spot on the photographic plate. The photographic plate is placed at right angles to the x-ray beam. The size of unit cell can be measured by this method.

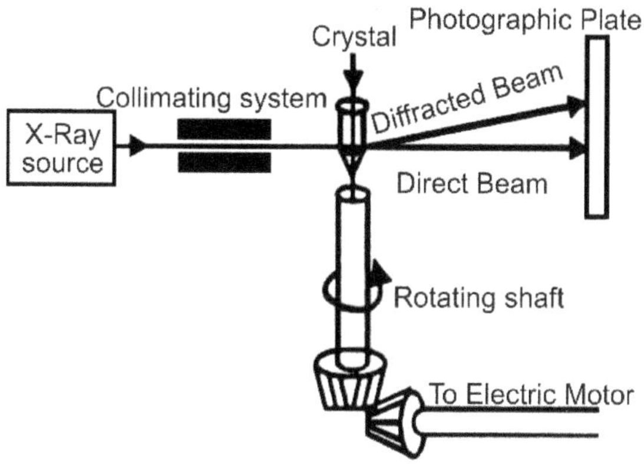

Diffraction can be recorded by two methods

(i) Complete rotation: In this method, a series of complete revolutions are performed, so that each set of plane is diffracted four times. A rectangular diffraction pattern is obtained.

(ii) Oscillation method: Here the crystal is oscillated through 15-20°C. The photographic plate also moves along with the crystal. Orientation of the crystal is indicated by the position of the spot on the plate.

4. Powder crystal method

The analyzed material is finely ground, homogenized, and average bulk composition is determined.

The x-rays from the source pass through the filter (monochromator) and made to fall on the powdered specimen P. Fine powder is struck on a hair with a gum, it is suspended vertically in the axis of a cylindrical camera. The photographic film surrounds the powder crystal in the form of circular arc. The x-rays after passing through the powder pass out of the camera through the film.

If the angle of incidence is θ then the angle of reflection will be 2θ

If the radius is r the circumference $2\pi r$ corresponds to a scattering angle of 360°

$$\theta = 360° \times 1/\pi r$$

From the above equation the value of θ can be calculated and substituted in Bragg's equation to get the value of d.

Applications of Powder crystal method

1. Used for cubic crystals.
2. Used for the detection of complex structures of metals and alloys
3. Used in differentiating allotropic modifications of substances.

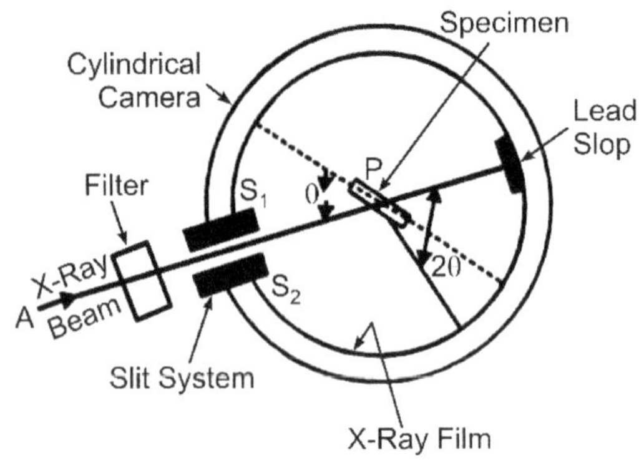

X-RAY DIFFRACTOMETER

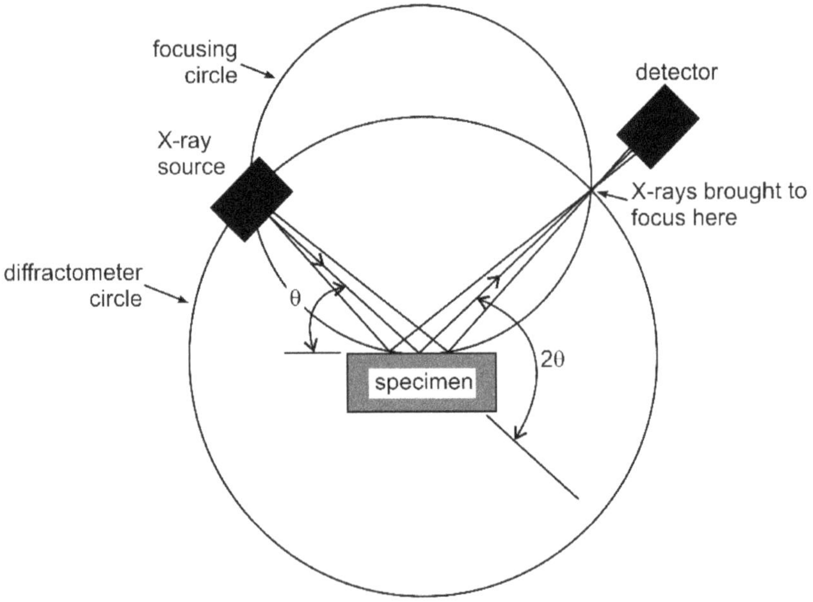

All the three components (x-ray source, sample holder and detector) lie on the same circle which is known as **focusing circle. The Bragg's** angle (θ) can be defined as angle between X-ray source and plane of the sample.

Angle between X-ray source and detector is given by 2 θ value.

In this geometry, detector moves via a range of angles, while X-ray source does not change its position. As the angle 2 θ increases, radius of the focusing circle also increases and 2θ lies between 0° to 170°. The 2θ range depends on the crystal pattern of the matter.

The detector and monochromatic x-ray source lies on the perimeter of the circle. The diffractometer circle is different from the focusing circle. The radius of the circle is fixed. The diffractometer circle of XRD has the sample holder. Source of X-ray and the detector are mounted on its arms. The diffractometer circle is mounted vertically in most of the powder diffractometer.

X-rays are generated by heating the filament in cathode ray tube. Then, these rays are accelerated with high voltage, and then bombarded onto the crystal lattice. Typical X-ray spectra are formed when electrons with sufficient energy dislocate the inner shell electrons. These λ of the rays produced are the characteristic of the targeted material. Monochromatic wavelength is produced using Crystal monochromator. The rays are made to incident on the sample crystal and the intensity of diffracted rays is recorded as the sample and the detector are rotated.

Constructive interference occurs when Bragg's Equation is satisfied and the peak is formed and recorded by the detector. The peak is converted to signal to a count rate by the detector and finally output is given to computer.

Advantages of XRD

1. Identification of unknown compounds, crystalline compounds and amorphous material
2. To determine 'D' spacing in crystals
3. Preparation of sample is easy.
4. Interpretation can be done with available patterns.
5. It is a non destructive method.

Applications

1. Structure of crystals

   XRD is used to find the orientation of crystals. Patterns are characteristic of particular compound and helps in identification of crystals. It is also used in determination of mixed crystals.

2. Polymer Characterization

   To find the degree of crystallinity of the polymer, the powder method is used. XRD is applied in polymer chemistry to study the nature of polymers.

3. Helps in determination of annealing states in metals.
4. Particle size determination is done with x-ray crystallography.
5. Used in determination of cis-trans isomerism.
6. Linkage isomerism can be determined using XRD.

CHAPTER 33

Thermal Methods

The physical and chemical changes experienced by a sample when it is heated is measured by thermal methods. The physical and chemical changes that take place during the heating of the unknown sample help in identifying the sample. Thermal analysis is a technique in which the physical change in the system is recorded as a function of temperature. By measuring the temperature at which such reactions occur and the heat involved in the reaction, the compounds present in the material can be characterized.

The various techniques available under thermal methods are Thermogravimetry (TG), Differential thermal analysis (DTA), Differential scanning calorimetry (DSC), and Thermomechanical analysis (TMA). In all these methods any one of the physical parameters is recorded against temperature. Some of the Thermal methods along with the property measured are given in the following table.

NAME	PROPERTY MEASURED	APPARATUS USED	GRAPH
Thermo gravimetry	Change in weight	Thermobalance	Mass vs Temperature
Differential Thermal Analysis	Heat absorbed or evolved (ΔT)	DTA apparatus	ΔT vs Temperature
Differential scanning calorimetry	DH/dt	Differential scanning calorimeter	DH/dt vs Temperature
Thermomechanical Analysis/Dilatometry	Volume or length	Dilatometer	Volume or length vs Temperature

The change in the thermal property with temperature is recorded by a thermogram.

For first-order transitions, such as melting, crystallization, sublimation, boiling, etc., integration of the curve gives the energy involved in the transition. Melting, boiling, sublimation, and desolvation are endothermic, which means they need energy. Crystallization is exothermic, which means that it supplies energy. Solid-to-solid phase transition and decomposition may be endothermic or exothermic. For second-order transitions, the signal gives the change in the specific heat; for example, in the glass transitions of amorphous materials.

The various thermal events are summarized as

A (S1) → A(S2) ------------ Solid to solid phase transition

A (S1) → A(l) -------------- Melting

A (S1) →A(g) -------------- Sublimation

A (S1) →B(s)+gases ------- Decomposition

A (S1) →Gases ------------ Decomposition

A (glass) → (A rubber) ---------------- glass transition

A (s)+ B (g) →C(s) --------------------- oxidation and tarnishing

A (s)+ B (g) → Gases ------------------ combustion, volatilization

A(s)+$(Gases)_1$ →A(s) + $(gases)_2$ ------ heterogeneous catalysis

A(s)+ B(s) →AB(s)-------------------- addition

AB(s)+CD(s) → AD(s)+CB(s) -------- double decomposition

DIFFERENTIAL THERMAL ANALYSIS (DTA)

INTRODUCTION

It is a comparison method in which the temperature difference created between a sample and reference is measured when both are treated with identical heat conditions like controlled heating or cooling program. In this analytical method, the difference in temperature (ΔT) between the sample and reference is recorded as a function of time/temp. Any change in specific heat or enthalpy of transition can be detected by DTA. If there is no temperature difference between the sample and the reference it means that the sample does not undergo any chemical or physical changes. The DTA curve is a fingerprint for qualitative identification.

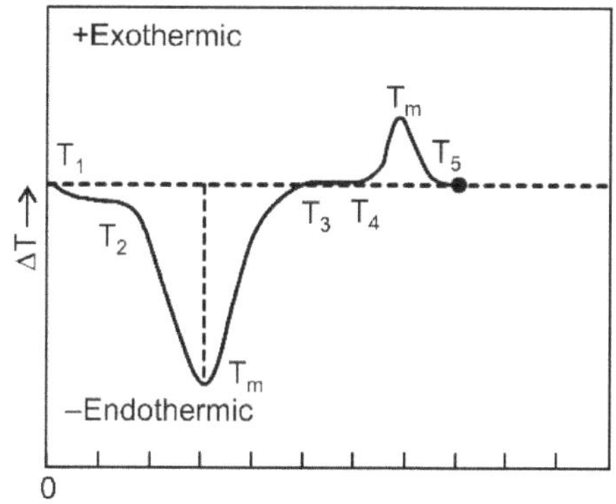

Differential thermogram

The technique involves the measurement of the difference in temperature between the sample and reference material against time or temp. Both the sample and reference are treated similarly in the same environment either heated or cooled at a controlled rate.

The differential thermogram (graph) consists of ΔT (differential temp between sample and reference) in the x-axis plotted as a function of time (t), sample temp (T_s), reference temp (T_r), or furnace temperature (T_f)

The figure shows an exothermic (emission of heat) and an endothermic (absorption of heat) peak. The peak size and shape give information about the nature of the test sample. A sharp endothermic peak shows changes in crystallinity or fusion and a broad endothermic peak shows a dehydration reaction. Physical changes lead to endothermic curves and chemical reactions like oxidation give exothermic curves. The endothermic or exothermic enthalpy changes are the energy difference between the products and the reactants or between two phases of the substance.

The DTA curve is parallel to the time/temp axis, as long as there is no change in the physical or chemical change state in the sample. When there is a change of state in the sample, at that temperature the additional heat flux leads to an increase in the temperature of the sample and there will be no change in the temperature of the reference.

The difference in temperature between the sample and reference is obtained as a differential signal (peak). After the completion of the change of state, the curve returns to the baseline. Thus, DTA can detect all physical and chemical changes even though there is no change in weight

FACTORS AFFECTING DTA CURVES

The various factors affecting die DTA curve are

(a) Environmental factors
(b) Instrumental factors
(c) Sample factors

(a) Environmental factors

It involves the gaseous atmosphere of the sample. For example, O_2 or air causes oxidation of the sample giving an exothermic peak. Hence in DTA studies, two types of gaseous atmospheres are used

(a) Static gaseous atmosphere
(b) Dynamic gaseous atmosphere

In both techniques, the shapes of curves are the same but the peak minimum temperature shifts to a lower temp in the dynamic gas technique.

Static gas atmosphere cannot be reproduced because the atmosphere surrounding the sample is constantly changing chemically due to evolved gases leading to errors in the study.

Dynamic gas atmosphere is maintained by using inert or reactive sweep gases in a controlled manner.

(b) Instrumental factors

(i) Sample holder: The material of construction of the sample holder may change the shape of the peaks, inception, and peak temperature.

Eg: Metal sample holders are made of high thermal conductivity materials and give sharp exothermic peaks but the endothermic peaks are flat with metal sample holders. With poor thermal conductivity materials like ceramic, the reverse happens.

The sample holder and sample size should be small to get better resolution.

(ii) Differential temperature sensing devices

The position and thickness of the wires in temperature sensing devices affect the peak height, peak temperature, and peak shapes. To get better results differential temperature is plotted against the same temperature.

(iii) Furnace characteristics

Uniformity in winding is important in DTA as it has a direct effect on DTA curves. If uniform winding is not there in the furnace, this leads to changes in base line.

(iv) Temperature program controller

Temperature program controllers are used to provide constant heating rate in DTA. High accuracy, control and precision should be maintained to measure small temperature differences.

(v) Thermal regime

Heating rates have great effect on DTA curves. Higher heating rates give high peak temperature and sharp peak with great intensity. Normally the heating rate employed is 10-20°C/min.

(vi) Recorder

The type of recorder, span chart speed, and pen response are the other factors which influence the DTA curves.

(c) Sample Characteristics

Physical properties

1. Degree of crystallinity of the sample affects DTA curves,
2. Increase in particle size of the sample decreases the area of the peak and the peak temperature shifts to higher values. This also increases the completion temperature

Chemical properties

The reactivity of the sample, sample holder, thermocouple material, gaseous environment, and diluent are the chemical factors that affect the DTA curves

Instrumentation

Components of the DTA apparatus are

1. Furnace- A heating device for the sample.
2. Sample holder- for holding samples and reference
3. Temperature controller –sensor, control element, and heater
4. Recorder- to record the DTA curve.

1. Furnace

Tubular furnace is used in DTA. The choice of construction material depends on the operation temperature and gaseous environments.

E.g. Silicon carbide, Tungsten

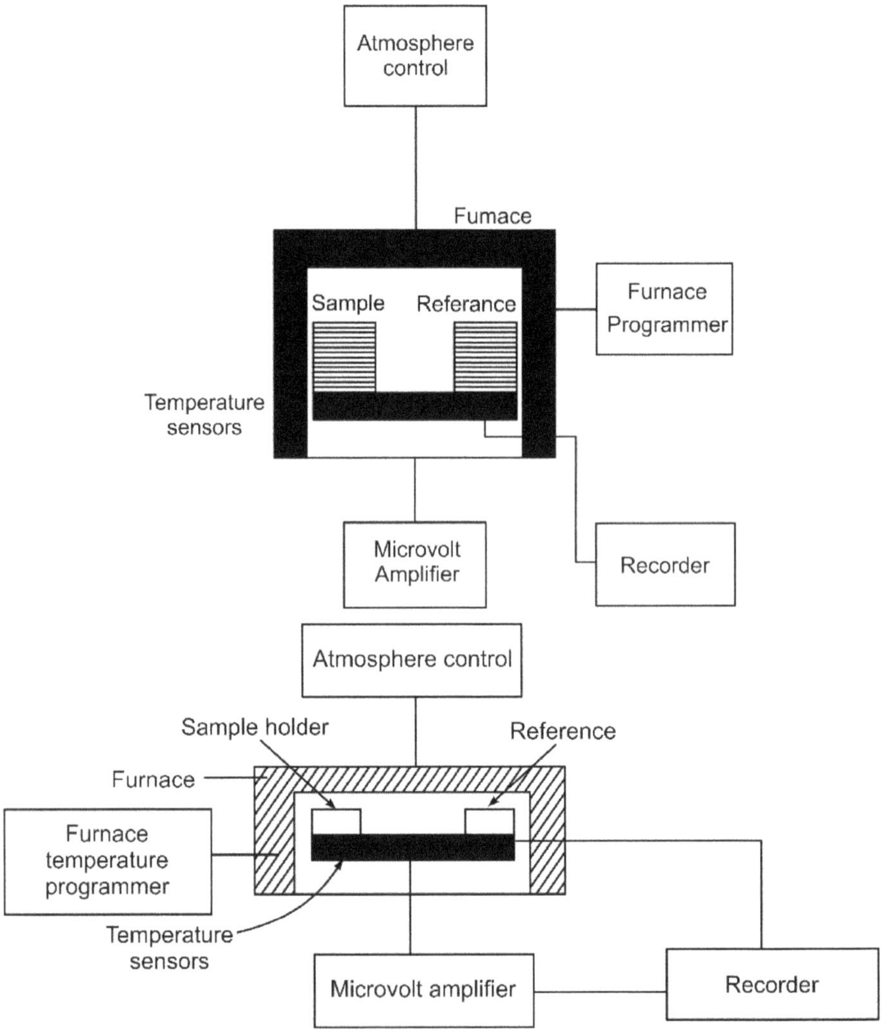

Block diagram of DTA apparatus

2. **Sample holder**

   Both metallic and non-metallic materials are used for construction. Eg. Metals used for construction -Nickel, Platinum, alloys and stainless steel

   Nonmetallic materials--glass, vitreous silica or sintered alumina. Generally cylindrical sample holders made of platinum are used.

3. **Temperature controller**

   The temperature controller consists of three elements. They are sensor, control element and heater.

Sensor- is located with respect to heater and mode of heat transfer and it senses the temp variation. **Thermocouples** serve as sensors. Material of construction is chromel P and aluel (Ni-chromium alloys) up to 1100° C. Above this temperature, pure platinum and platinum-rhodium alloy wires are used.

Control element- matches the heat input requirement with the heat loss from the system.

Proportional controllers (temp) are used and they can minimize the input temperature progressively as the temperature reaches the desired value.

Temperature Programming

It is a time dependent temperature cycling of the furnace. Temperature programming ensures uniform rate of heating. It is the uniform rate in change of temperature at specific time intervals. For example, 5 °C/min

Recorder

The signal is recorded as a trace on paper or film by ink or optical beam.

Applications of DTA

(i) **Heat of reaction**

Peak area of DTA is a linear function of heat of reaction (ΔH). This principle is used to determine the heat of reaction in DTA.

(ii) **Specific heat**

The heat transfer between sample and reference and the sample holder is used to find the specific heat of the substances like naphthalene.

(iii) **Thermal diffusivity**

It is determined by measuring temperature difference between centre and surface of sample, which is heated at a uniform rate.

(iv) **Qualitative analysis**

1. Identification of substances using DTA curves. DTA curves are fingerprint for each substance.
2. Identification of products in a reaction
3. Determination of melting point to check the purity of the substance.

(v) **Quantitative analysis**

This analysis is based on the principle that the area of DTA peak is proportional to the weight of the sample

(vi) Quality control of variety of substances like cement, glass, soil, textiles etc are carried out using DTA

(vii) Thermal stability of inorganic compounds and complexes are studied using DTA

(viii) Identification and purity determination of polymers, explosives, pharmaceuticals, oils, fats and other organic compounds are carried out using DTA.

DIFFERENTIAL SCANNING CALORIMETRY (DSC)

It is a thermal technique in which the energy required to establish zero temperature difference between sample and reference is measured as a function of temperature or time, where both the sample and reference are heated or cooled at predetermined rate

$\Delta H/\Delta T$ is plotted against transition temperature in DSC. The total energy transfer from or to the sample is given by the area of the peak

COMPARISON OF DTA AND DSC TECHNIQUE

S. No	Property	DSC	DTA
1	Size of sample	2-10 mg	50-20.0 mg
2	Sensitivity of measurement of heat of transition	A few joule/mol	0.5 kj/mole
3.	Heating and cooling cycles	Programmed heating and cooling possible	Generally programmed heating
4.	Second-order phase transition	observed with a sample size of 200mg	It is not observed
5.	Specific heat measurement	Accurate	Not accurate
6.	Graph	dH/DT vs. temperature	ΔT vs. Temperature
7.	Parameter measured	Heat absorbed or liberated during heating or cooling	The temperature difference is measured during heating or cooling

DSC is the most widely used method of thermal analysis in the pharmaceutical field. When an endothermic transition happens, the energy absorbed by the sample is counter-reacted by increasing the energy input to the sample, so that zero temperature difference is maintained. Since the input energy is equal to the energy absorbed, a direct calorimetric measurement of transition is obtained.

In the DSC chart, the abscissa indicates transition temperature, and the area of the peak measures total energy transfer from or to the sample

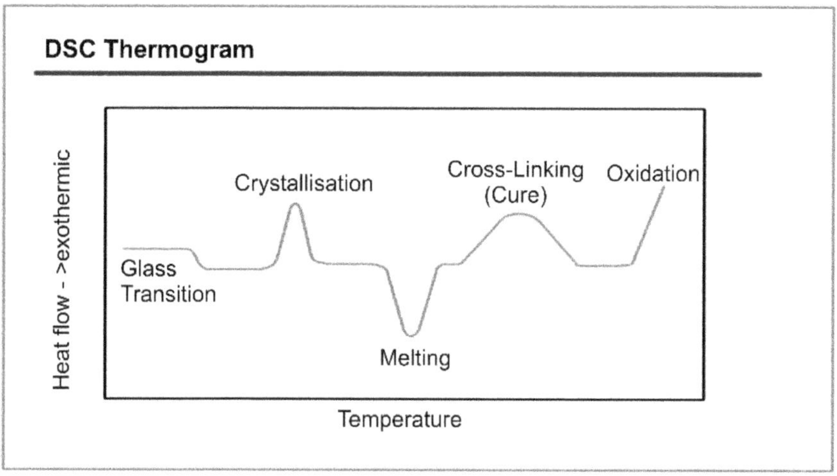

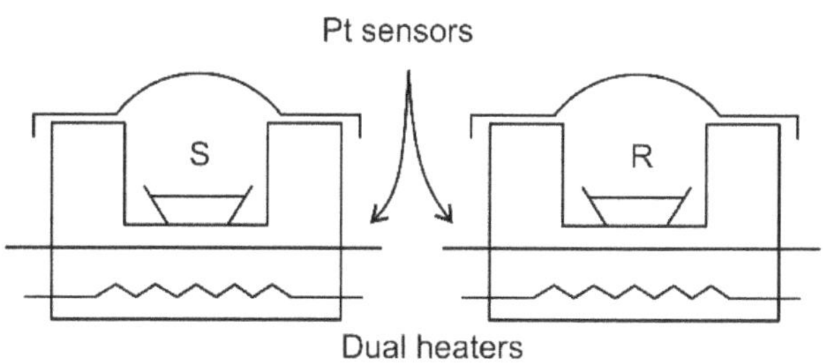

Power compensated DSC

Heat Flux DSC

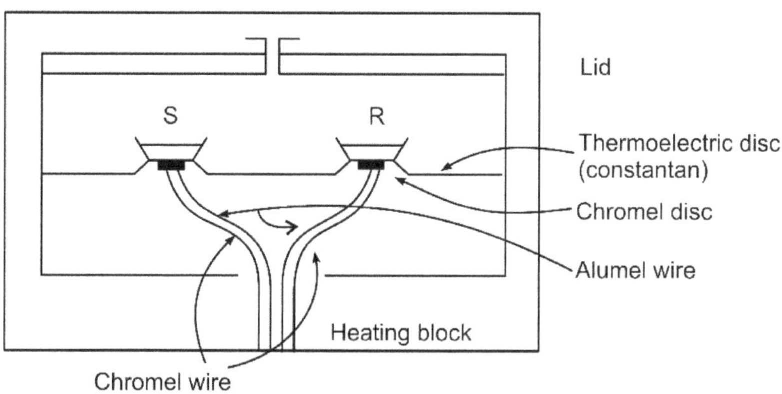

DSC is a thermo analytical technique in which the amount of heat required to maintain the sample and reference at the same temperature is measured.

DSC is classified as

(i) Heat flux DSC
(ii) Power compensated DSC

In heat flux DSC, the differential temperature between sample and reference is measured using single large metal furnace. Both the sample and reference are heated at a constant rate and detectors used are thermocouples

In power compensated DSC, the energy is applied or removed from the furnace to compensate the energy changes between reference and the sample. Whenever an exothermic or endothermic change happens in the sample, an energy difference occurs between sample and reference. By compensating the energy difference, a thermal null state is maintained. The amount of the power required to maintain thermal null state is proportional to energy changes. In power compensated DSC, individual heaters with separate furnaces are used for sample and reference.

INSTRUMENTATION

(a) Thermo balance
(b) Sample holder
(c) Sensors
(d) Furnace
(e) Temperature controller

(a) Thermo balance

There are two types of thermo balances

1. Deflection thermo balance
2. Null thermo balance

In deflection thermo balance, any change in the sample mass is shown as a deflection of the beam. The imbalance in the photodiode current is amplified and recorded

In null thermo balance, the deviation of the balance beam from its null position is detected by the sensor. This deviation is directly proportional to the weight change. The current needed to null balance the thermo balance is recorded

(b) Sample holder

The material of construction of the sample holder (pan) may be aluminium, platinum, or stainless steel; the sample for DSC can be solid or liquid. Solids may be in the form of powder, crystals, granules, or foil.

(c) Sensors

Usually, thermocouples are used as sensors. The temperature difference between the hot and the cold junction is measured.

(d) Furnace

It is made up of high-quality metal to handle temperature ranges from 1000-2000°C. Separate blocks are used for sample and reference

(e) Temperature controller

Controls the rise in temperature and measures the temperature difference between the sample and the reference. The reference material used is an inert material like alumina. An empty pan with a lid can also be used as a reference.

DSC instrumentation consists of two circuits. The left half contains the differential temperature control circuit and the right half contains the average temperature control circuit

In an average temperature control circuit, the programmer generates an electrical signal proportional to the dialed temperature of the sample and reference holder.

In the differential temperature control circuit, the temperature of the sample and reference are compared. The differential power input to both the sample and reference heaters is zero, then there is no reaction in the sample. When there is a reaction taking place in the sample ($\Delta H \neq 0$) a differential power is given as input to the heaters. A signal proportional to the differential power is recorded. The peak area gives the energy changes in the sample.

ENVIRONMENT

The DSC measurements are carried out in the presence of the purging gases like nitrogen, helium, Air/Oxygen at a flow rate of 20-30ml/min

Factors affecting DSC curves

1. **Sample shape**

   The shape of the sample plays an important role in qualitative analysis. Samples are used in the form of disc film or power spread on a pan.

2. **Sample size**

   About 0.5 to 10mg is used. A small sample size gives faster scanning, better resolution, and good-shaped peaks.

   In a large sample size, precision is greater.

3. **Heating rates**

   Faster heating rates increase sensitivity but decrease resolution whereas the slow heating rate decreases sensitivity but increases resolution

   Heating rates usually start at 10° C /min. Other factors which affect DSC curves are type of pan, nature of samples, particle size distribution, packing, and porosity.

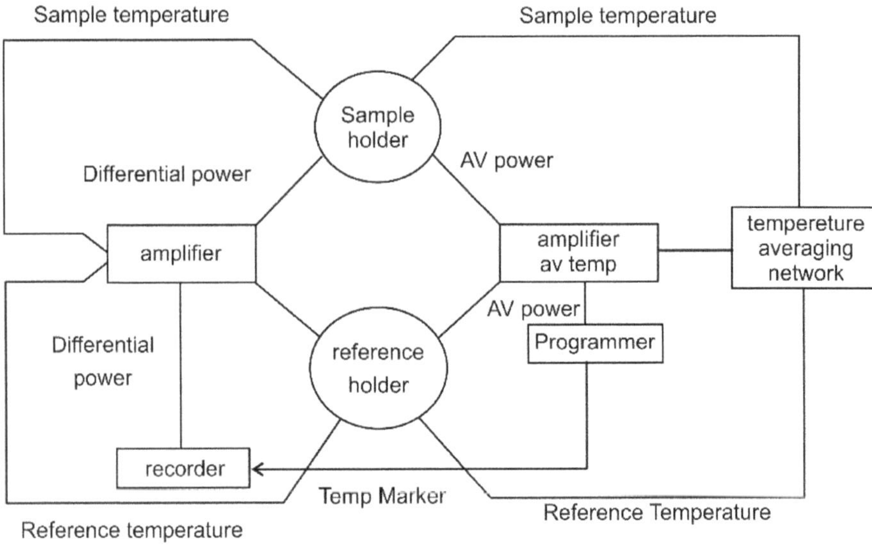

Block diagram for DSC instrument

Advantages

1. Small sample size
2. Better resolution

Applications of DSC

1. Determination of crystallinity in a polymer
2. Purity analysis
3. Analysis of spray dried system
4. Study of liquid crystals
5. Compatibility studies.
6. Preparation of synthetic polymer blends.

www.ingramcontent.com/pod-product-compliance
Ingram Content Group UK Ltd.
Pitfield, Milton Keynes, MK11 3LW, UK
UKHW021322190726
13845UKWH00003B/18

9 789349 562011